Psychopathology

Psychopathology

A CASE-BASED APPROACH

DAVID A. SCOTT
Clemson University

MICHELLE GRANT SCOTT
Lander University

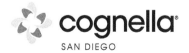
cognella®

SAN DIEGO

Bassim Hamadeh, CEO and Publisher
Amy Smith, Senior Project Editor
Alia Bales, Production Editor
Emely Villavicencio, Senior Graphic Designer
Stephanie Kohl, Licensing Coordinator
Natalie Piccotti, Senior Marketing Manager
Kassie Graves, Vice President of Editorial
Jamie Giganti, Director of Academic Publishing

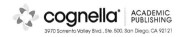

cognella® ACADEMIC PUBLISHING
3970 Sorrento Valley Blvd., Ste. 500, San Diego, CA 92121

Dedicated to our always supportive parents and to our daughters Taylor Grace and Caroline.

You inspire us every day.

BRIEF TABLE OF CONTENTS

CONTENTS

CHAPTER 1

INTRODUCTION AND OVERVIEW OF PSYCHOPATHOLOGY   1
David A. Scott and Michelle Grant Scott

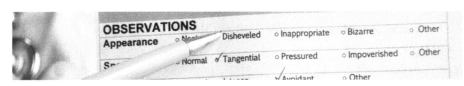

CHAPTER 2

ASSESSMENT, DIAGNOSING, AND THEORY   19
Liz Boyd, Melanie Burgess, Sonja Lund, and David A. Scott

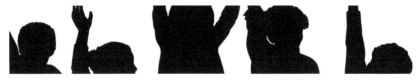

CHAPTER 3

CHILDHOOD DISORDERS   39

Chadwick Royal, Regina Gavin Williams, Kyla Maria Sawyer-Kurian, Taheera Blount,
Jennifer Barrow, and David A. Scott

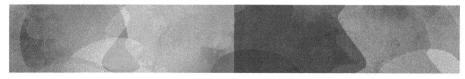

CHAPTER 4

SCHIZOPHRENIA AND OTHER PSYCHOTIC DISORDERS   67

Andy J. Flaherty, David A. Scott, and Michelle Grant Scott

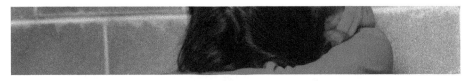

CHAPTER 5

MOOD DISORDERS   89

David A. Scott and Michelle Grant Scott

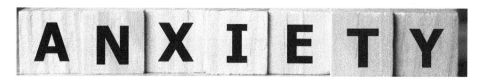

CHAPTER 6

ANXIETY DISORDERS   111

Michelle Grant Scott and David A. Scott

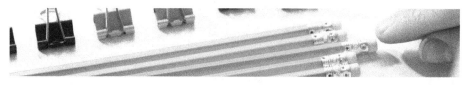

CHAPTER 7

OBSESSIVE-COMPULSIVE DISORDER AND RELATED DISORDERS   127

Michelle Grant Scott and David A. Scott

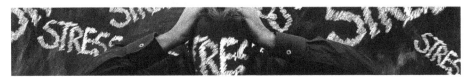

CHAPTER 8

TRAUMA AND STRESSOR-RELATED DISORDERS   141

Brooke Wymer, Christopher J. Hipp, Liz Boyd, and David A. Scott

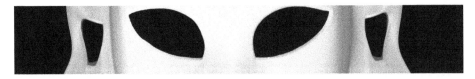

CHAPTER 9

SOMATIC SYMPTOM AND DISSOCIATIVE DISORDERS   161

Theresa C. Allen and David A. Scott

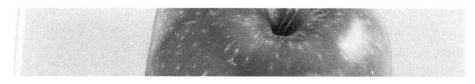

CHAPTER 10

FEEDING AND EATING DISORDERS   175

Melanie Burgess, Liz Boyd, and David A. Scott

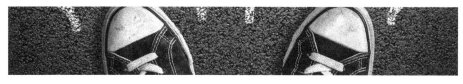

CHAPTER 11

SEXUAL DISORDERS AND GENDER DYSPHORIA   191

Sonja Lund, T'Airra Belcher, and David A. Scott

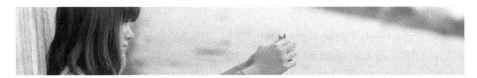

CHAPTER 12

DISRUPTIVE, IMPULSE-CONTROL, AND CONDUCT DISORDERS   219

Robin Moody, Theresa C. Allen, and David A. Scott

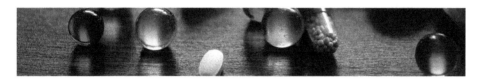

SUBSTANCE-RELATED AND ADDICTIVE DISORDERS

Andy J. Flaherty, David A. Scott, and Michelle Grant Scott

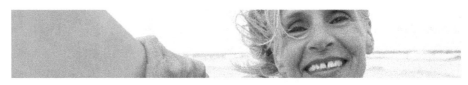

CHAPTER 14

NEUROCOGNITIVE DISORDERS   267

David A. Scott, Michelle Grant Scott, and Robin L. Moody

PERSONALITY

CHAPTER 15

PERSONALITY DISORDERS   285
Chadwick Royal and David A. Scott

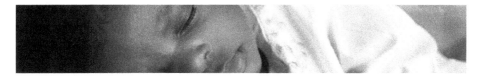

CHAPTER 16

SLEEP-WAKE DISORDERS   305
David A. Scott and Michelle Grant Scott

PREFACE

Within the mental health field, treating mental disorders in the absence of the required knowledge and skills may prove to be both unethical and illegal. This text, *Psychopathology: A Case-Based Approach,* serves as a springboard toward the requisite knowledge base and skill sets essential to the role of mental health professionals engaged in the process of helping treat abnormal behavior. More specifically, *Psychopathology: A Case-Based Approach* provides the mental health field with an understanding of the multifaceted and often interconnected constructs and dynamics inherent within the treatment of mental disorders. *This text will work to integrate appropriate treatment models, competencies, and best practices for students and mental health professionals being trained in counseling, social work, psychology, human services, and marriage and family programs.* One of the main goals of this book was to bring in the expertise of authors from various disciplines within the mental health field. We have contributing authors with years of clinical experience and backgrounds in counselor education, social work, and psychology.

This text is designed to address specific competencies identified as essential to knowing the etiology, the diagnostic process and nomenclature, treatment, referral, and prevention of mental and emotional disorders. This book will provide a framework for all mental health professionals who are interested in providing services to those with mental disorders and students who aspire to do so in their careers.

Specifically, the goals of this text are to

a. provide the reader with an understanding of mental disorders, including sections on effective evidence-based treatment;

b. recognize the importance of family, social networks, and community systems in the treatment of mental and emotional disorders;

c. understand current literature that outlines theories, approaches, strategies, and techniques shown to be effective when working with specific populations of clients with mental and emotional disorders;

d. provide an overview of the *Diagnostic and Statistical Manual of Mental Disorders, 5th Edition (DSM-5)* and *International Statistical Classification of Diseases (ICD-10[11])* and how they interrelate with listed mental disorders;

e. review and provide a clear description and analysis of relevant historical and contemporary research supporting the study of abnormal behavior;

f. provide an overview of psychotropic medications and their effectiveness with specific mental disorders; and

g. review the ethical, legal, and practical guidelines for counselors working with clients who have mental disorders.

Features

Becoming a mental health professional is a developmental process involving personal and professional awareness of the simplicity and complexity of counseling's clinical, procedural, and relational elements. The text is designed to ensure that students and mental health practitioners alike remain attuned to the requisite knowledge, skills, and experiences necessary to encourage mastery of the practice and understanding of mental disorders and relevant treatment options. Simply reading the current version of the *ICD* or *DSM* is not enough to fully understand the multiple facets of mental illnesses. While the *DSM* and *ICD* provide a list of coding and the steps to make appropriate diagnoses, they lack the in-depth exploration a text specific to psychopathology can provide. *Psychopathology: A Case-Based Approach* goes beyond the taxonomy of the *DSM* and *ICD* and provides rich exploration of mental disorders by

- examining current and relevant issues related to mental disorders,
- reviewing current treatment approaches,
- offering an overview of disorders using the *DSM* and *ICD* in a collaborative manner,
- teaching through real-life examples of abnormal behaviors,
- including chapter exercises and vignettes, and
- bringing all of these resources together for comprehension, analysis, application, and overall knowledge.

Mental health professionals working with mental disorders should expect to encounter and be able to adapt to the concerns and needs of an increasingly diverse range of clients and their issues. The ultimate goal of this addition is to provide the mental health professional with the broadest knowledge base on psychopathology to ensure that they can compete in an increasingly diverse marketplace. More and more mental health professionals are being asked to diagnose clients in professional settings or at least possess a working knowledge of mental disorders. Mental health professionals must take adequate coursework to be able to function in this role and understand the diagnosis-treatment connection. With this responsibility comes the need for these professionals to understand the ethical, legal, and practical implications associated with being called upon to diagnose and treat clients in various settings. Thus after completing a psychopathology course, clinicians should be well equipped to organize information and make meaning of experiences in a more comprehensive, integrated, and differentiated manner, thereby broadening their potential to effect positive change in a variety of settings.

ACKNOWLEDGMENTS

We would like to thank the editors and staff at Cognella for all of their help and support. This book would not have been possible without the encouragement and guidance of Kassie Graves and Amy Smith. We are extremely grateful for the expertise and clinical experiences shared by our contributing authors. These contributions not only strengthened our book but also provided outstanding viewpoints from professionals in various disciplines within the field of mental health. A special thanks goes to our outside reviewers whose comments provided us with fresh perspectives on the chapters: Travis A. Cos, PhD, La Salle University; Wendy R. Dragon, PhD, Wright State University; Jeff Driskell, PhD, LICSW, Salem State University; and Jennifer C. Hughes, PhD, MSW, LISW-S, Wright State University.

We would like to thank several of our former graduate students for contributing case studies and vignettes used throughout the book, including Katie Haldeman, Tierra Nunn, Katlyn McCormick, Zack Butterfield, Julia Kate, Devin Evans, and Amanda Tuttle.

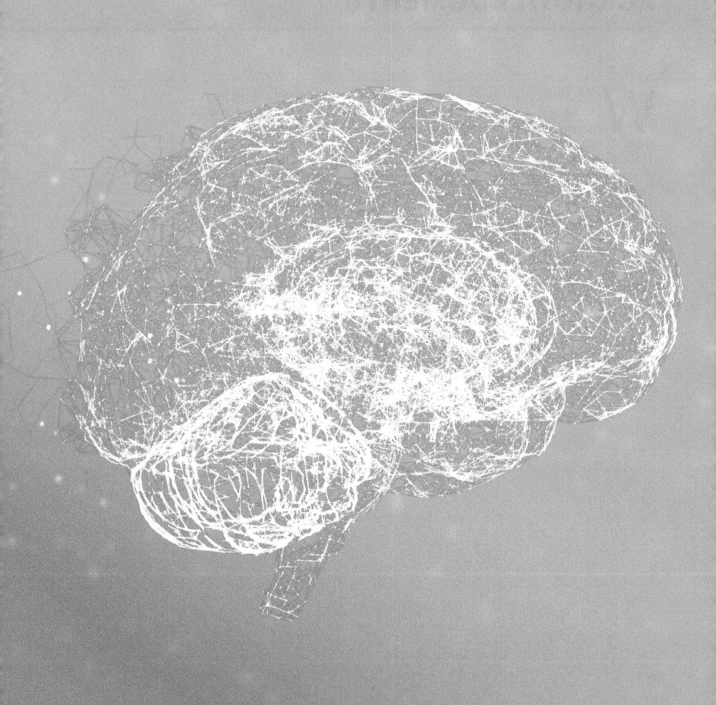

CHAPTER ONE

INTRODUCTION AND OVERVIEW OF PSYCHOPATHOLOGY

David A. Scott and Michelle Grant Scott

What Makes Behavior Abnormal?

We have all heard the term *abnormal behavior*. We have probably all used the term at some point in our lives to describe someone's behavior that just seems, to us, a little odd or different. Professionals have been trying to formulate a concise definition of abnormal behavior for centuries. The challenge is behaviors and defining those behaviors continue to change and evolve. Also, what is considered odd or abnormal to one culture may be considered completely typical (or *normal*) to another culture.

Can you think of a behavior/activity that you or your family practices that may seem odd to others?

A critical piece to working as a mental health professional is that we must take into account all aspects of a person's behavior before we jump to diagnosing a mental disorder. Being able to discern typical behaviors for a person or culture versus behaviors that may constitute the need for professional help will be a requirement for you as you enter the field of mental health. On top of trying to define abnormal behavior, we can also add the term *psychopathology*.

Before we begin to define abnormal behavior and psychopathology, take a few minutes and think about what those words mean to you. Getting in touch with our own thoughts and preconceived biases about psychopathology can be helpful in our development into culturally competent clinicians.

Who do you see as the imaginary client? Do they look like you? Do they look different than you? How so? Can you tell by looking at someone if they have a mental illness?

The following is a list of common terms used by mental health professionals and their definitions:

> *Any Mental Illness.* Any emotional, behavioral, or mental disorder. Severity can range from no impairment, mild, moderate, to severe (NIMH, 2019).

Did You Know?

- One in four people in the world will be impacted by mental illness in their lifetime (World Health Organization [WHO], 2019a).
- Only half of those dealing with mental illness ever receive treatment (National Institute of Mental Health [NIMH], 2018).
- Most low- to middle-income countries spend less than $2 per person per year for the treatment of mental disorders (WHO, 2015).
- Mental illness will cost the global economy $16 trillion by 2030 (Patel et al., 2018).

Mental Health. "A state of well-being in which every individual realizes his or her own potential, can cope with the normal stresses of life, can work productively and fruitfully, and is able to make a contribution to her or his community" (WHO, 2019).

Serious Mental Illness. Any emotional, behavioral, or mental disorder that significantly affects a person's life and their daily activities (NIMH, 2019).

Abnormal Behavior. Any behavior that is statistically uncommon within a specific culture. This behavior can negatively affect a person's daily living/functioning (American Psychological Association, 2020).

While some of the definitions seem very cut and dry, often researchers would question how and why we even needed these types of definitions. Szasz (1960) postulated that society's definition of abnormal was incorrect and the true issue for most was a person struggling to find their niche or problems with living. Szasz (1960) suggested these definitions were merely used to try to control or change individuals to meet society's standards.

What do think about Szasz's thoughts on not trying to define abnormal behaviors?

The World Health Organization (WHO, 2019b) defines mental disorders as "a broad range of problems, with different symptoms. However, they are generally characterized by some combination of abnormal thoughts, emotions, behavior and relationships with others. Examples are schizophrenia, depression, intellectual disabilities and disorders because of drug abuse. Most of these disorders can be successfully treated."

The *Diagnostic and Statistical Manual of Mental Disorders, 5th Edition* (DSM-5; American Psychiatric Association, 2013) stipulates in Box 1.2 that the following elements need to be included to qualify for the definition of a mental disorder:

Box 1.2 *DSM*-5 Definition of a Mental Disorder

- Clinically significant disturbance(s) in cognition or behavior
- These disturbances are manifested by distress or disability in various areas of a person's life (career, social interactions, relationships)
- These disturbances are not a normal part of a specific culture
- Typically, the disturbances are not related to political, sexual, or religious behaviors

One way to view and understand mental health is by using the **biopsychosocial (BPS)** model. Developed by George Engel in 1977, the BPS model viewed treatment in a more holistic way and improved upon the existing biomedical model that was used at the time (Engel, 1977). One of the main deficits of the prevailing biomedical model was the dehumanization and disempowerment of clients (Borrell-Carrió et al., 2004). The BPS model encourages clinicians to view clients as potentially being impacted by biological, psychological, and/or social factors. Understanding the relationship each component can play in a person's life can help the clinician have a clearer view of the client. The *biological* component involves factors associated within the client's body, such as genetics, health, and nutrition issues, which may be categorized in this section. Any physical changes to body organs or accidents that affect a person's daily functioning can fall into this category. The *psychological* area covers issues that originate from the brain and internal stressors (i.e., self-defeating thoughts, stress, cognitive issues). This category also contains our thoughts, behaviors, and emotions.

The third area, *social*, involves factors that are in the environment, including living conditions, political strife, economy, and relationships. Clinicians often add a spiritual component to the social area or elsewhere in their assessment process. Spirituality for clients can be defined in a variety of ways but typically relates to religious faith, morals, and values or existential beliefs.

One final issue to explore is if a person's particular behavior or experiences significantly interfere with a person's daily activities. During an assessment, clinicians need to ask, *Do the behaviors or experiences (symptoms) cause significant distress?* Exhibiting unusual behaviors does not necessarily constitute abnormal behavior or a diagnosis (it makes us who we are!). It is when these behaviors and symptoms affect a person's life in a maladaptive manner that we consider a mental health diagnosis.

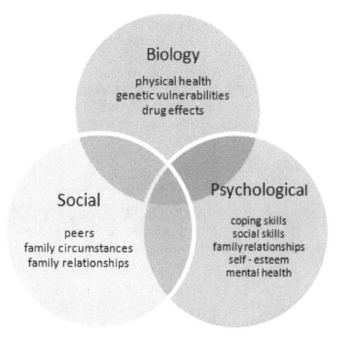

Image 1.2

Multicultural/Diversity Issues

For hundreds of years, culture was typically not included in the diagnostic process. We now see culture and its effect on the diagnosing and treatment of clients. Trying to determine abnormal behavior without a thorough investigation of a client's culture and background could be considered negligent on behalf of the mental health professional. Culturally sensitive assessments and practices will be a critical component. Something for us to keep in mind is that not all behaviors can fit neatly into the *International Statistical Classification of Diseases (ICD)* or *DSM* categories. In fact, back in the 1930s, Benedict (1934) urged caution against viewing "strange cultural expressions with psychological manifestations." Also, getting to know our clients and their customs is a fantastic way to broaden our horizons and worldviews. Taking the time to try to understand a client's worldview will help us see how the client views themselves in the world and community. This will also allow clinicians to understand how the clients view their surroundings (i.e., other people, nature, religion) and ways in which they have been influenced in the development of their personalities. Understanding how external forces (socioeconomic, political events, religion, discrimination, environment) intersect with race and gender will enable the clinician to be better prepared to make an informed diagnosis. Minority groups are typically exposed to a higher number of risk factors that could lead to mental health issues. An example is that there is a higher risk for suicide in the lesbian, gay, bisexual, transgender, and queer or questioning plus community because of higher levels of discrimination, social exclusion, and victimization (Moleiro, 2018).

This book cannot cover every ritual or custom that would be considered abnormal outside of a specific culture. Each chapter will, however, provide sections and information discussing the role of diversity and multiculturism. Along with each chapter's discussion, Table 1.1 provides some brief examples of different types of behavior. Relationships with family and friends can also play an important role in abnormal behaviors. Ayan and Calliess (2005) discussed how personality disorders seem to be more frequent in industrialized countries where social isolation is more common and there is less connectedness.

Of note is that traditional Western-oriented psychotherapy may not be appropriate for many cultures and populations. Strong ties and commitment to family and the community may hinder the ability of Western-oriented therapies that include individualism and not a strong emphasis on religion or spirituality.

TABLE 1.1 Behaviors

REGION/CULTURE	NAME/BEHAVIOR	REASON
Central and South American Native Tribes	Cutting arms and wrists	Viewed as an ancient initiation ritual
Southeast Asia	*Amok*: non-premeditated violent attack on people or objects	Reaction to an insult or disrespect
Cambodia	*Khyâl cap*: dizziness, shortness of breath, etc., similar to anxiety attack	Believe there is a wind-like substance in the body
Greece	Spitting on the bride at weddings	Believed to ward off the devil
Denmark	Spending leisure time in local cemeteries	Socially acceptable to convert this into usable space
United States	Laughing with your mouth open	In Japan, this is considered impolite

Historical Perspectives

Treatment of those struggling with mental health disorders has truly come a long way. Since so little was known about the brain and mental illness, many *experts in the field* seemed to treat mental disorders with whatever they could come up with at the time. Some would rely on religious practices, and others would use current science practices. Most of the treatments would subject the clients to pain and suffering as bad or worse than the actual disorder. The following is a list of some of the "techniques" commonly used throughout history to attempt to treat mental illness. Table 1.2 provides a brief overview of mental health treatment through the ages.

Trephination. Considered one of the oldest forms of neurosurgical treatment, trephination involved literally drilling a hole in the skull of the patient to relieve pressure. An interesting aspect of this procedure was that the use of trephination was widespread throughout the world at different times in history.

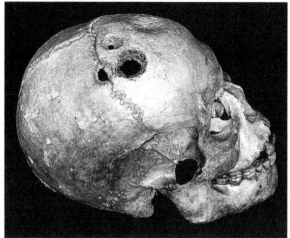

Bloodletting and Purging. The popular practice of bloodletting and purging started around 3,000 years ago. Hippocrates believed that a person suffering with a mental illness had an imbalance of the four humors (blood, phlegm, black bile, and yellow bile). By removing an excessive amount of one of the four humors (blood), he postulated that this would reduce the person's mental illness. Bloodletting procedures would include the typical needle, scraping the skin, or using leeches to suck the blood out. The practice of bloodletting and purging continued for centuries until it was finally debunked in the late 19th century (Greenstone, 2010). Although most forms of bloodletting and purging are no longer used, the practice of cupping (considered a form of bloodletting) regained popularity with athletes in the 2000s.

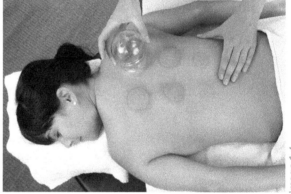

Lobotomy. In 1946, an aspiring psychiatrist, Dr. Walter Freeman, desperate to make a name for himself, decided that the best way to regulate overactive emotions and mental illness was to perform a transorbital lobotomy (severing connections to the prefrontal cortex). The procedure begins by shocking the patient unconscious and then inserting a tool similar to an ice pick through the orbit of the eye into the frontal lobes of the brain. He would then move the pick back and forth and do the procedure on both sides (Norris, 2005). As barbaric as the procedure sounds, it actually became very popular in the United States. Since there were really no reliable medications and no other procedures, the practice of lobotomies was the standard. It wasn't until Dr. Freeman had performed more than 2,500 lobotomies that his practice finally came to an end when his final patient died of a brain hemorrhage in 1967 after more than 20 years of these procedures.

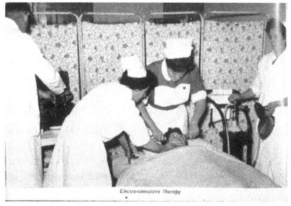

Electro-convulsive Therapy

Electroconvulsive Therapy. Electroconvulsive therapy (ECT) started back in the 1940s in an effort to treat mental health issues when almost all other options had failed. We have probably all watched or know about how ECT is depicted in television shows or in movies, such as *One Flew Over the Cuckoo's Nest*. Patients were initially strapped to a hospital bed while a doctor sent high-level electric current through their brains. Early on, patients were provided with very little in the way of anesthesia and would violently convulse/seize during the procedure. The electrical current is believed to be like a reset button for the brain, activating neurons and chemicals in the brain to reduce depression and psychosis. ECT is still widely used today, but advances in humane treatment now allow the patient to be under general anesthesia and sleep through the procedure. New advances in brain stimulation treatment, such as transcranial magnetic stimulation, vagus nerve stimulation, and deep brain stimulation, have taken this type of treatment to new and more effective levels.

Asylums. Widely used throughout the world, early asylums offered little in the way of treatment. With limited therapies and treatment for mentally ill patients, many in the medical field and communities favored placing these patients in facilities where they could be controlled. For centuries, mental illness was considered a moral or spiritual issue and the best remedy was punishment and shame (Ozarin, 2017). One of the first hospitals to treat mental illness opened in 1247 in London. The Bethlehem Hospital (aka Bedlam) treated "lunatic people." In the 1750s, the Quakers opened up the basement in the Pennsylvania Hospital for people suffering from mental illness. The mode of treatment consisted of chaining patients to the wall in the basement, and they were subjected to various trials of treatment. They went on to open up a separate hospital named Pennsylvania Hospital for the Insane, which operated until 1998. Stays in these types of asylums continued to lack ethical and appropriate services for many years. Dorothea Dix was credited for being one of the first to advocate for ethical and humane care for people with mental illness. She is responsible for opening up 32 state mental hospitals in the United States (Ozarin, 2017).

TRUE LIFE 1.1

Elizabeth Mary Jane Cochran

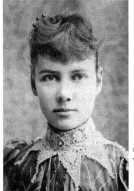

Image 1.6

Born May 5, 1864, American born journalist, industrialist, and inventor Elizabeth Mary Jane Cochran (AKA ... Nellie Bly) was widely recognized as a woman of many talents. She traveled the globe in record fashion at 72 days, 6 hours, 11 minutes, and 14 seconds after having read *Around the World in 80 Days* and was a very popular columnist. Cochran's columns combatted the negative perceptions of women in newspapers during her time and harped on what we know today as feminism. One of Cochran's best known exposés involved her feigning mental illness so as to uncover the truth behind the maltreatment endured by mentally ill patients in mental institutions (Biography.com, 2020).

Elizabeth Cochran was challenged by her editor to go undercover in one of New York's most well-known hospitals, the Women's Lunatic Asylum, to investigate reports of brutality and neglect. Cochran had herself committed to the asylum by taking the following steps. She checked herself into a boarding home, *Temporary Homes for Females*. Instead of going to sleep as she normally would, she stayed up the duration of the night so as to give herself the appearance of a wide-eyed and disturbed woman. Cochran went on to make absurd accusations that the other residents were insane and claimed to one of the assistants that, "There are so many crazy people about, and one can never tell what they will do." Between her accusations and distraught appearance, Cochran instilled a sense of fear and unease in the other residents so much so that the police were called (Norwood, 2017).

After being examined by a doctor and receiving a dementia diagnosis along with other psychological illnesses, she was committed to Blackwell Island where patients were not afforded privacy. Outsiders were permitted to visit patients to curb their craving of excitement of those deemed "mad." Undercover, Bly went on to document the horrors that patients fell victim to: forced to take ice-cold baths and remain in wet clothes for hours, leading to frequent illnesses; forced to sit still on benches, without speaking or moving, for stints lasting 12 hours or more; patients were tethered together with ropes (Biography.com, 2020).

Bly's biggest discovery lay in her learning that many of the patients committed were not mentally ill but rather were without family, poor, or of immigrant status. And if they were not mentally ill prior to their commitment, the treatment from the asylum's staff inflicted psychological damage which led to their prolonged stay. Nellie Bly went on to publish her 10-day experience in her book, *Ten Days in a Mad-House*. The launch of her book helped propel forth a bill which increased funding for mental institutions upwards of $1 million. Bly's courageousness helped to ignite mental health reformation (Norwood, 2017).

TABLE 1.2 Mental Illness Throughout History

400 BC
Hippocrates declares mental illness as a disease. Suggests an imbalance in the four humors.
Middle Ages
Establishment of asylums. Mentally ill were either provided some support or treated as demons and witches.
1407
The first European facility to treat mental illness is opened in Valencia, Spain.
1600s
Mentally ill patients are being treated inhumanely. Being chained to a wall is one form of treatment.
Late 1700s
French physician Philippe Pinel takes over the Bicêtre insane asylum and forbids the use of chains and shackles. He removes patients from dungeons and allows them to exercise on the grounds. Mistreatment of patients is still rampant in other parts of the world.

(*continued*)

TABLE 1.2 *(Continued)*

1840s
Dorothea Dix advocates for more humane conditions for the mentally ill. Establishes 32 state psychiatric hospitals in the United States.

Late 1800s
State mental hospitals are overcrowded and conditions worsen. Nellie Bly, a reporter for *New York World*, poses as a patient and exposes the woeful conditions within these hospitals.

Early 1900s
Pioneer theorists like Sigmund Freud and Carl Jung develop theories and techniques to work with mentally ill patients.

1908
After spending a year in a mental hospital, Clifford Beers writes *A Mind That Found Itself* and goes on to found the National Committee for Mental Hygiene.

1930s
Psychotropic medications are now being used to treat mental illness. Most medications have severe side effects. Lobotomies, insulin-induced comas, and bloodletting are common treatment options. The drug Camphor is first used to treat schizophrenia.

1940s
President Truman signs the National Mental Health Act and creates the National Institute of Mental Health. Psychiatrist Dr. John Cade is one of the first to use lithium to treat psychosis.

1950s
First generation drugs are developed and used to treat psychosis. Thorazine is one of the first antipsychotic drugs.
Behavioral therapy is developed.

1960s
Begins the deinstitution movement. While numbers in the hospitals drop, a surge in the homeless population is a direct result of the lack of treatment on an outpatient level.
Money was provided for community-based services because of the passage of the Mental Retardation Facilities and Community Mental Health Centers Construction Act.

1970s
The National Alliance for the Mentally Ill is created. This agency will provide mental health services across the country.

1980s
There is continued growth in psychotropic medications, along with the creation of the National Alliance for Research on Schizophrenia and Depression.

Source: PBS, 2019

Professional Licensing Standards

Mental health professionals who diagnose and treat clients come from a variety of educational backgrounds. There are varying paths to take for one to become a mental health professional or *clinician* (a reciprocal term also used in this book). Clinicians typically hold a master's or doctorate degree in clinical mental health counseling, social work, psychology, marriage and family therapy, or other disciplines. As an example, programs such as most master of social work programs will provide students with a focus area, such as in mental health/health-related social work or a specific tract to prepare graduates for careers in clinical work. Most graduate clinical programs share some commonalities, including studying theories guiding clinical practice and courses/internships designed to teach client assessment and treatment skills. Each discipline has its own version of clinical licensure, required at the state and national levels for clinical or private practice and its own guiding *code of ethics*. In addition to the completion of a related master's and/or doctorate degree, most disciplines require passing a clinical licensure examination and two or more years of clinically supervised practice experience to become clinically licensed. There are variations of preliminary or provisional licenses offered in some states. Box 1.3 provides helpful websites to learn more about professional associations and clinical licensure.

Box 1.3 Professional Organizations

- American Counseling Association: www.counseling.org
- National Association of Social Workers: https://socialworkers.org
- American Psychological Association: https://.apa.org
- Association of Marriage and Family Therapy: https://amftrb.org/
- American Psychiatric Association: https://www.psychiatry.org

---

While most mental health professionals are required to have at least a master's degree, there are a large number of mental health paraprofessionals who are meeting the many needs of clients in various settings. These paraprofessionals assist in providing personal care and transportation, implementing treatment plans, and providing case management and behavior management plans. The majority of these careers do not require an advanced degree (master's or PhD).

Table 1.3 provides a quick reference for the different types of mental health professionals.

TABLE 1.3 Mental Health Professionals

Clinical mental health counselor	Requires either a master's degree, PhD, or EdD, typically in counselor education with a concentration in clinical mental health counseling. Most states require licensure, and counselors will have the ability to provide counseling services and make diagnoses and assessments. Primary service is counseling with individuals and groups. Counselor education curriculums also typically contain coursework in career counseling.
Clinical social worker	Requires completion of a master's degree (MSW) and/or a doctorate (PhD or DSW) and earning a clinical license. Clinical social workers provide services such as clinical assessment, professional counseling, and mental health diagnosing. Social work program curriculums may also provide coursework in medical social work, which lends itself to practice in hospitals, hospices, and other medical settings. Social work curriculums also contain an emphasis on social justice.
Marriage and family therapist	Requires completion of either a master's or PhD in marriage and family therapy. They take a holistic approach to care and have at least two years of clinical experience. They are able to treat the full range of mental health issues (AAMFT, 2020).

(continued)

TABLE 1.3 *(Continued)*

Psychologist	Requires completion of a PhD, PsyD, or EdD. Clinicians with a master's degree in psychology are usually considered psychological associates who require supervision throughout their careers. Psychologists are trained to work with various mental health issues, make diagnoses, and conduct testing and assessments. Some states allow psychologists with advanced training to prescribe medication.
Psychiatrist	Requires completion of medical school, MD or DO, and specialization in mental health. They are qualified to assess and treat mental health and physical issues. They can treat, diagnose, and administer psychological tests and assessments. They can also prescribe medications used in the treatment of mental health conditions.
Mental health paraprofessional	Requires at a minimum a high school diploma but typically prefers a two- or four-year degree. Other job titles can include mental health technician, psychiatric technician, or aide. They provide case management, psychoeducational programs, monitor patient's conditions, and assist in daily activities.

Psychopathology for Mental Health Professionals

Some students have asked questions about why studying pathology is important, especially if a clinician has strong counseling skills and compassion for helping clients. As noted earlier, there are varying ways to become clinically licensed. One thing the disciplines all share, however, is the agreement that understanding both typical development and psychopathology is valuable in properly treating clients. If clinicians can correctly identify symptoms and disorder patterns in clients, it greatly assists in choosing an appropriate diagnosis and intervention with the client. Of course, we as clinicians see our clients as *people* first, not their diagnosis. But having an accurate and workable diagnosis is often necessary to help our clients get the help they want and need.

Understanding how to interpret and use diagnostic tools and manuals well will equip clinicians to diagnose more accurately, which may ultimately assist clients in recovering faster. For example, according to the National Institute of Mental Health (2016), there are bodies of research that indicate clients who meet criteria for major depressive disorder will often benefit from cognitive behavioral therapy and, in some cases, the use of specific antidepressant medications. Thus a clinician trained to accurately diagnose a client with major depressive disorder may then feel confident suggesting cognitive behavioral therapy to the client as a possible treatment option. If the client's symptoms were more fitting with a typical grief reaction, however, the clinician may suggest a supportive counseling approach or bereavement support group.

As readers journey through the chapters, they are encouraged to take notice not only of the symptom criteria but also the "Clinicians Corner" and "Did You Know?" sections, all designed to give students and budding clinicians more practical insight.

The Legal and Ethical Considerations

In almost all cases, the mental health professionals referred to in this book are mandated by law to report suspected abuse or neglect of a minor or an elderly person. Although maintaining a client's privacy is very important to mental health professionals, such clinicians are also required to report a client's risk of harm to self or others if the risk is seen as imminent. Specific laws vary based on the state, so it is important for a clinician to know the state laws in which they practice, especially as they apply to the delivery of clinical services. Furthermore, states differ with regard to details such as how long clinical files are to be kept by the clinician after discharging clients from services and other specifics. For reasons like this, it is important for clinicians, especially those in private practice, to seek consult from their national associations or legal advisors about laws that guide their practices.

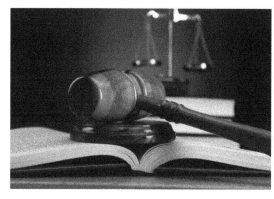

Image 1.7

As noted in this book, mental health professionals are strongly encouraged to be familiar with their specific discipline's code of ethics. Most state licensing boards will expect licensed clinicians to uphold the ethics of said discipline. The state licensing boards typically also have the authority to suspend or discontinue clinical or practice licenses if proof of unethical behavior is confirmed. In many cases, state and federal laws and ethical standards related to serving clients will overlap. Clinicians should be aware, however, that just because a behavior is **legal** does not necessarily mean it would be considered **ethical** or in the best interest of the client. For example, it may be legal in some states for a clinician to have a social relationship or be Facebook friends with a client, but most licensing boards would highly discourage this behavior to avoid dual relationships.

Codes of ethics are in place to not only protect the clients being served but also to give guidance on how clinicians should conduct themselves with colleagues and in the community. With regard to colleagues, clinicians are encouraged to show professional respect and courtesy when sharing client cases or giving and receiving referrals to one another. Finally, it is advisable for clinicians to be aware of ethical standards specific to their areas of practice. For example, the National Association of Social Workers Code of Ethics has specific ethical guidelines for social workers in clinical practice that may differ slightly from those guidelines for practicing in a health-care setting (NASW, 2017).

What Do You Know?

As you progress through your course and this book, we wanted to provide you with a brief pre- and post-assessment tool. We recommend that you try to answer these questions at the beginning of the course and then at the end to evaluate your growth in the area of psychopathology.

Self-Assessment Pretest and Posttest

1. Name one professional mental health association.
2. In 1946, an aspiring psychiatrist, Dr. Walter Freeman, desperate to make a name for himself, decided that the best way to regulate overactive emotions and mental illness was to perform a _____.

3. Explain the biopsychosocial model:

4. _____ advocated for more humane conditions for the mentally ill. Established 32 state psychiatric hospitals in the United States.

5. To be diagnosed with attention deficit hyperactivity disorder, the core symptoms of inattention and/or hyperactive-impulsive behavior must be present prior to age _____.

   a. 4 years
   b. 6 years
   c. 10 years
   d. 12 years

6. _____ is an elimination disorder and is the voiding of urine (either involuntary or intentional) into the bed or clothes.

   a. Urinalysis
   b. Encopresis
   c. Enuresis
   d. Dysgraphia

7. Which personality disorder cluster is characterized by its odd and eccentric behavior?

   a. Cluster A
   b. Cluster B
   c. Cluster C
   d. Cluster D

8. Which of the following personality disorders is labeled by the World Health Organization as "emotionally unstable personality disorder"?

   a. Antisocial personality disorder
   b. Borderline personality disorder
   c. Narcissistic personality disorder
   d. Schizoid personality disorder

9. Which disruptive, impulse-control, and conduct disorders are most prevalent in men?

   _____

10. Which disruptive, impulse-control, and conduct disorders have a strong genetic predisposition?

11. What are the two most commonly used manuals for diagnosing mental health disorders?

12. Which is considered to be the earliest theoretical approach?

   a. Person-centered therapy
   b. Psychodynamic/psychoanalysis therapy
   c. Solution-focused therapy
   d. Behavior therapy

13. Lithium is considered an effective psychotropic drug for what mental health conditions?

   _____

14. What are the four main components of a treatment plan?

   _____

15. Explain the importance of assessment in the counseling process.

16. Of the following treatment modalities, which has not been found to be effective in clients with post-traumatic stress disorder?

   a. Cognitive processing therapy
   b. Pharmacological interventions
   c. Eye movement desensitization and reprocessing therapy
   d. Exposure therapy

17. When children experience prolonged exposure to trauma, this area of the brain can diminish in size:

   a. Hippocampus
   b. Amygdala
   c. Prefrontal cortex
   d. Basal ganglia

18. What is the primary difference between post-traumatic stress disorder and acute stress disorder?

19. What is controversial about the diagnosis of reactive attachment disorder?

20. What are the four categories of sexual dysfunction?

21. What is one form of treatment for female sexual interest/arousal disorder?

22. What is the most common sexual dysfunction that affects men?

23. Which of the following paraphilic disorders involves deriving pleasure by inflicting pain on others?

   a. Sexual sadism disorder
   b. Sexual masochism disorder
   c. Frotteurism disorder
   d. Transvestic disorder

24. Which of the following eating and feeding disorders presents earliest in life and is characterized by the unintentional regurgitation of food?

   a. Pica
   b. Binge-eating disorder
   c. Rumination disorder
   d. Anorexia nervosa

25. All of the following eating and feeding disorders are mutually exclusive, except for which disorder?

   a. Binge eating disorder
   b. Pica

    c. Bulimia nervosa
    d. Avoidant/restrictive food intake disorder

26. Please describe what modalities you might include in a treatment plan for a child client diagnosed with avoidant/restrictive food intake disorder.

    _____

27. The most commonly diagnosed of the depressive disorders is _____.
28. The chronic version of a major depressive episode is called _____.
29. The *ICD-10* describes symptoms of _____ disorder as clients who present with recurrent and frequent physical symptoms that last two years or more.
30. _____ disorders are a group of disorders that are characterized by a break with reality, sometimes as a response to a traumatic event.
31. A _____ is a condition in which the brain function has become impaired and functioning is distinguished from the premorbid condition.
32. Probably the most well-known neurocognitive disorder is _____ disease.
33. One of the most common types of neurocognitive disorders is _____.
34. The basic definition of _____ is a disorder where people have problems falling asleep and/or staying asleep.
35. _____ are sleep disorders that involve unwanted experiences or behaviors, such as sleep terrors, sleepwalking, nightmares, bedwetting, sleep talking, and sleep-related eating episodes.
36. Individuals who struggle with _____ may be described as having "perfectionistic" tendencies or a "type A" personality.
37. A person diagnosed with _____ shows persistent difficulty in discarding items of little value, experiences significant distress related to parting with such items, and strongly feels the need to save the items.
38. _____ is characterized by the compulsive desire and habitual behavior of pulling out one's own hair.
39. _____ are the most commonly diagnosed mental disorders in the United States.
40. _____ is an extremely intense fear and avoidance of a specific object or situation.

Pre-and Post-Assessment Key

1. American Counseling Association
   National Association of Social Workers
   American Psychological Association
   Association of Marriage and Family Therapy
   American Psychiatric Association
2. Transorbital lobotomy
3. The BPS model encourages clinicians to view clients as potentially being impacted by biological, psychological, and/or social factors.
4. Dorothea Dix
5. d
6. c
7. a
8. b
9. Conduct disorder, antisocial personality disorder, and pyromania

Intermittent explosive disorder, conduct disorder, and antisocial personality disorder

10. Intermittent Explosive Disorder, Conduct Disorder, and Antisocial Personality Disorder
11. *ICD-10* and *DSM-5*
12. b
13. Mania and bipolar
14. Problem identification, setting goals and objectives, and progress evaluation
15. Assessment procedures involve collecting meaningful data from clients to better understand them from a holistic perspective.
16. b
17. a
18. Post-traumatic stress disorder can't be diagnosed until one month after exposure to the traumatic event but acute stress disorder can.
19. Previous versions of the *DSM-5* and *ICD-10* (11) have included both attachment and social behaviors that often led to misdiagnosis.
20. Sexual desire/interest, arousal, orgasm, and sexual pain
21. Narrative therapy, the medication Filbanserin (Addyi), along with therapy, or Concurrent therapy.
22. Erectile dysfunction
23. a
24. c
25. b
26. Treatment methods for Avoidant/Restrictive Food Intake Disorder include pharmacotherapy, psychological treatment, and multimodal methods to meet a wide range of needs.
27. Major depressive disorder
28. Dysthymic disorder
29. Somatization
30. Dissociative disorders
31. Neurocognitive disorder
32. Alzheimer's
33. Traumatic brain injury
34. Insomnia
35. Parasomnias
36. Obsessive-compulsive disorder
37. Hoarding disorder
38. Trichotillomania
39. Anxiety disorders
40. Specific phobia

Guided Practice Exercises

Each chapter will have several exercises to expand your knowledge. These exercises will select various mental health issues in each chapter. As you read through the chapters, you will begin to get a sense of possible diagnoses for each case example. Each case was intentionally left with some room for discussion and clinical interpretation. We feel that having the ability to explore various possibilities will assist you in deciding on possible diagnoses.

Web-Based and Literature-Based Resources

American Counseling Association: www.counseling.org

National Association of Social Workers: www.socialworkers.org

American Psychological Association: www.apa.org

American Association for Marriage and Family Therapy: www.aamft.org

World Health Organization: www.who.int

References

American Association for Marriage and Family Therapy (AAMFT). (2020). *About marriage and family therapists*. https://www.aamft.org/About_AAMFT/About_Marriage_and_Family_Therapists.aspx

American Psychological Association. (2020). *APA dictionary of psychology*.

American Psychiatric Association. (2013). *Diagnostic and statistical manual of mental disorders* (5th ed.).

Ayan, S. J., & Calliess, T. (2005). Abnormal as norm. *Scientific America*. https://www.scientificamerican.com/article/abnormal-as-norm/

Benedict, R. (1934). Culture and the abnormal. *Journal of General Psychology,10*, 59–82.

Biography.com. (2020). *Nellie Bly Biography*. A&E Television Networks. https://www.biography.com/activist/nellie-bly

Borrell-Carrió, F., Suchman, A. L., & Epstein, R. M. (2004). The biopsychosocial model 25 years later: Principles, practice, and scientific inquiry. *Annals of Family Medicine, 2*(6), 576–582. https://doi.org/10.1370/afm.245

Engel, G. (1977). The need for a new medical model: A challenge biomedicine. *Science, 196*, 129–136.

Greenstone, G. (2010). The history of bloodletting. *BC Medical Journal, 52*, 12–14.

Moleiro, C. (2018). Culture and psychopathology: New perspectives on research, practice, and clinical training in a globalized world. *Frontiers in Psychiatry, 9*, 366. https://doi.org/10.3389/fpsyt.2018.00366

National Association of Social Workers (NASW). (2017, August). *Code of ethics*. https://www.socialworkers.org/About/Ethics/Code-of-Ethics

National Institute of Mental Health (NIMH). (2016, November). *Psychotherapies*. https://www.nimh.nih.gov/health/topics/psychotherapies/index.shtml

National Institute of Mental Health. (NIMH). (2018, January). *Mental health information: Statistics*. https://www.nimh.nih.gov/health/statistics/index.shtml

National Institute of Mental Health (NIMH). (2019, February). *Mental illness*. https://www.nimh.nih.gov/health/statistics/mental-illness.shtml

Norris, M. (2005, November). 'My lobotomy': Howard Dully's journey. *NPR's All Things Considered*. https://www.npr.org/2005/11/16/5014080/my-lobotomy-howard-dullys-journey

Norwood, A. R. (2017). *Nellie Bly*. National Women's History Museum. https://www.womenshistory.org/education-resources/biographies/nellie-bly

Ozarin, L. (2017). *Diseases of the mind: Highlights of American psychiatry through 1900*. U.S. National Library of Medicine.

Patel, V., Saxena, S., Lund, C., Thornicroft, G., Baingana, F., Bolton, P., Chisholm, D., Collins, P. Y., Cooper, J. L., Eaton, J., Herrman, H., Herzallah, M. M., Huang, Y., Jordans, M. J. D., Kleinman, A., Medina-Mora, M. E., Morgan, E., Niaz, U., Omigbodun, O., ... UnÜtzer, Jü. (2018). The Lancet Commission on global mental health and sustainable development. *Lancet (London, England), 392*(10157), 1553–1598. https://doi.org.libproxy.clemson.edu/10.1016/S0140-6736(18)31612-X

Public Broadcasting System (PBS). (2019). *Treatments for mental illness*. https://www.pbs.org/wgbh/americanexperience/features/nash-treatments-mental-illness/

Szasz, T. S. (1960). The myth of mental illness. *American Psychologist, 15*(2), 113–118. https://doi.org/10.1037/h0046535

World Health Organization (WHO). (2001). *Mental disorders affect one in four people*. https://www.who.int/whr/2001/media_centre/press_release/en/

World Health Organization (WHO). (2015). *Mental health ATLAS 2014*.

World Health Organization (WHO). (2019a). *WHO urges more investments, services for mental health*. https://www.who.int/mental_health/who_urges_investment/en/

World Health Organization (WHO). (2019b). *Mental disorders*. https://www.who.int/mental_health/management/en/

Credits

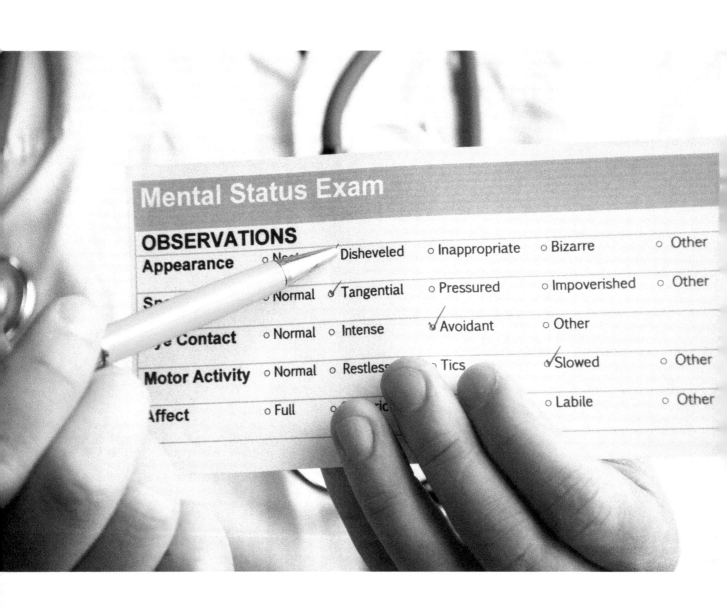

CHAPTER TWO

ASSESSMENT, DIAGNOSING, AND THEORY

Liz Boyd, Melanie Burgess, Sonja Lund, and David A. Scott

CASE STUDY 2.1 Nia has been suffering with panic disorder and is wanting to see some changes in her life. She is unable to drive her adolescent son to and from school because of the fear that she and her son may be involved in a car accident if she has a panic attack. This leaves her son, who does not possess a driver's license, to drive himself to and from school, and he runs the risk of being pulled over by a police officer. Nia also has not been attending work consistently because of her anxiety surrounding her panic attacks, so her boss laid her off and suggested she return when she is able to work as expected.

Nia and her counselor are in the process of creating her treatment plan, which her counselor explains as a map to help her reach her desired destination. Her therapist explains that it is Nia's responsibility to choose her goals, for it places her in a position to be more accountable for her progress and because it is more meaningful if she herself chooses what it is that she wants to better about herself. Nia chooses three goals: (1) notice the signs that an attack is emerging, (2) develop coping skills that will help reduce the sensations associated with the panic attacks, (3) combat the intrusive negative thoughts surrounding her panic attacks. Upon looking at her goals, Nia doubts her ability to achieve, in her words, "such impossible goals." Nia's counselor helps her to set objectives for her to work toward so that they can measure her progress. Once Nia sees the multiple objectives under each of her overall goals, she views them as less intimidating and has a more positive view of her ability to accomplish them.

Did You Know?

- Psychopharmacology is a billion-dollar industry with the United States leading in usage.
- In the United States, almost one out of every five people have a mental health diagnosis (Center for Behavioral Health Statistics and Quality, 2016).
- Lithium has had many uses, including to treat gout and even as a salt substitute.
- Many drugs contain the letter X, Y, or Z to make us think they are effective.

Introduction

Chances are high that if you are reading this text, you are already a natural helper. You may be the person friends or family call when they need to talk through an issue, make a decision, or need a shoulder to cry on. This chapter will begin to walk you through the shift from being a natural helper to a mental health professional. This transition involves learning to systematically identify client concerns and create treatment plans through a series of steps (Neukrug & Schwitzer, 2006). This chapter will provide you with an overview of client assessment, diagnosing, theoretical orientations, and treatment planning. In addition, we will discuss current research related to psychopharmacology and neuropsychological issues.

Assessment

Assessment procedures involve collecting meaningful data from clients to better understand them from a holistic perspective. These procedures include a variety of methods, from informal techniques and observations to clinical interviews and psychometrically sound formal tests. As practitioners gather information about their clients, assessments can assist them in their client conceptualization, goal setting, and treatment planning. In addition, practitioners may select certain assessments to acquire information from specific domains, such as intellectual/cognitive functioning, career and specific aptitudes, and clinical assessments, such as objective and projective personality tests.

Tests of Intelligence and Cognitive Functioning

To better understand the cognitive capabilities of our clients, or the way they think, practitioners may choose to use intelligence tests. The concept of intelligence has been around for more than a century; however, there are many different models regarding how we define intelligence as a construct (Neukrug & Fawcett, 2015). Intelligence tests aim to measure what a client is capable of, and practitioners use these tests to identify cognitive impairments, assess for giftedness, and/or track changes in functioning over time.

Currently, the Weschler scales of intelligence are the most widely used intelligence tests. These scales are divided into select age groups, including the Weschler Preschool and Primary Scale of Intelligence (WPPSI), the Wechsler Intelligence Scale for Children (WISC), and the Wechsler Adult Intelligence Scale (WAIS). These instruments have been researched extensively over the years, undergoing multiple revisions that demonstrate excellent reliability and good validity (Wechsler, 2003). These intelligence tests consist of developmentally appropriate subscales that form composite scores, such as the verbal comprehension index and processing speed index on the WISC (Wechsler, 2003). Since these instruments require verbal ability, the Wechsler Nonverbal Scale of Ability (WNV) addresses linguistically diverse populations (Pearson, n.d.). No matter what instrument is used to assess intelligence, practitioners are cautioned about drawing firm conclusions about intellectual capabilities without taking instrument limitations and cultural differences into context.

Career and Specific Aptitude Assessments

Career interest inventories and special/multiple aptitude tests are used to uncover client strengths and interest areas that may translate into vocational and academic paths. Practitioners can use these assessments to assist clients throughout their lives; however, they may be especially beneficial during transitional periods, such as adolescence and emerging adulthood, graduating from postsecondary schooling, and during career shifts. Several notable instruments include the Strong Interest Inventory (SII), the Self-Directed Search (SDS), and the Occupational Information and Network (O*NET).

Many career inventories are built on the work of John Holland, the creator of the Holland codes. Holland codes include six personality types that exist in a hexagonal model: realistic (R), investigative (I), artistic (A), social (S), enterprising (E), and conventional (C; see Figure 2.1). Upon taking a career inventory that uses Holland codes, a client is given a three-letter Holland code representing the client's strongest personality types. This result can be compared to repositories of more than 12,000 occupational codes that may align with your client's score, essentially linking their score with occupations that most closely align with their personality type. For example, the Holland code for "counselor" is SAE: social, artistic, and enterprising. Ultimately, research has shown that individuals in occupations that align with their Holland codes have moderate to high job satisfaction (Neukrug & Fawcett, 2015; Rottinghaus et al., 2009).

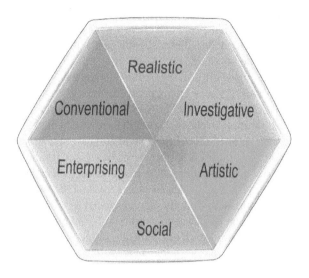

FIGURE 2.1 Holland's Hexagonal Model

Other popular instruments that use Holland codes include the Strong Interest Inventory, Self-Directed Search, and O*NET. The Strong Interest Inventory, the most common career assessment, is a 291-item instrument used in individual or group settings and provides results that include general occupational themes and scales, basic interests, personal style scales, and a general response summary (Herk & Thompson, 2011; Neukrug & Fawcett, 2015). In addition, the Self-Directed Search is a self-administered and self-scored instrument that aims to measure interests using Holland codes but also estimates client self-report of ability (PAR, inc., 2009). Several formats of the Self-Directed Search exist, including ones for children, adolescents and emerging adults, adults with limited reading ability, and professional-level employees. The Self-Directed Search can help practitioners support realistic goal setting with clients by identifying interests but also recognizing client competencies that link with their interests to better prepare them for jobs that they might find fulfilling. Lastly, O*NET is a free online tool and database that includes self-assessments (e.g., Ability Profiler, Interest Profiler, Work Importance Profiler) and occupational classifications based on Holland code results (O*NET, n.d.). This resource can be helpful as practitioners and clients explore career options after reviewing career inventory results.

Clinical Assessment

In terms of clinical assessment, practitioners rely on clinical interviews and instruments to aid in diagnosis, client conceptualization to provide greater insight, and treatment planning. As such, one of the first, and continuous, informal assessments counselors use is the mental status exam. The mental status exam relies on information and behaviors observed by the counselor and typically includes attitudes, use of speech and language, cognitive functioning, thought processes, and emotional expression, as well as suicidality and homocidality (Schwitzer & Rubin, 2015).

In addition, counselors may use objective personality tests or pencil-and-paper tests that have multiple choice or true/false questions to analyze different aspects of a client's personality. Frequently used objective personality tests include the Minnesota Multiphasic Personality Inventory (MMPI), which assists in the diagnosis of a range of mental health disorders and aspects of a client's personality, and the Myers-Briggs Type Indicator (MBTI), which classifies a client's personality and perceptions based on Carl Jung's theory of personality.

Additional frequently used clinical measures include the Substance Abuse Subtle Screening Inventory (SASSI), Beck Depression Inventory (BDI), and Beck Anxiety Inventory (BAI; Peterson et al., 2014). The SASSI is used by practitioners to identify adults who may have a substance-related disorder (Lazowski et al., 2016). The SASSI-A2 is a modified version of the SASSI for children and adolescents between the ages of 12 and 17. The instrument is composed of nine subscales that contain scaling questions related to substance use and frequency. The BDI and BAI are both well-established brief instruments that use rating scales to assess for and determine the severity of clients' self-reported depression and anxiety, respectively (Beck et al., 1961, 1988). While these instruments have evidence of validity and reliability, BDI and BAI scores have a relatively high correlation with one another, suggesting that there is some difficulty distinguishing between the two constructs of depression and anxiety (Neukrug & Fawcett, 2015). As always, instruments should be used in combination with other criteria to determine diagnoses and assess client progress.

In contrast to objective personality tests, projective personality tests present clients with ambiguous stimuli that elicit a wide range of responses. Projective tests lack validity and reliability because of the nature of open-ended responses and interpretation; however, they can prompt valuable information beyond objective tests concerning your clients' perspectives, emotions, conflicts, and underlying personality traits. Two of the more common projective tests include the Rorschach Inkblot Test and the Thematic Apperception Test (TAT; Neukrug & Fawcett, 2015). The Rorschach Inkblot Test is a popular projective test that encourages clients to describe what they see when looking at ambiguous symmetrical splattered ink on cards. In addition, the Thematic Apperception Test involves having children and adults develop a story based on a set of cards depicting vague images. While these assessment procedures have received critiques for their lack of standardization, validity, and reliability, the clients' descriptions and storytelling may reveal important facets of their worldviews in combination with other assessment methods.

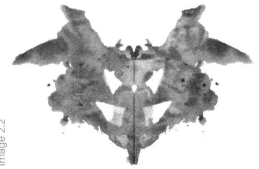

Image 2.2

Diagnosing

Counselors across the world rely on diagnostic manuals to appropriately identify and describe client issues and concerns. Throughout this text, we will explore the most recent editions of two widely used diagnostic handbooks: the *Diagnostic and Statistical Manual, 5th Edition* (DSM-5; American Psychiatric Association [APA], 2013) and the *International Classification of Diseases, 10* (ICD-10; World Health Organization [WHO],

2016). These manuals provide all health professionals with nomenclature, a common language, for psychopathology. Broadly speaking, the *DSM* is most commonly used by mental health professionals in North America to diagnose mental health disorders, whereas the *ICD* is a global publication that includes both medical and mental health diagnoses.

DSM-5

The forerunner to the first edition of the *DSM* was published in 1844 and provided a classification system for mental health patients. Since World War II, five editions have been published, each containing research-based expansions from the last. The overarching goal of the *DSM* is to provide guidelines for diagnosing and treating individuals with mental health disorders (APA, 2013). The *DSM-5* provides mental health and medical professionals with more than 900 pages of guidance related to diagnostic criteria, prevalence rates, groups for research, and public health statistics (e.g., morbidity and mortality). The manual is used across many clinical settings, including inpatient, outpatient, hospitals, and medical practices in the United States.

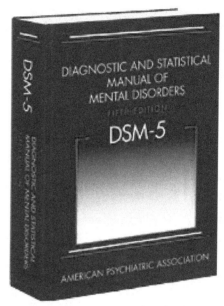

DSM-5
2013

Image 2.3

The book itself can be both overwhelming and exhilarating to novice counselors, as it contains hundreds of mental health diagnoses. Understanding the overall organization of the *DSM-5* will make it more user-friendly. The chapters follow the life span from infancy to older adulthood. The first two chapters focus on neurodevelopmental and schizophrenia-related disorders, most of which manifest early in life. The next few chapters focus on disorders that often manifest in adolescence, such as anxiety, depressive, and bipolar disorders. The manual ends with neurocognitive disorders that tend to develop later in life. The disorders within each chapter are closely aligned with the life span as well.

The APA group that worked to update the most recent version of the *DSM* collaborated with members of the WHO to harmonize the classifications between the manuals. At the time of publication of the *DSM-5*, the *ICD-9* was in use. The *ICD-10 Clinical Modification* was then adapted in the United States in 2014. When using the *DSM-5*, you will notice codes for both the *ICD-9* and *-10*, with *-10* in parentheses. The *DSM* relies on *ICD* codes for billing and reporting purposes. With all this in mind, the revision committees from APA and WHO chose to align the *DSM-5* with the *ICD-11*, which is scheduled to be released for use in early 2022. While the dates of release of these manuals do not line up perfectly, it is helpful to know that the two associations work closely together to identify disorders and determine how to best track mortality and morbidity.

ICD-10 (11)

The WHO organizes diagnoses through the *ICD*. The *ICD-10 2019 edition* is currently in use, with the expectation that the *ICD-11* will be adapted in the United States in early 2022. A key feature of the *ICD-11* is its compatibility with virtual health-care reporting systems, in keeping up with advances in technology. Specifically related to mental health, the mental health program became involved in improving the classifications and descriptions of mental and behavioral health in the early 1960s, with the first improvements featured in the eighth version of the *ICD*. The current version has a chapter dedicated to mental health titled "Mental and Behavioural Health," whereas the proposed new version has four chapters dedicated to mental health. The proposed chapters include mental, behavioral, and neurodevelopmental disorders; sleep-wake disorders; diseases of the nervous system; and conditions related to sexual health.

The *ICD* is the international standard used for systematically classifying and diagnosing symptoms and disorders. There are many purposes for a numeric classification system, including record keeping, data management, and analyses. Health professionals may not use the exact same language to describe symptoms, whereas using the *ICD* requires them to choose a code that is linked to specific symptoms or disorders. This allows medical researchers to quickly find and analyze data. For example, in 2020, the *ICD* created emergency codes for the COVID-19 pandemic. There are codes for suspected cases and cases confirmed by testing, and both codes can be used to describe mortality. The common codes that are used by medical professionals throughout the world allow researchers to best determine rates of infection in specific areas, establish trends, and shape future projections. The use of the *ICD* codes through the pandemic has been imperative to learning about the virus to support the safety of the world's population. The same concept relates to mental health disorders. Clinicians and researchers use the data in similar ways to describe and identify symptoms and track data related to prevalence, mortality, and morbidity. The data collected allows researchers to identify health trends and statistics worldwide.

Theoretical Options

In the mental health field, theories are used to guide our therapeutic work with clients. Some practitioners may choose to identify with one theory; however, flexibility in our approach is important. At times, we may choose to integrate, or combine, theories for optimal client outcomes. Often, the client's current diagnosis will influence the theory we implement throughout treatment. While certain patterns exist among disorders, each client will present with unique concerns, contextual/environmental factors, and multicultural backgrounds. Taking all of these factors into account when selecting our approach often creates the best outcomes and ability to connect with our clients. Using evidence-based, or research-supported, treatment is also important not only to increase the likelihood of successful outcomes but also for ethical practice. To understand theories and their application fully, they should be studied in-depth. This section reviews the application of a few select theories but is not an extensive exploration of all theories.

Psychoanalysis/psychodynamic theory is one of the earliest approaches to mental health treatment. Associated with Sigmund Freud, this theory is rooted in the belief that unconscious forces drive human behavior. Historically, treatment from this perspective was long-term, lasting years for some individuals. A more modern psychodynamic approach uses short-term treatment. Research has found psychodynamic psychotherapy to be effective in the treatment of depression, social anxiety, and some personality disorders (Bogels et al., 2014; Leichsenring et al., 2004).

Humanistic approaches focus on helping clients reach their highest potential. Carl Rogers's person-centered, or client-centered, therapy is a nondirective humanistic approach. Person-centered therapy uses empathy, unconditional positive regard, and genuineness. It is not uncommon to integrate this theory with other theoretical approaches. Person-centered therapy embraces many of the qualities needed for effective therapy, including active listening and building rapport with the client. As such, a person-centered approach can be effective for a variety of client concerns. Existential therapy is another human-istic approach. This theory emphasizes concepts such as freedom, death, responsibility, and isolation (Neukrug, 2018). Living an authentic life is an important part of this theory. Therapeutic techniques include acceptance, con-frontation, and encouragement. While not appropriate for all clients, short-term existential psychotherapy has been found to be effective in the treatment of depression and anxiety (Rayner & Vitali, 2016). Further, long-term results have been relatively positive and client dropout rates are typically low.

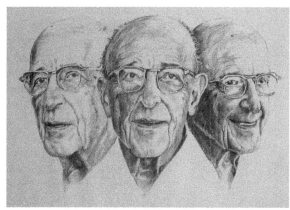

Image 2.4

Behavior therapy, often associated with B. F. Skinner, examines the effect of operant conditioning, classical conditioning, and modeling on human behavior, along with the ways conditioning can be used to assist in client change (Neukrug, 2018). While conditioning is a complex process, modern behaviorists also believe that our thoughts, or cognitions, can be conditioned. Applied behavioral analysis (ABA) is a behaviorally rooted approach commonly used in the treatment of autism (Roane et al., 2016). This approach examines the relationship between a specific behavior and the environment in which it occurs. Applied behavioral analysis is specifically useful with the autistic population because it focuses on eliminating atypical behaviors and acquiring various skills. Other applications of behavior therapy include the treatment of post-traumatic stress disorder (PTSD). Modern therapeutic techniques associated with behavior therapy that are effective in post-traumatic stress disorder treatment include exposure therapy and eye movement desensitization and reprocessing (EMDR; Watts et al., 2013). Evidence also exists for the efficacy of cog-nitive approaches in the treatment of post-traumatic stress disorder.

As behavioral therapy has evolved, concepts such as mindfulness, acceptance, and emotional expression have been integrated into practice, along with a movement toward cognitive behavioral therapy (CBT). One modern behavioral approach includes dialectical behavior therapy (DBT). While personality disorders are often challenging in terms of therapeutic treatment, DBT is commonly used in the treatment of borderline personality disorder with relatively successful outcomes (Kliem et al., 2010). Skills training is common in DBT treatment; however, there is also a focus on awareness of behaviors and cognitions, acceptance of emotional distress, and emotional regulation. DBT places an emphasis on reducing suicidal gestures and self-injurious behaviors, which are commonly seen in those with borderline personality disorder. Acceptance and commitment therapy (ACT), another behavioral spin-off, is a mindfulness-based approach that emphasizes nonjudgmental acceptance of the here and now (Hayes, 2006). Commitment to action is a major tenant of the approach and involves making mindful decisions about living a meaningful life. While most research on the efficacy of acceptance and commitment therapy is preliminary, evidence exists for its useful-ness in treating depression, psychosis, substance use disorders, and eating disorders. CBT is a popular theoretical approach because of its evidence-based effectiveness with a variety of diagnoses. Pioneered by Aaron Beck, CBT examines how a person's thoughts affect their feelings and behaviors. Core and automatic thoughts that are often irrational or distorted are examined and challenged and replaced with rational ones. CBT has been found to be most effective in the treatment of anxiety disorders, somatoform disorders, and bulimia (Hofmann et al., 2012).

Postmodern therapeutic approaches include narrative and solution-focused therapies. Narrative therapy is a positive, future-oriented, and strength-based theoretical approach (Neukrug, 2018). Much of the focus is on where the client wants to go rather than where they have been. This theory examines the multiple "stories" that we live by, along with how they are currently affecting us. Clients can identify and break down their problem-saturated stories and re-story, or re-author, their lives. The goal is to separate the person from the problem and develop healthier stories. This can be particularly helpful in the treatment of depression and eating disorders (Lopes et al., 2014; Weber et al., 2006). Solution-focused brief therapy (SFBT) is typically conducted in six sessions or less and thus is a cost-effective option for many clients. Viewing the client as the expert, SFBT focuses on client strengths and solutions rather than deficits and problems (Neukrug, 2018). Much of the existing research has examined the effectiveness of depression treatment. Results indicate that SFBT is effective in the treatment of depression and is comparable to other established alternative treatments (Gingerich & Peterson, 2013).

Theories help define the client-therapist relationship, the therapeutic process, and various techniques used in treatment. Research supports the use of certain theoretical approaches over others in the use of treating specific disorders. Possessing a well-rounded knowledge of theories and being flexible in one's approach to treatment based on individual client factors will likely lead to optimal outcomes. As research continues to emerge regarding theories and treatment, it is important for practitioners to continually examine the literature to increase their competence.

Treatment Planning

Once we have conducted an assessment, made a diagnosis, and gotten our feet under our own theoretical orientation, we can begin to create a treatment plan *with* our client. Working with a client to establish the elements of the treatment plan can further enhance therapeutic alliance and allow the counselor to better understand the problems from the client's viewpoint. Counselors should take individualized characteristics, such as symptoms, problems, needs, background, family history, strengths, and areas for improvement, into consideration when determining a treatment plan with a client (Jongsma et. al, 2014). Next, we will discuss the major elements of a treatment plan, including problem identification, setting goals and objectives, and progress evaluation.

The first step, *problem identification*, is essentially an overview and confirmation of the problems identified through formal and informal assessments. Once these problems are identified and agreed upon by the counselor and client, they can begin to *set goals* together. Begin by asking the client what they want to accomplish through counseling. The answer to this will provide a baseline for the goals, and the *objectives* will help further determine how the goals will be achieved. When setting goals, keep in mind that they should be realistic, meaning that the goal is something that the client has the means to accomplish. It is also important to be specific about a time line. With the client, you should also consider what is reasonable. For example, if the client's goal is to secure new housing, a month may be a more realistic time line than a week. The more specific the goals and objectives are, the easier it will be to measure the client's progress.

Evaluation of a client's progress is an essential part of the treatment plan. There are many ways to measure progress, so you should work with the client to determine the best method based on the goals and objectives. The client could report the progress through self-reports to the counselor during sessions or bring journals or logs to share. The counselor could also administer assessments at certain intervals to compare pre- and post-scores. This could be especially helpful for someone working to reduce their substance use (SASSI) or reduce levels of depression (BDI).

Recall the case with Nia. The counselor asked her to identify her goals. Nia was able to do this, yet she was still concerned about whether she would be able to accomplish them. Together, Nia and the counselor worked to identify objectives that helped to break each goal down into more manageable tasks.

If you were working with Nia, what objectives could you suggest to help her make her goals more attainable? What forms of measurement would you use to determine her progress toward accomplishing her goals?

Now let's look at another client and counselor interaction. While reading through the script, work to identify the problem(s), the goal(s), and the measures of progress.

Client-Counselor Transcript

Client: I can't believe I was fired from my job. I honestly didn't see it coming. Things at work were going fine, and I thought I was well liked and respected. It just hurts to be let down like this. And I'm scared about finances and the impact on my family. When will I find a new job? Will I be able to match my previous salary? I just have so many questions.

Counselor: You really did not expect this change in employment and have been left with a lot of unanswered questions. Specifically, you've mentioned the shock from losing your job and the uncertainty of the future. Would you like to focus on either of those today?

Client: Yeah, honestly, I think I want to talk about the future. I'm just so scared that I won't be able to provide for my family.

Counselor: All right, let's think together about this problem. What are the most pressing implications related to the change in finances?

Client: Well, I have six months' severance, so realistically, I have a little time. I'm just worried time will slip away.

Counselor: It makes sense to be concerned about this, even ahead of time. How can we ensure that you don't let time slip away?

Client: Hmm. I guess I just need to keep myself motivated to look for new jobs.

Counselor: That sounds like an excellent step. It might help to make it more specific. How often do you want to look for jobs?

Client: I should probably check job boards at least once a day. I think I could commit to at least looking at potential jobs for an hour every day of the week.

Counselor: Okay great. What happens if you see a job you are interested in?

Client: I guess I should set some time aside for job applications too. I'll plan to apply for at least two jobs a week. If I see more that I'm interested in, I'll apply for more than two during that week.

Counselor: I think these are strong goals. To reiterate, you plan to (1) check job boards for at least an hour every day and (2) apply for at least two jobs every week. Does that sound correct?

Client: Absolutely. I think these are attainable and realistic.

Counselor: How would you like to check in regarding your progress? We could have an informal check-in during your weekly sessions, or you could keep a journal about your progress that we review together every week. Or do you have another idea?

Client: Let's try weekly check-ins. I'll keep my own journal just so I know what I've seen and applied for, but I'd appreciate checking in with you briefly each week just for accountability's sake.

Counselor: That sounds like a strong plan moving forward. We can always reevaluate and make changes as we need to.

You will notice in the client-counselor interaction that the client comes in with a couple of problems to explore. They are upset about losing their job and concerned about the financial effect of the change in employment. Notice that the counselor works with the client to narrow down the focus of the session and then subtlety moves the client toward goal setting. The client is receptive and eager to establish some goals and report back during the next session. Of course, not all clients will be this easygoing, and this process could take longer than what is shown here. What is most important to pick up out of this interaction is the open dialogue. The counselor allows the client space to lead the conversation, using questions and prompts to guide and support the goal-setting process. As you continue through this text, challenge yourself to think about treatment plans that could work for clients with specific disorders.

Psychopharmacology

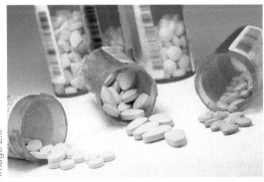

Image 2.5

If you were to ask a non-mental health professional what comes to mind when asked about possible treatment for mental health issues, what do you think they would say? There would be a high probability that one of the first things they would say is medication. The inclusion of medication in the treatment of mental health issues has been one of the most dramatic factors in the last 50 years. Without medications, many people would never be able to live productive lives. At the same time, many believe that we have become too dependent on medications, using meds to solve our problems. "Just take this pill, everything will be fine" is sometimes our philosophy for treating mental illness. While taking a pill may make us feel better, it does not change our environment, working conditions, or overall situation. Most believe that a combination of mental health therapy and medication is the optimal treatment plan. Box 2.2 will start the conversation around medications. Each chapter in this book will detail the most common medications used for each set of mental health disorders. Table 2.1 provides a quick reference of the types of medications used for different disorders.

Box 2.2

Take a moment and think about your viewpoints on using medications to help treat mental illness. Discuss the following in class:

1 Ways in which medications can be used
2 Times when medications should not be used
3 Thoughts on general practitioners writing prescriptions for psychotropic meds

TABLE 2.1 Medications

MENTAL HEALTH DISORDERS	TYPES OF MEDICATIONS	NAMES OF MEDICATIONS (BRAND NAMES)
Depression	Serotonin reuptake inhibitors (SSRIs) Serotonin and norepinephrine reuptake inhibitors (SNRIs) Atypical antidepressants	Fluoxetine (Prozac) Sertraline (Zoloft) Paroxetine (Paxil) Venlafaxine (Effexor) Duloxetine (Cymbalta) Bupropion (Wellbutrin)
Anxiety	Benzodiazepines Anxiolytics	Alprazolam (Xanax) Lorazepam (Ativan) Buspirone (BuSpar)
Attention deficit hyperactivity disorder (ADHD)	Stimulants	Methylphenidate (Ritalin) Dextroamphetamine (Dexedrine)
Psychosis	Antipsychotics First generation Second generation	Haloperidol (Haldol) Chlorpromazine (Thorazine) Perphenazine (Trilafon) Risperidone (Risperdal) Olanzapine (Zyprexa) Aripiprazole (Abilify) Lurasidone (Latuda)
Bipolar, mood swings, mania	Mood stabilizer/ antimanic Anticonvulsants	Lithium (Eskalith) Valproic Acid (Depakote) Carbamazepine (Tegretol) Lamotrigine (Lamictal)

Source: (NIMH, 2020)

Two of the most influential psychotropic medications used today are lithium and Prozac. Their beginnings and road to widespread use give us insight into how medications are developed and approved for use in the general public.

Story of Lithium

Lithium can be considered one of the most impactful mental health medications of all time. Lithium's ability to successfully treat individuals diagnosed with mania and bipolar disorders has allowed countless patients to regain a semblance of their normal daily activities where this was not even comprehensible before lithium treatment. Lithium has been around for years and was even used as a salt substitute—with deadly results. Corcoran, Taylor, and Page (1949) warned of the use of lithium in low-sodium diets and suggested that lithium no longer be used in this manner. Stories of the beneficial use of lithium sprang up in different parts of the United States. From the Mineral Wells in Texas labeled as "crazy waters" (Fowler, 1991) to the use and even bottling of lithium water from the lithium springs of Lithia Springs, Georgia. In 1887, a congress of physicians recommended using the lithium water to treat everything from kidney stones, typhoid fever, indigestion, and "diseases of delicate women" (May, 1989).

Lithium has been used in the medical field for years. Initially used to treat gout, the value of lithium to treat manic depression and mania was rediscovered by Australian John Cade. Even though Dr. Cade supported the use of lithium, the more mainstream use came after psychiatrist Mogens Schou published his results in 1954 (Shorter, 2009). Schou randomized his study using a coin flip to determine control or placebo. Lithium quickly become the medication of choice to treat mania over the use of barbiturates and electroconvulsive therapy (ECT).

The Story of Prozac

With depression being one of the most common mental health disorders worldwide (WHO, 2019), there was a critical need to find effective options for treatment. Yet early treatment options were far and few between. Over 50 years, researchers discovered that clients with depression have low levels of serotonin, norepinephrine, and dopamine. This is when the monoamine hypothesis was developed (Bunney & Davis, 1965). With constant trial and error, two types of medications led the treatment of depression: monoamine oxidase inhibitors and tricyclic antidepressants (Hillhouse & Porter, 2015). Unfortunately, monoamine oxidase inhibitors (MAOs) and tricyclic antidepressants (TCAs) have some severe side effects. Thus the search for a more effective treatment with less serious side effects continued. Tucked away in a lab at the pharmaceutical company Eli Lilly was a drug compound named fluoxetine that was at times being used to treat high blood pressure and served as an antiobesity drug (Moore, 2007). It took several more years for Ray Fuller, Bryan Molloy, and David Wong to develop and secure the Food and Drug Administration's approval for fluoxetine hydrochloride (aka Prozac) to be used to treat depression on a worldwide stage. Prozac revolutionized the medical treatment of depression. Prozac went on to be labeled as one of the breakthrough drugs of the century and earned Eli Lilly $2.8 billion in 1998 (peak annual sale; Wong et al., 2005).

The Future of Psychotropic Medications

While the development and use of psychotropic medications in the 1950s to 1990s was prolific, the development of new medications has dramatically decreased. There was a 70% decrease in investments in the development of psychotropic medications in the past decade (O'Hara & Duncan, 2016). Factors such as fewer incentives, complexity of the brain, and increased difficulty of getting new drugs approved have contributed to this reduction in new drugs. It typically takes roughly nine to 15 *years* for a drug to make it from preclinical trials to market with a cost to the manufacture from $1.3 to $1.7 *billion* (O'Brien et al., 2014). As is with all drugs, the patent usually lasts around 20 years. After this time period, other companies are allowed to produce generic versions of the drugs, continuing to cut into the profits of the original manufacturer. With the effectiveness of many psychotropic drugs in question, the motivation to spend billions of dollars to produce novel psychotropic meds may continue to wane until we know more about the brain and how medications can treat mental illness.

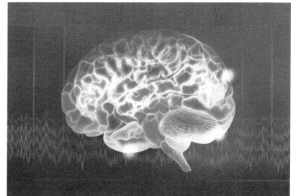

Image 2.6

Current Research on Neuropsychological Issues

As you will read throughout this text, psychopathology tends to focus on behaviors, signs, and symptoms of mental health disorders. Neuroscience takes the diagnostic process to another level, seeking to understand the "why" behind the signs and symptoms (Ray, 2017). Beeson (2017) defined neuroscience broadly as "the scientific study of the nervous system." Initial work with neuropsychology, a branch of neuroscience, focused on the psychological effect of traumatic brain injuries from accidents and developmental delays. Current research has broadened to investigate neurological markers related to mental health disorders. As we discussed earlier in this chapter, the diagnostic process helps mental health professionals to align symptoms with diagnoses to create an effective treatment plan. The field of neuropsychology is working to determine the neurological reasons that two clients with the same disorder may present differently. For example, perhaps you have two clients who have schizophrenia. One shares experiences with auditory hallucinations, whereas the other reports visual hallucinations. While both experiences are valid and lead us to the same diagnosis, neuroscientists suggest that there could be differences in the brains of these clients that cause the different experiences of hallucinations. Brain imaging techniques, such as magnetic resonance imaging, functional magnetic resonance imaging, electroencephalography, and magnetoencephalography, are used to compare brain functioning to gain a deeper understanding of mental health signs and symptoms (Ray, 2017).

Research in neuropsychology has substantially increased over the past 30 years. In 1992, the American Psychological Association established a journal specifically dedicated to the topic called *Neuropsychology*, which has published more than 2,200 articles. More recently, there has been a shift to integrate this research into the counseling field. Around 2013, neuroscience interest networks were founded in the American Counseling Association and the American Mental Health Counselors Association. The

American Mental Health Counselors Association's neurocounseling interest network has more than 800 members, which is more than in any other the organization's interest networks (Beeson, 2017).

Neurocounseling

Russell-Chapin (2016) defined neurocounseling as "the integration of neuroscience into the practice of counseling by teaching and illustrating the physiological underpinnings of many of our mental health concerns" (p. 93). Neurocounseling provides counselors with ways to better understand current practices, conducts brain-based studies that evaluate processes and outcomes, and provides counselors with new brain-based techniques to use with clients, such as neurofeedback (Beeson, 2017). Neurofeedback is a therapeutic technique that uses a computerized system to monitor brain activity. When brain-wave patterns are within the desired range, the program uses visual or auditory signals to retrain or reorganize the client's brain activity (Sirkin & Manzi, 2019). Neurofeedback is a common intervention for individuals of all ages with behavioral disorders, stress-induced disorders, and developmental delays.

Neurocounseling can be easily integrated into a traditional counseling environment. Russell-Chapin (2016) shared an example of this. Consider the introductory handshake that a counselor typically shares with a new client. This handshake has often been the first step in building rapport. A counselor who is practicing neurocounseling would look for information in that handshake. Was the client's hand hot or cold, dry or balmy, firm or limp? The counselor would consider all the factors and begin to make mental notes about a client's possible anxiety or stress level. What are other examples of neurocounseling in sessions?

Most research on neuroscience exists within related helping fields, primarily psychology, and is generalized to the counseling field (Beeson, 2017). While the generalizations provide a solid basis of understanding and knowledge, there is a need for empirically based research specific to the counseling field. The Research Domain Criteria Initiative provides an organization system that offers structure for neuroscience research (Beeson & Aideyan, 2016). The initiative has created an incredible opportunity for counselors and counselor educators to enhance the field through research and publications. Counselors and counselor educators are working every day to find new ways to implement neurocounseling into their work with clients and counselors in training.

Case Study Summary

This chapter's case study reviewed the behaviors of Nia. As you process the story and examine possible diagnostic criteria, take a few minutes to answer the following questions:

1. What would be the correct diagnosis for Nia?

    _____

    _____

2. What are the specific symptoms or criteria that led you to this diagnosis?

    _____

    _____

3. What other possible disorders might you diagnose Nia with and why?

_____

_____

4. Briefly discuss what types of treatment may be beneficial for Nia. Could you see using a certain counseling theory and/or medication?

_____

_____

Guided Practice Exercises

Scenario 1

Ben is a 7-year-old boy who has been diagnosed with attention deficit hyperactivity disorder, hyperactive-impulsive type. For several months now, he has attended counseling bimonthly to better develop his social skills and attentiveness. Based on feedback from Ben's mother and his teachers, it seems that Ben is not able to transfer the skills that he practices in therapy into the school or home environment. Ben's mother is concerned and asks his therapist what more can be done to help assist her son. The counselor shares that in his past experience and based on available research, medication and therapy have proven to be the most effective means of treatment when combined. Based on the look of worry, the counselor offers to schedule Ben and his mother for an appointment with the agency's psychiatrist to further discuss the option of medication.

Two months have passed since Ben and his mother saw the psychiatrist, and he was prescribed a dosage of Focalin. Ben shared with his therapist that now he receives smiley faces in his folder at least 4 days a week and that he does not get out of his seat as much. Ben's mother reported that she is very pleased with the progress of her son since he began taking medication, as well as attending therapy. She says that Ben's teacher calls her weekly and describes the improvement she has seen in Ben. Ben appears to understand boundaries with peers more, so he is not horseplaying as much. He also is able to sit on the carpet without moving around and without touching anyone while paying attention to his teacher's instructions. He also does not have nearly as many verbal outbursts as he used to during class. Ben's mother shares that based on his treatment plan, she signed Ben up for baseball so that he may exert some of that excess energy he possesses. It appears as if the client and mother are accepting of the suggested treatment and plan to continue forward with it.

> Take a minute to think about the pros and cons of taking stimulants for attention deficit hyperactivity disorder. Briefly write down your thoughts (pros and cons) about using a stimulant medication to treat attention deficit hyperactivity disorder.
>
> _____
>
> _____

Scenario 2

Taylor is a 13-year-old transgender female. After a recommendation from her best friend, she had her mother take her to counseling to better cope with her depression and anxiety. Taylor shared with her counselor that she really wants help but does not think that her counselor will set realistic goals to help with depression and anxiety. Upon hearing this, Taylor's counselor assures her that it is not his responsibility to set goals for her but rather that is her responsibility. Taylor's counselor assures her that he will help her to the best of his ability, but it ultimately comes down to what effort Taylor is willing to put into counseling, both in and out of session. Taylor goes on to explain to her counselor that she has lacked enthusiasm for some of her favorite activities and lost motivation to perform well in school. Since she began to identify as a transgender female 3 months ago, Taylor has not spoken to any of her friends about her thoughts concerning her identity and has stopped participating in after-school activities.

In making Taylor's treatment plan, her therapist asks, "If you woke up tomorrow and your problem(s) were gone, how would you know?"

Taylor replies, "I would not have a panic attack when I see others whispering. I would be hanging out with my friends after school instead of locking myself in my room. I would not struggle with communicating my thoughts and feelings to others."

Taylor's therapist informs her that she just established her own goals for therapy and together they could decide on some objectives for her to meet her goals. This pleased Taylor, and she was happy to move forward.

> *Get in groups to develop a working treatment plan for Taylor. After you work on the treatment plan, share with the class in group discussion.

Web-Based and Literature-Based Resources

DSM-5 Assessment Measures: https://www.psychiatry.org/psychiatrists/practice/dsm/educational-resources/assessment-measures

The *ICD-10* Classification of Mental and Behavioural Health Disorders: Clinical Descriptions and Diagnostic Guidelines-https://www.who.int/classifications/icd/en/bluebook.pdf

References

American Psychiatric Association (APA). (2013). *Diagnostic and statistical manual of mental disorders* (5th ed.).

Bunney, W. E., Jr., Davis, J. M. (1965). Norepinephrine in depressive reactions: A review. *Archives of General Psychiatry, 13*, 483–494. https://doi.org/10.1001/archpsyc.1965.01730060001001

Beck, A. T., Ward, C. H., Mendelson, M., Mock, J., & Erbaugh, J. (1961). An inventory for measuring depression. *Archives of General Psychiatry, 4*, 561–571.

Beck, A. T., Steer, R. A., & Garbin, M. G. (1988). Psychometric properties of the Beck depression inventory: Twenty-five years of evaluation. *Clinical Psychology Review, 8*(1), 77–100.

Beeson, E. T. (2017). Neurocounseling: A new section of the journal of mental health counseling. *Journal of Mental Health Counseling, 39*(1), 71–83. https://doi.org/10.17744/mehc.39.1.06

Beeson, E. T., & Aideyan, B. (2016). The research domain criteria initiative: Implications for neurocounseling. *Counseling Today, 59*(5), 18–21.

Bogels, S. M., Wijts, P., Oort, F. J., & Sallaerts, S. J. M. (2014). Psychodynamic psychotherapy versus cognitive behavior therapy for social anxiety disorder: An efficacy and partial effectiveness trial. *Depression and Anxiety, 31*, 363–373. https://doi.org/10.1002/da.22246

Center for Behavioral Health Statistics and Quality. (2016). *Key substance use and mental health indicators in the United States: Results from the 2015 national survey on drug use and health* (HHS Publication No. SMA 16-4984, NSDUH Series H-51). http://www.samhsa.gov/data/

Corcoran, A. C., Taylor, R. D., & Page, I. H. (1949). Lithium poisoning from the use of salt substitutes. *Journal of the American Medical Association, 139*(11), 685–688. https://doi.org/10.1001/jama.1949.02900280001001

Fowler G. (1991). *Crazy water: The story of mineral wells and other Texas health resorts*. Texas Christian University Press.

Gingerich, W. J., & Peterson, L. T. (2013). Effectiveness of solution-focused brief therapy: A systematic qualitative review of controlled outcome studies. *Research on Social Work Practice, 23*(3), 266–283. https://doi.org/10.1177/1049731512470859

Hayes, S. C. (2006). Acceptance and commitment therapy, relational frame theory, and the third wave of behavioral and cognitive therapies. *Behavior Therapy, 35*(4), 639–665. https://doi.org/10.1016/S0005-7894(04)80013-3

Herk, N. A., & Thompson, R. C. (2011). *International technical brief for the strong interest inventory assessment*. https://shop.themyersbriggs.com/Pdfs/Strong_Intl_Tech_Brief.pdf

Hillhouse, T. M., & Porter, J. H. (2015). A brief history of the development of antidepressant drugs: From monoamines to glutamate. *Experimental and clinical psychopharmacology, 23*(1), 1–21. https://doi.org/10.1037/a0038550

Hofmann, S. G., Asnaani, A., Vonk, I. J. J., Sawyer, A. T., & Fang, A. (2012). The efficacy of cognitive behavioral therapy: A review of meta-analyses. *Cognitive Therapy and Research, 36*, 427–440.

Jongsma, A. E., Peterson, L. M., & Bruce, T. J. (2014). *The complete adult psychotherapy treatment planner* (5th ed.). John Wiley & Sons.

Kliem, S., Kröger, C., & Kosfelder, J. (2010). Dialectical behavior therapy for borderline personality disorder: A meta-analysis using mixed-effects modeling. *Journal of Consulting and Clinical Psychology, 78*(6), 936–951. https://doi.org/10.1037/a0021015

Lazowski, L. E., Kimmell, K. S., & Baker, S. L. (2016). *The adult substance abuse subtle screening inventory-4 (SASSI-4) user guide & manual*. The SASSI Institute.

Leichsenring, F., Rabung, S., & Leibing, E. (2004). The efficacy of short-term psychodynamic psychotherapy in specific psychiatric disorders: A meta-analysis. *Achieves of General Psychiatry, 61*, 1208–1216.

Lopes, R. T., Goncalves, M. M., Machado, P. P., Sinai, D., Bento, T., & Salgado, J. (2014). Narrative therapy vs. cognitive-behavioral therapy for moderate depression: Empirical evidence from a controlled clinical trial. *Psychotherapy Research, 24*(6), 662–674. https://doi.org/10.1080/10503307.2013.874052

May, L. (1989, December 4). Business is bubbling again as lithium-water drinkers swear by its healing powers. *Los Angeles Times*. https://www.latimes.com/archives/la-xpm-1989-12-04-mn-156-story.html

Moore, A. (2007, May 13). Eternal sunshine. *The Guardian*. https://www.theguardian.com/society/2007/may/13/socialcare.medicineandhealth

National Institute of Mental Health (NIMH). (2020). *Mental health medications*. https://www.nimh.nih.gov/health/topics/mental-health-medications/index.shtml#part_149867

Neukrug, E. (2018). *Counseling theory and practice* (2nd ed.). Cognella.

Neukrug, E. S., & Fawcett, C. R. (2015). *Essentials of testing and assessment: A practical guide for counselors, social workers, and psychologists* (3rd ed.). Cengage. ISBN-13: 978-1285454245

Neukrug, E. S., & Schwitzer, A. M. (2006). *Skills and tools for today's counselors and psychotherapists: From natural helping to professional helping*. Wadsworth/Thompson/Brooks/Cole.

O'Brien, P. L., Thomas, C. P., Hodgkin, D., Levit, K. R., & Mark, T. L. (2014). The diminished pipeline for medications to treat mental health and substance use disorders. *Psychiatric Services, 65*(12), 1433–1438. https://doi-org.libproxy.clemson.edu/10.1176/appi.ps.201400044

Occupational Information and Network (O*NET). (n.d.). *O*NET online*. https://www.onetonline.org/

O'Hara, M., & Duncan, P. (2016). Why 'big pharma' stopped searching for the next Prozac. *The Guardian*, 27. www.theguardian.com/society/2016/jan/27/prozac-next-psychiatric-wonder-drug-research-medicine-mental-illness

Pearson. (n.d.). *Wechsler nonverbal scale of ability (WNV)*. https://www.pearsonassessments.com/store/usassessments/en/Store/Professional-Assessments/Cognition-%26-Neuro/Wechsler-Nonverbal-Scale-of-Ability/p/100000313.html?tab=product-details

Peterson, C., Lomas, G., Neukrug, E., & Bonner, M. (2014). Assessment use by counselors in the United States: Implications for policy and practice. *Journal of Counseling and Development, 92*, 90–98.

Psychological Assessment Resources (PAR, inc.). (2009). *Self-Directed Search*. https://www.parinc.com/Search-Results?Search=Career

Ray, W. (2017). *Abnormal psychology* (2nd ed.). SAGE Publications.

Rayner, M., & Vitali, D. (2016). Short-term existential psychotherapy in primary care: A quantitative report. *Journal of Humanistic Psychology, 56*(4), 357–372. https://doi.org/10.1177/0022167815569884

Roane, H. S., Fisher, W. W., & Carr, J. E. (2016). Applied behavior analysis as treatment for autism spectrum disorder. *Journal of Pediatrics, 175*, 27–32. https://doi.org/10.1016/j.jpeds.2016.04.023

Rottinghaus, P. J., Hees, C. K., & Conrath, J. A. (2009). Enhancing job satisfaction perspectives: Combining Holland themes and basic interests. *Journal of Vocational Behavior, 75*(2), 129–151. https://doi.org/10.1016/j.jvb.2009.05.010

Russell-Chapin, L. A. (2016). Integrating neurocounseling into the counseling profession: An introduction. *Journal of Mental Health Counseling, 38*(2), 93–102. https://doi.org/lo.17744/m ehc.38.2.ol

Schwitzer, A. M., & Rubin, L. C. (2015). *Diagnosis and treatment planning skills: A popular culture casebook approach* (2nd ed.). SAGE Publications.

Shorter, E. (2009). The history of lithium therapy. *Bipolar Disorders, 11*, 4–9. https://doi.org/10.1111/j.1399-5618.2009.00706.x

Sirkin, M. I. & Manzi, A. (2019). Phase: Mindfulness and neuroscience: An integrated approach to positive counseling. In G. M. McAuliffe (Ed.), *Positive counseling: A guide to assessing and enhancing client strength and growth* (pp. 307–332). Cognella.

Watts, B. V., Schnurr, P. P., Mayo, L., Young-Xu, Y., Weeks, W. B., & Friedman, M. J. (2013). Meta-analysis of the efficacy of treatments for posttraumatic stress disorder. *Journal of Clinical Psychiatry, 74*(6), 541–550. https://doi.org/10.4088/JCP.12r0822

Weber, M., Davis, K., & McPhie, L. (2006). Narrative therapy, eating disorders and groups: Enhancing outcomes in rural NSW. *Australian Social Work, 59*(4), 391–405. https://doi.org/10.1080/03124070600985970

Wechsler, D. (2003). *WISC-IV administration and scoring manual.* Harcourt.

Wong, D., Perry, K., & Bymaster, F. (2005). The discovery of fluoxetine hydrochloride (Prozac). *Nature Reviews Drug Discovery 4*, 764–774. https://doi.org/10.1038/nrd1821

World Health Organization (WHO). (2016). *International statistical classification of diseases and related health problems, 10th revision (ICD-10).*

World Health Organization (WHO). (2019, November 28). *Mental disorders.* https://www.who.int/news-room/fact-sheets/detail/mental-disorders

Credits

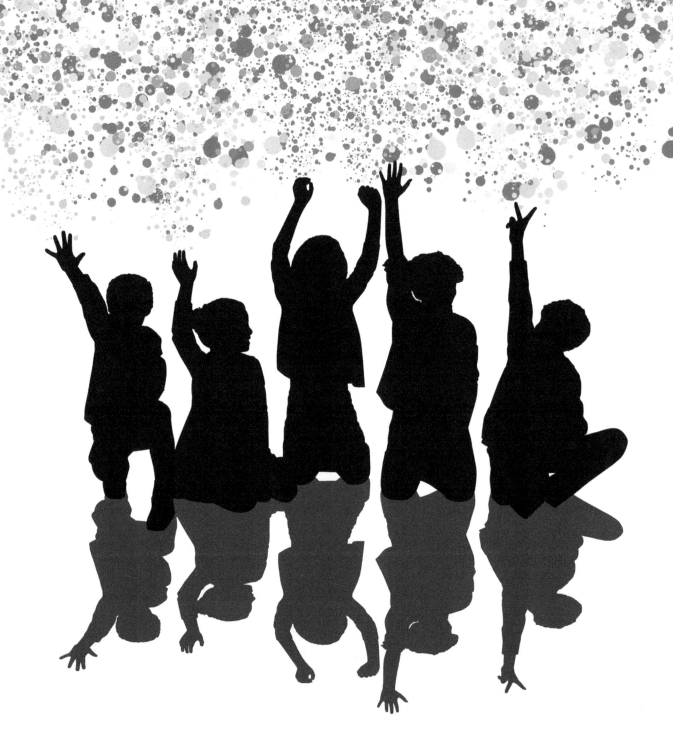

CHAPTER THREE

CHILDHOOD DISORDERS

Chadwick Royal, Regina Gavin Williams, Kyla Maria Sawyer-Kurian, Taheera Blount, Jennifer Barrow, and David A. Scott

CASE STUDY 3.1 Selena is a 7-year-old currently attending second grade at a public elementary school. She has struggled a bit in school and is a bit behind—not working at a pace to remain at grade level. Her teacher has noticed that Selena often makes careless mistakes in her work and misses details that might have helped her to solve some math problems in particular. When reading aloud, Selena often makes errors by either leaving some words out or reading a word incorrectly (e.g., substituting words incorrectly because she is not paying close enough attention). During class instruction time, Selena is often seen doing something unrelated to the task or looking elsewhere in the classroom, and she has to be called on to capture her attention. During small-group instruction time, Selena still has difficulty remaining focused on the teacher or her fellow group members.

Selena does not get into much trouble at school. She is pleasant and cooperative, and she does not get in trouble for being out of her seat or other behavioral issues. However, it is common for Selena to miss playground time because she is asked to stay inside to finish some schoolwork that was not completed during the day, or she has to clean up her unusually messy desk. She usually completes her homework but says sometimes that she loses it somewhere between home and turning it in at school. Over the last year or two, Selena has repeatedly voiced that she has started to dislike school.

Overview

Disorders first present in childhood can have a major effect on normal physical and psychological development (Willis, 2014). A child who experiences significant problems related to psychopathology can have difficulty with achieving developmental milestones, experience social difficulties (difficulty making friends), and possibly encounter significant academic or behavioral problems in school. Any one of these problems can have a lasting effect on the rest of their life.

The *Diagnostic and Statistical Manual for Mental Disorders, 5th Edition* (*DSM-5*: American Psychiatric Association [APA], 2013a) and the *International Statistical Classification of Diseases* (*ICD-10*: World Health Organization [WHO], 1992) both have sections that describe disabilities or disorders that are first present in childhood. The *DSM-5* labels this overall category as "neurodevelopmental disorders," while the *ICD-10* has three subsections specific to "Intellectual Abilities" (F70-F79), "Pervasive and Specific

Did You Know?

- One of the most common childhood mental disorders is attention deficit hyperactivity disorder (Centers for Disease Control and Prevention [CDC], 2019).

- One in 160 children has autism spectrum disorder (World Health Organization, 2019).

- About 6.1 million children aged 2–17 have been diagnosed with attention deficit hyperactivity disorder (CDC, 2019).

- Females are more likely to be diagnosed with anxiety, while males are more likely diagnosed with conduct disorder, attention deficit hyperactivity disorder, and autism (Whiteford et al., 2013).

Developmental Disorders" (F80-F89), and "Behavioral and Emotional Disorders with Onset Usually Occurring in Childhood and Adolescence" (F90-F98; WHO, 1992). In this chapter, we won't cover all childhood disorders, but we will review some of the disorders that are more likely to be encountered in practice. We will explore childhood disorders, including intellectual disabilities, attention deficit hyperactivity disorder (hyperkinetic disorders), autism spectrum disorders (pervasive developmental disorders), learning and communication disorders (specific developmental disorders of speech and language and scholastic skills), motor disorders (motor function, tic disorders), and elimination disorders (other behavioral and emotional disorders).

Intellectual Disabilities

CASE STUDY 3.2 Kamlai is a 14-year-old girl who has been in self-contained classrooms for the majority of her educational years. At age 6, Kamlai was struggling with completing her schoolwork, which her teachers said was something that would work itself out. After much complaining from Kamlai's mother, the school finally decided to evaluate Kamlai. She was administered the Woodcock-Johnson IV Test of Achievement and received results that placed her in the 15% percentile of kids her age who took the test. This result predicted that Kamlai would have a harder time than most kids in academic adjustment. The school psychologist, principal, social worker, and Kamlai's teacher and mother came together to create an Individualized Education Plan (IEP) so as to have an outline to follow to help Kamlai be as successful as possible in school.

At 12, Kamlai took the WISC-R and scored a 58. With this score, her report reflected that her working memory and verbal comprehension skills were very much below average. Meanwhile, her math skills were low average. Kamlai is wanting to transition into regular education classrooms, but because of consistent test scores reflecting her low academic capabilities, she is being kept in special education classrooms for the time being.

At home, Kamlai does not have the best social life. She is an only child, and her parents seldom interact with her because they work all the time. Growing up, it was always Kamlai and her nanny. She never had playdates nor attended daycare, which may also help explain her poor social skills.

Intellectual Disability (Intellectual Developmental Disorder)

> **Mild (F70) (317)**
> **Moderate (F71) (318.0)**
> **Severe (F72) (318.1)**
> **Profound (F73) (318.2)**
> **Global Developmental Delay (F88) (315.8)**

Intellectual disability, also known as intellectual developmental disorder, is a disorder that has a childhood onset and is distinguished by intellectual function limitations (e.g., learning, reasoning, problem solving, abstract thinking), making it difficult to perform daily life functions (American Heritage Dictionary of Medicine, 2015). According to the American Association on Intellectual and Developmental Disabilities (AAIDD; 2010), intellectual disability is defined as having significant limitations in intellectual functioning and in both practical and social skills to adaptively function, which have originated prior to the age of 18 years old.

For an individual to be diagnosed with an intellectual disability, they must have a deficit in intellectual functioning (e.g., problem solving, judgment, academic learning, reasoning; criterion A), a deficit in adaptive functioning as a result of not meeting the sociocultural and developmental standards that are associated with social responsibility and individual independence (criterion B), and childhood onset of deficits related to intellectual and adaptive functions (criterion C; American Psychiatric Association, 2013a). The levels of severity of intellectual disability, classified according to adaptive functioning, are located in Box 3.2.

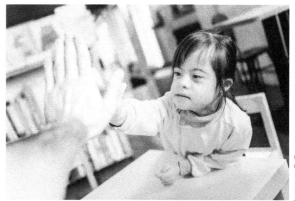

Image 3.2

Would you diagnosis Kamlai with an intellectual disability?

Box 3.2 Levels of Intellectual Disability

- Mild: *ICD-10* code, F70 (317)
- Moderate: *ICD-10* code, F71 (318.0)
- Severe: *ICD-10* code, F72 (318.1)
- Profound: *ICD-10* code, F73 (318.2)

In contrast to the previous version of the *DSM*, the *DSM-IV*, absolute IQ cutoffs do not define these areas of adaptive functioning for learning disability in the *DMS-5* (Marrus & Hall, 2017). They are instead classified within a range of IQ scores. The three domains of adaptive functioning for intellectual disability are as follows:

1. Conceptual domain (i.e., memory, knowledge, and language)
2. Social domain (i.e., social judgment, ability to follow rules, and empathy)
3. Practical domain (i.e., daily living skills, organization, and self-care; Marrus & Hall, 2017)

There is a frequency of co-occurring disorders (i.e., physical, medical, mental, and neurodevelopmental) in intellectual disability. Some of these disorders include attention deficit hyperactivity disorder, anxiety disorder, bipolar disorder, depressive disorders, and autism spectrum disorder. Furthermore, presentation of intellectual disability varies with both age and cause, such as late attainment of developmental milestones or identification of academic difficulties in the school setting (Simpson et al., 2016).

Think about our case study of Selena. Is Selena exhibiting some of these symptoms?

Treatment Options

Intellectual disability has been recognized as a challenge when it comes to implementing inclusive and effective practices (Ferreira et al., 2016). The treatment interventions for intellectual disability depends on the level of severity. Appropriate assessments (e.g., the mental status examination) should be administered to establish whether an individual has an intellectual disability and its cause, as well as to identify whether the individual will need any supports or interventions (Simpson et al., 2016). Administering a physical examination can also be useful for individuals who report any physical symptoms or for those who cannot communicate their symptoms.

In a follow-up to assessment results, a multidisciplinary approach to treatment is needed. The areas to focus treatment options on can be reviewed in the following areas:

- *Biological.* Physical conditions can be treated with psychotropic medication prescribed by a doctor or psychiatrist. These conditions must be treated optimally since they may account for either some or all on one's physical symptoms.
- *Psychological.* Cognitive behavioral therapy techniques can be used depending on the language skills of an individual. Minimal language-dependent therapies, such as anger management or behavioral activation, can also be used. Psychosocial interventions, such as antecedents, behavior, consequences, can also be used to identify reinforcers or triggers to any problem behaviors.
- *Developmental.* Individuals presenting with developmental concerns can benefit from interventions such as skill-building programs or speech and language training. This, in turn, can help to build confidence, as well as form therapeutic alliances.
- *Social.* Environmental modifications, such as creating a predictable routine, can help to reduce anxiety one may experience. In addition, providing meaningful and structured activities daily, providing quieter settings for noise sensitivity, and making adaptions to improve sensory impairments can be helpful. Safety and suitability of the home environment should also be considered (Simpson et al., 2016).

Attention Deficit Hyperactivity Disorder (ADHD)

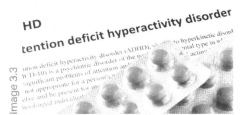

Image 3.3

Attention Deficit Hyperactivity Disorder (F90.X) (314.0X)

One of the most common mental disorders affecting children is attention deficit hyperactivity disorder. This disorder is a chronic condition that is characterized by attention difficulty (not being able to keep focus), hyperactivity (excess movement that is not fitting for the setting), and impulsiveness (hasty acts that occur in the moment without thought). The onset of this disorder is in childhood and can persist into the adult years. Attention deficit hyperactivity disorder may contribute to (a) difficulty in school or in the workplace, (b) low self-esteem, and (c) challenges within relationships with others (American Psychiatric Association, 2019; Mayo Foundation for Medical Education and Research, 2019a). There are more than three million cases of attention deficit hyperactivity disorder per year (Mayo Foundation for Medical Education and Research, 2019a), and there is an estimated 8.4% of children and 2.5% of adults who are diagnosed with the disorder. Because attention deficit hyperactivity disorder leads to disruption in the classroom or problems with schoolwork, this disorder is often first detected in school-aged children. It is found more commonly among boys than girls; however, it can also affect adults. The cause of attention deficit hyperactivity disorder is not certain. There is evidence that suggests genetics (a relative having the disorder), being born prematurely, brain injury, and the mother smoking, using alcohol, or having extreme stress during pregnancy may contribute to the development of attention deficit hyperactivity disorder (APA, 2019).

According to the Mayo Foundation for Medical Education and Research (2019), a child should not receive a diagnosis of attention deficit hyperactivity disorder unless two circumstances occur: (1) the core symptoms (i.e., inattention and hyperactive-impulsive behavior) of attention deficit hyperactivity disorder start before age 12, and (2) the symptoms create significant problems at home and at school on a regular and consistent basis. There is no specific test for attention deficit hyperactivity disorder, but making a diagnosis will likely include the items listed in Table 3.1.

TABLE 3.1 Attention Deficit Hyperactivity Disorder Assessment

- Medical exam that would help rule out other possible causes of symptoms
- Gathering information, such as any current medical history and any issues, family medical history, and school records
- Family members, the child's teachers, or other people who know the child well, such as caregivers, babysitters, and coaches, would participate in interviews or answering questionnaires
- Attention deficit hyperactivity disorder rating scales to help collect and evaluate information about the child
- Attention deficit hyperactivity disorder criteria from the American Psychiatric Association *DSM-5*

According to the *DSM-5*'s (2013) criteria, there are five diagnostic criteria, which include (Criterion A) a persistent pattern of inattention and/or hyperactivity impulsivity that interferes with functioning or development. There are specific symptoms, nine each, associated with inattention and hyperactivity impulsivity. For Criterion A to be met, there needs to be six or more inattention symptoms and/or six or more hyperactivity-impulsivity symptoms that have persisted for at least 6 months to a degree that is inconsistent with the developmental level of the child and that have negatively affected social and academic activities. (*Please note that older adolescents and adults [over age 17 years] must present with five symptoms.*) The second criterion for attention deficit hyperactivity disorder (Criterion B) includes several inattentive or hyperactive-impulsive symptoms that were present prior to 12 years old. The third criterion (Criterion C) includes several inattentive or hyperactive-impulsive symptoms that are present in two or more settings (e.g., at home, school, or work; with friends or relatives; in other activities). Criterion D, the fourth criterion, includes clear evidence that the symptoms interfere with, or reduce the quality of, social, academic, or occupational functioning. Lastly, Criterion E, the fifth criterion, requires that the symptoms do not occur exclusively during the course of schizophrenia or another psychotic disorder and are not better explained by another mental disorder (e.g., mood disorder, anxiety disorder, dissociative disorder, personality disorder, substance intoxication or withdrawal).

When criteria have been met, a diagnosis will be assigned. The *ICD-10-CM* for attention deficit hyperactivity disorder includes the information located in Box 3.3.

> ## Box 3.3 *ICD-10* for Attention Deficit Hyperactivity Disorder
>
> - Attention deficit hyperactivity disorder, predominantly inattentive type, F90.0 (314.00)
> - Attention deficit hyperactivity disorder, predominantly hyperactive type, F90.1(314.01)
> - Attention deficit hyperactivity disorder, combined type, F90.2 (314.01)
> - Attention deficit hyperactivity disorder, other type, F90.8
> - Attention deficit hyperactivity disorder, unspecified type, F90.9

In addition to the attention deficit hyperactivity disorder presentation, *DSM-5* further classifies the severity of the disorder's present symptoms as "mild," "moderate," or "severe" (APA, 2013a).

Could Selena be diagnosed with attention deficit hyperactivity disorder?

Treatment Options

When a child is diagnosed with attention deficit hyperactivity disorder, parents often have concerns about which treatment is appropriate for their child. With the right treatment, attention deficit hyperactivity disorder can be managed. There are a myriad of treatment options for the disorder. The treatment option that works best can depend on the individual child and family. To find the option that best meets the needs of the child and the family, it is recommended that parents team up with others involved in the life of their child, including health-care providers, therapists, teachers, coaches, and other family members (CDC, 2019). Standard treatments for attention deficit hyperactivity disorder include medication, counseling, behavioral therapy, and educational services and interventions. While these interventions are effective in relieving many symptoms of attention deficit hyperactivity disorder, they do not cure the disorder (Mayo Foundation for Medical Education and Research, 2019a).

Treatment recommendations for children vary depending on age. The American Academy of Pediatrics (AAP, 2019) recommends parent training in behavior management as the first line of treatment for children with attention deficit hyperactivity disorder younger than 6 years old. Behavioral management is recommended before medication is tried. If behavioral interventions do not provide significant improvement and problems persist with the child, medication may be used.

Conversely, AAP recommends that children 6 years of age and older include medication and behavior therapy together. Specifically, the behavioral therapy should include training for parents in behavior management (for children up to age 12) and other types of behavior therapy and training for adolescents. An important component of treatment is done through teaming with the teachers and administration at school. AAP recommendations also include adding behavioral classroom intervention and school supports.

CLINICIAN'S CORNER 3.1

Working with children can be a vastly different experience from working with adults, and this can have an effect on both diagnosis and treatment. When it comes to diagnosis, you have to take into account potential differences in presentation. Some symptoms may manifest themselves differently in children than they do in adults. For example, the symptoms of depression in children may look quite different than they do in adults. Some children may act out and display aggression toward others, whereas the adult may display aggression toward themselves. Cognitive development plays a large role in this difference. Some children may not yet have developed the self-awareness or the language to be able to express themselves in the same way that an adult would. The depression (that you think you see) could be related to other problems (e.g., attention deficit hyperactivity disorder, learning differences).

The more important thing that you must realize as a practitioner, in my opinion, is how treatment may be very different for children. Because of the differences in cognitive development and potential limited ability to articulate or express themselves, your efforts as a clinician will need to be geared toward the child's level of development. It may take more time to establish rapport, determine needs, and focus your work on developmentally appropriate goals. You may need to be creative, and engage in artistic, recreational, or play therapy activities to find out information from your client and direct your intervention efforts. Because of this difference, you will see insurance companies, for example, typically authorize more initial sessions for a child than for an adult.

Chadwick Royal, PhD, LPCS, CCCE

The Food and Drug Administration (2016) has approved two types of medications for the treatment of attention deficit hyperactivity disorder—stimulants and nonstimulants—to help reduce the symptoms and improve functioning in children as young as 6 years of age. It may seem counterintuitive, but despite the name, stimulants, which contain various forms of methylphenidate (for example, methylphenidate [Concerta, Ritalin, others] and dexmethylphenidate [Focalin]), amphetamine (for, example, dextroamphetamine [Dexedrine], dextroamphetamine-amphetamine [Adderall XR, Mydayis], and lisdexamfetamine [Vyvanse]), actually have a calming effect on hyperactive children diagnosed with attention deficit hyperactivity disorder. These stimulants are believed to increase brain levels of dopamine, a neurotransmitter associated with motivation, attention, and movement. Furthermore, the Food and Drug Administration has also approved three nonstimulants to treat the symptoms of attention deficit hyperactivity disorder: Strattera (atomoxetine), Intuniv (guanfacine), and Kapvay (clonidine). These provide a useful alternative for children who do not tolerate stimulants well.

Do you think Selena would respond well to these types of medications?

Good treatment plans, which may include behavior therapy and/or medication, will include close monitoring of whether and how much the treatment helps the child's behavior, as well as making changes as needed along the way.

Autism Spectrum Disorder

TRUE LIFE 3.1

Temple Grandin

Mary Temple Grandin—Autism Spectrum Disorder

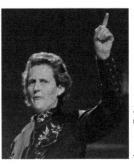

Image 3.4

One of the first individuals to ever record her own personal experience as an individual on the autism spectrum, Mary Temple Grandin has taken the world by storm. Since her birth on August 29, 1947, she has constantly had to overcome obstacles. Growing up, she was teased and bullied because of her speech impairment. Grandin's teachers had to teach her how to take turns when playing games with her peers. These negatives were shortly followed by greatness.

As a child, Mary Temple Grandin was never diagnosed with autism. Doctors attributed her lagging abilities to brain damage. As a child with high anxiety, Grandin craved to have her nerves settled, but she was unable to find a solution. One day as a teenager, she watched cattle being branded in a squeeze chute, and she noticed that as soon as pressure was administered to the cattle, they calmed down. Grandin (1992) thought that this could help reduce her high nerves, which led to her creation, "the Hug Box" (Edelson, n.d.). Now, Grandin's creation is used as a form of treatment of those with autism because her machine has proven time and time again that it does give users a calming effect after utilization.

Not only has Grandin had an effect on the autism community but on animal science as well. Grandin is responsible for more than 60 peer-reviewed scientific papers on animal behavior. Grandin serves as a consultant for livestock handling, equipment design, and animal welfare. She also serves as a professor of animal science at Colorado State University (Grandin, n.d.).

Grandin has written two books on her experience as an adult with autism: *Emergence Labeled Autistic* and *Thinking in Pictures*. These books give readers an inside look into how anxiety took over Grandin's life and how deep pressure ultimately helped reduce the severe anxiety she experienced. As a young child, Grandin sought after deep pressure but was unable to receive it from people because they would either give her too much or too little pressure. This led to Grandin crawling between sofa cushions or wrapping herself in blankets (Edelson, n.d.) until she created the Hug Box.

From a tiny girl who did not speak until she was 3-and-a-half years to a prominent speaker on animal behavior and autism, Grandin has shown what the possibilities are for some individuals living on the autism spectrum.

Autism Spectrum Disorder (F84.0) (299.00)

Autism spectrum disorder is considered a neurodevelopmental condition in individuals. Although all causes of the disorder are unknown, there are environmental and hereditary influences that are considered to make an individual more likely to have autism spectrum disorder (Callaghan & Sylvester, 2019; Centers for Disease Control and Prevention, 2018). A diagnosis of autism spectrum disorder can result in communication, behavioral, and social barriers. Furthermore, there has been a growing prevalence of autism spectrum disorder diagnosis among children. According to the Centers for Disease Control and Prevention (2019), the rate of children identified with autism spectrum disorder has increased from 1 in 150 to 1 in 68 children since 2000 (Centers for Disease Control and Prevention, 2019).

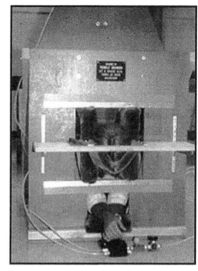

Image 3.5

Autism was previously included in the *DSM-IV* as a subtype of pervasive developmental disorder. Now classified as autism spectrum disorder in the *DSM-5*, it is included under neurodevelopmental disorders. The *ICD-10* includes this disorder under F84.0. Any individual who was previously diagnosed with autistic disorder, pervasive developmental disorder not otherwise specified or Asperger's disorder under the *DSM-IV* should now be given a diagnosis of autism spectrum disorder. According to the *DSM-5* (APA, 2013a), to be diagnosed with autism spectrum disorder, a person must have deficits in social communication, which includes social and emotional reciprocity, nonverbal communication taking place during social interactions, and developing, understanding, and maintaining relationships with others (Criterion A). A person diagnosed with autism spectrum disorder will also display both repetitive and restrictive patterns of interests and activities or behavior in at least two (either currently or in history) out of four of the following specified contexts (Criterion B):

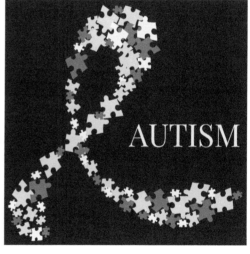

Image 3.6

- Repetitive and stereotyped movements, speech, or use of objects.
- Inflexibility as it relates to adhering to routines, the desire for sameness, or verbal or nonverbal ritualized patterns.
- Interests that are highly fixated, restricted, and considered atypical as it relates to attention or intensity.
- Possessing an unusual interest in sensory environmental aspects or hyperactivity or hyporeactivity as it relates to sensory input. (APA, 2013a)

CASE STUDY 3.3 Carlos is 5 years old. He presents with a flat affect where one is unable to read his facial expressions or any other body language. Aside from not presenting any emotion, he appears to be a content young boy with few things that bother him. When Carlos is on the playground, he tends to chase behind the other kids while quacking like a duck. He does not make conversation with the other kids and mostly enjoys being on his own. When he comes inside from recess at his after-school program, he sits in the same chair at the same table each day. If someone is sitting in his seat, Carlos will begin to throw a tantrum until he receives attention from an adult. He will then point to whomever is in his seat, indicating that he wants them to move. If the student does not move, Carlos does tend to become aggressive and needs to be separated from the other children.

Carlos does not engage in conversation with other kids nor does he interact much with the staff at his after-school program. He is a quiet kid who does not like to be disturbed from his activities. When staff members attempt to talk to Carlos about his day, he stares at the table and gives a one-word response. Occasionally, Carlos will approach staff members and share his knowledge on the different types of dinosaurs that existed. For a 5-year-old, he is able to give great details regarding how big the different dinosaurs were, what type of food each one ate, and where they tended to live. He also knows interesting facts that others would not know about different animals found in the jungle.

Persons with autism spectrum disorder (ASD) have symptoms that are present earlier in their development but perhaps do not become evident until later in life or until social demands become increasingly difficult to manage because of limited capacities (Criterion C). In addition, symptoms caused by autism spectrum disorder can impair important areas of current functioning on a clinically significant level, such as social and occupational functioning (Criterion D). Furthermore, individuals diagnosed with autism spectrum disorder cannot be more appropriately explained by a global developmental delay or by an intellectual disability. In frequent cases, autism spectrum disorder and intellectual disability may co-occur (Criterion E). To individualize an autism spectrum disorder diagnosis and provide a better clinical description, the diagnosis is accompanied by a specifier to account for individual clinical characteristics (e.g., with or without accompanying structural language impairment). Individual characteristics are also noted through specifiers that explain symptoms of autism (e.g., severity). There are three severity levels that describe the symptomatology of autism spectrum disorder ranging from *requiring support* (level 1) to *requiring very substantial support* (level 3). The onset of symptoms of autism spectrum disorder may be present in the first year of life, between age 12 and 24 months, or more subtle symptoms may be seen later than 24 months.

Would you diagnose Carlos with autism spectrum disorder?

Treatment Options

There is currently no pharmacological intervention to treat symptoms related to autism spectrum disorder. However, behavioral, educational, and developmental evidence-based treatment options can help to improve the functioning and overall quality of life of individuals diagnosed with this disorder (Alateeqi & Maria, 2019). Some of these options are listed in table 3.2.

To provide the most appropriate intervention, clinicians must be aware of the evidence related to it and use interventions that may specifically address a difficulty affiliated with autism spectrum disorder (e.g., social skills group intervention to address social skills difficulties).

TABLE 3.2 Autism Spectrum Disorder Treatment Options

- Applied behavior analysis
- Discrete trial training
- Early intensive behavioral intervention
- Social skills intervention (e.g., social skills groups, video modeling, social stories)
- The developmental, individual difference, relationship-based model (i.e., DIRFloortime®)
- The early start Denver model
- Sensory integration therapy
- The teaching and education of autistic and communication handicapped children autism program
- Alternative augmentative communication
- The picture exchange communication system
- Speech-generating devices
- Auditory integration training
  (Alateeqi & Maria, 2019)

Learning and Communication Disorders

Learning Disorders (F81.X) (315.XX)

A learning disorder, also called learning disability, is an information-processing difficulty that prevents an individual from learning a skill and using it effectively. Generally speaking, learning disorders affect individuals of average or above-average intelligence. As a consequence, the disorder manifests as a gap between expected skills, based on age and intelligence, and academic performance. Common learning disorders affect a child's abilities in reading, written expression, math, or nonverbal skills. Unfortunately, school-aged children with learning disorders often struggle with schoolwork long before being diagnosed. This struggle can affect a child's self-esteem and motivation (Mayo Foundation for Medical Education and Research, 2019b).

Learning disabilities are diagnosed using both educational and medical perspectives (Cortiella & Horowitz, 2014). From an educational perspective, the most commonly used definition can be found in the federal special education law, the Individuals with Disabilities Education Act. The medical perspective on learning disorders is expounded upon in the *DSM-5* (previously the *DSM-IV*) published by the American Psychiatric Association (APA, 2013a).

Reading learning disabilities are usually based on difficulty perceiving a spoken word as a combination of distinct sounds. This can make it challenging to understand how a letter, or letters, represents a sound and how letter combinations make a word. Difficulties with working memory, which is the ability to retain and manipulate information in the moment, contribute to the issues related to learning disabilities. Even when foundational reading skills are mastered, children may have real challenges with the following skills: (a) reading at a typical pace, (b) understanding what they read, (c) recalling accurately what they read, (d) making inferences based on their reading, and (e) spelling.

Dyslexia, a learning disorder in reading, is the term that is usually used, but some specialists may use the term dyslexia to describe only some of the information-processing problems that can cause difficulty with reading (Mayo Foundation for Medical Education and Research, 2019b). It is important to note here that the *ICD-10-CM* for dyslexia and alexia (known as word blindness) is R48.0 and is *not elsewhere classified*.

Do you think Selena has a learning disability?

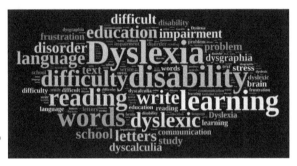

Image 3.7

Dysgraphia is a learning disability that affects writing skills and abilities (WedMD, 2019). The ability to write requires complex visual, motor, and information-processing skills. A learning disorder in written expression may cause the following: "a) slow and labor-intensive handwriting; b) handwriting that's hard to read; c) difficulty putting thoughts into writing d) written text that's poorly organized or hard to understand; and e) trouble with spelling, grammar, and punctuation" (Mayo Foundation for Medical Education and Research, 2019b, para. 8).

A learning disorder as it relates to math or *dyscalculia* may cause challenges with the following skills: "a) understanding how numbers work and relate to each other, b) calculating math problems, c) memorizing basic calculations, d) using math symbols, e) understanding word problems and f) organizing and recording information while solving a math problem" (Mayo Foundation for Medical Education and Research, 2019b, para. 9).

According to the National Academy of Sciences (2015), a diagnosis is made based on a clinical review of an individual's history, teacher reports, academic records, and responses to interventions. Furthermore, in the *DSM-5* (APA, 2013), the diagnosis of a specific learning disorder includes the following symptoms:

A. An individual has persistent challenges in reading, writing, arithmetic, or mathematical reasoning skills during schooling. The symptoms may include imprecise or labored and effortful reading, poor written expression that lacks lucidity, challenges in remembering number facts, or imprecise mathematical reasoning. Symptoms need to have persisted for at least 6 months, despite any interventions that have been provided that target the difficulties.

B. The individual's current academic abilities must be well below the average range of scores in culturally and linguistically appropriate reading, writing, or mathematics tests. Consequently, an individual who is dyslexic must read with great labor and not in the same way as those who are reading at the appropriate grade level.

C. A student's learning challenges begin during the school-age years.

D. The student's challenges must not be better explained by psychosocial adversities or other intellectual, developmental, sensory (vision or hearing), neurological, or motor disabilities. In addition, the challenges must significantly interfere with academic success, occupational performance, or day-to-day living activities (APA, 2013a).

The diagnostic codes for the *ICD-10* are listed in Box 3.4.

TREATMENT OPTIONS

While learning disabilities have no cure, great improvement can occur. The key to addressing a learning disorder is early intervention, which can lessen its effects. Individuals with learning disabilities can develop ways to manage their disabilities. Early interventions increase the chances of success in school and later in life (NIH, 2018). If learning disabilities continue to be untreated, a child may begin to feel frustrated, which can lead to low self-esteem and other problems.

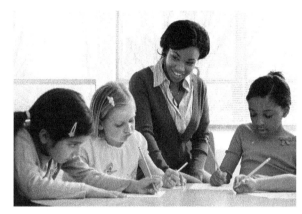

Image 3.8

Experts can assist a child with learning skills by building on the child's strengths and discovering ways to compensate for the child's weaknesses. Interventions vary depending on the nature and extent of the disability. Treatment options may include extra help (i.e., a reading specialist or math tutor), individualized education programs, classroom accommodations (i.e., more time to complete assignments or tests), therapy (i.e., fine motor skills or speech language), or even medication (Mayo Foundation for Medical Education and Research, 2019).

The following are a select number of the ways teachers and administrators can help children with specific learning disabilities. Students who have dyslexia can be helped with intensive teaching techniques, such as step-by-step methods of instruction, including small-group or one-on-one instruction. Further, teachers can make modifications to classroom activities, such as extra time to finish tasks and allowing students to use technology. For students who have dysgraphia, teachers can provide special tools, such as oral exams or allowing a child to use computer software to produce written text. Further, teachers can provide preprinted study sheets. Students with dyscalculia can benefit from memory aids, computer drills, and visual techniques, such as drawing pictures to represent word problems (NIH, 2018).

Communication Disorders (F80.XX) (315.XX)

Many disorders can affect individuals' speech and communication. The effects range from saying sounds incorrectly to being completely unable to speak or understand speech. Causes of communication disorders include (a) hearing disorders and deafness; (b) voice problems, such as dysphonia or those caused by a cleft lip or palate; (c) speech problems, such as stuttering; (d) developmental disabilities; (e) learning disabilities; (f) autism spectrum disorder; (g) brain injury; and (h) stroke. Some problems associated with speaking and communicating may be a result of genetics. Oftentimes, the causes are unknown. About 5% of children have noticeable speech disorders by the first grade.

The following describes the various types of communication disorders. According to the U.S. National Library of Medicine (2019), a phonological disorder is a kind of speech sound disorder. Patients with speech sound disorders have an inability to correctly form the sounds of words. Speech sound disorders also include articulation disorder, disfluency, and voice disorders. Patients, specifically children, with phonological disorder do not use some or all of the speech sounds to form words as expected for children the same age. Second, Bressert (2019) stated that the essential feature of expressive language disorder is an impairment in expressive language development in a child. This is determined by scores on standardized individually administered tests, which measure both nonverbal intellectual capacity and receptive language development. The difficulties may occur in communication involving both verbal language and sign language. Third, patients who have mixed receptive-expressive language issues have difficulty understanding and using spoken language (Understood, 2020). Fourth, speech and language development delays because of hearing loss are best described as listening challenges because hearing loss or auditory processing problems continue to be at risk for developmental delays (American Speech-Language Hearing Association, 2015). Fifth, stuttering or stammering is a common disorder also known as *childhood-onset fluency disorder.* A multifactorial speech disorder, it is normally seen with recurrent prolongations, reverberations, or blocks of sounds, syllables, phrases, or words (Maguire et al., 2012). Sixth, and finally, *social (pragmatic) communication disorder* refers to "individuals who have significant problems using verbal and nonverbal communication for social purposes, leading to impairments in their ability to effectively communicate, participate socially, maintain social relationships, or otherwise perform academically or occupationally" (APA, 2013a). It is important to note that autism spectrum disorder must be ruled out before social (pragmatic) communication disorder can be diagnosed (APA, 2013b).

The *ICD-10-CM* codes for communication disorders are as provided in Box 3.5.

Box 3.5 *ICD-10* for Communication Disorders

- F80 Specific developmental disorders of speech and language
  - F80.0 Phonological disorder
  - F80.1 Expressive language disorder
  - F80.2 Mixed receptive-expressive language disorder (315.32)
  - F80.4 Speech and language development delay because of hearing loss
  - F80.8 Other developmental disorders of speech and language
  - F80.81 Childhood-onset fluency disorder (315.35)
  - F80.82 Social pragmatic communication disorder
- F80.89 Other developmental disorders of speech and language
- F80.9 Developmental disorder of speech and language, unspecified

TREATMENT OPTIONS

There are a varied number of interventions to treat communication disorders. Treatment plans may include one or more of the following types of interventions:

- The first of those interventions includes *speech therapy* to help children learn new vocabulary, organize their thoughts and beliefs, and correct grammatical or word errors.
- Second, *behavior therapy* is designed to increase patients' use of desirable communication behaviors, decrease their unwanted problem behaviors and use of maladaptive coping strategies, and promote their development of useful interpersonal skills. Changes occur via a program of systematic reward and reinforcement. For example, children may be encouraged to use mnemonic strategies (adaptive coping behavior) to help them remember facts relevant to their school performance. Remembering the word "HOMES" can trigger the names of the five great lakes: Huron, Ontario, Michigan, Erie, and Superior.
- Third, some clinicians may also recommend the use of *stimulant medications* as an option for treatment for any impulsivity or hyperactivity symptoms that may be reported by the patient. This type of treatment is a variation on a common intervention typically used for treating attention deficit hyperactivity disorder.
- Fourth, other modifications, such as *environmental modification*, can also be an important part of treatment for communication disorders. For example, children with communication disorders can be given extra time during schoolwork or oral test situations to formulate responses more adequately. Rates of success for communication disorder treatments based on methods such as those just described are typically reported to be high, with around 70% of treated children benefiting. Follow-up treatment is sometimes necessary when relapses occur (MentalHealth.net, 2019).

Motor Disorders

Developmental Coordination Disorder (F82.0) (315.4)

Developmental coordination disorder is defined as a distinct motor disorder, which is categorized under a broader heading of neurodevelopmental disorders in the *DSM-5* (APA, 2013a). Developmental coordination disorder affects approximately 5%–6% of children ages 5–11 years old (APA, 2013a). This disorder is characterized by marked impairment in motor coordination for the child's age and opportunity for learning (APA, 2013a). The deficits that exist within children who have been diagnosed with developmental coordination disorder cannot be attributed to intellectual disability, visual impairment, or neurological conditions that affect motor skills (APA, 2013a). Developmental coordination disorder does not have a single presentation, as fine motor skills and/or gross motor skills can be affected (Visser, 2003; Zwicker et al., 2012).

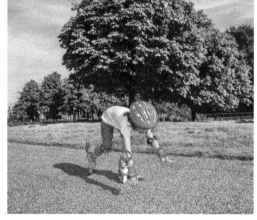

Image 3.9

Children with developmental coordination disorder are frequently thought to be "clumsy" and experience difficulty performing activities of daily living (Harris et al., 2008). This could be attributed to their slowness and inaccurate performance of motor activities, such as handwriting and participating in sports (APA, 2013a). Delays in motor learning are associated with poor performance, which in turn leads to a decrease in participation in activities of daily living in children with developmental coordination disorder (Van der Linde et al., 2015). These difficulties contribute to depression, social isolation, and motor activity avoidance, as well as low levels of physical activity participation in adulthood (Mandich et al., 2003; Rasmussen & Gillberg, 2000). Moreover, children with developmental coordination disorder participate less frequently in organized recreational and physical activities and spend more time performing activities individually than typically developing children (Christiansen, 2000; Poulsen et al., 2007; Poulsen et al., 2008; Zwicker et al., 2013). Furthermore, developmental coordination disorder influences multiple domains of quality of life, including physical, psychological, and social functioning (Zwicker et al., 2013).

According to the *DSM-5* (APA, 2013a), for an individual to be diagnosed with a developmental coordination disorder, the diagnosis must be based on a clinical synthesis of the history (developmental and medical), physical examination, school or workplace report, and individual assessment using psychometrically sound and culturally appropriate standardized tests. In addition, the motor skills deficits are not explained by intellectual disability or visual impairment and are not attributable to a neurological condition affecting movement. The *DSM-5* (APA, 2013a) established diagnostic criteria for individuals with developmental coordination disorder:

> *Criterion A.* Varies with age; young children may be delayed in achieving motor milestones (i.e., sitting, crawling, walking). There may be a delay in developing skills (i.e., pedaling, buttoning shirts, completing puzzles). With older children and adults, there may be slow speed or slow speed with motor activities. The motor skills within this category significantly and persistently interfere with activities of daily living.

> *Criterion B.* Is diagnosed only if the impairment in motor skills significantly interferes with performance of or participation in a daily activity in family, social, school, or community life.

> *Criterion C.* The onset of symptoms must be in the early developmental period. Typically, not diagnosed before the age of 5.

> *Criterion D.* Is made if the coordination difficulties are not better explained by visual impairment or attributed to a neurological condition. Visual function examination and neurological examination must be included in the diagnostic evaluation.

TREATMENT OPTIONS

Treatment for children with developmental coordination disorder can consist of occupational therapy to work on motor control; physical therapy to help with muscle strength, balance, and coordination; and for children who have attention deficit hyperactivity disorder, drug therapies (e.g., methylphenidate) have been used (Harris et al., 2015). There is a new contemporary model approach called cognitive orientation to daily occupational performance, which is an individualized method that focuses on identifying the strategies required for successful task performance (Miller et al., 2001).

Stereotypic Movement Disorders (F98.4) (307.3) (SMD)

Stereotypic movement disorder is known as repetitive, purposeless motor behavior that occurs in a specific pattern and is often distractible (Tan et al., 1997). Primary simple motor stereotypes occur roughly in 20%–70% of typically developing children, whereas complex motor stereotypes occur roughly in 3%–4% of typically developing children (APA, 2013a; Robinson et al., 2016). Common simple stereotypic movements include leg shaking, body rocking, head nodding, body rocking, hair twirling, and nail-biting (MacKenzie, 2018; Singer, 2011). The repetitive movements interfere with social, academic, or other activities and may result in self-injury (APA, 2013a). The age onset of stereotypic movements typically appears before the age of 3 and has a chronic course (Harris et al., 2008). Stereotypic movement disorders are classified as "primary," indicating their presence in an otherwise typically developing child, or "secondary" if another of the aforementioned neuropsychiatric disorders are present (APA, 2013). The *DSM-5* (APA, 2013a) has established diagnostic criteria for individuals with stereotypic movement disorder:

> *Criterion A.* The movements are repetitive and seemingly driven by purposeless motor behavior.

> *Criterion B.* States that stereotypic movements interfere with social, academic, or other activities and in some children, may result in self-injury.

> *Criterion C.* Onset is in the early developmental period.

> *Criterion D.* The repetitive motor behavior is not attributed to the physiological effects of a substance or neurological condition and is not better explained by another neurodevelopmental or mental disorder (i.e., trichotillomania, obsessive-compulsive disorder).

TREATMENT OPTIONS

There are several options that are available for the treatment of stereotypic movement disorder. Researchers indicate that behavioral techniques, including differential reinforcement of other behavior (Ringdahl et al., 2002; Taylor et al., 2005), response interruption, and redirection, may reduce the frequency of stereotypic movements (Miguel et al., 2009). Other forms of treatment that may be beneficial consist of habit-reversal training, function-based assessment and intervention, and use of a behavioral reward system, which has proven to show reductions in stereotypic movements (Ricketts et al., 2013).

Tic Disorders (F95.2) (307.23)

Tics is defined as the presence of sudden, rapid, recurrent, nonrhythmic motor movement or vocalizations that appear before age 18 years and last for more than 1 year (APA, 2013a). Tics that are often disruptive and are not embedded in a certain context but can be inhibited on demand (Ganos et al., 2014). The estimated prevalence of Tourette's disorder for all tic disorders in pediatric populations consist of 3% in pediatric populations (Knight et al., 2012). Males are more commonly affected than females (APA, 2013a). Tic disorder is classified into four categories that are hierarchical in nature. These include Tourette's disorder, persistent (chronic) motor or vocal tic disorder, provisional tic disorder, and the other specified and unspecified tic disorders. The *DSM-5* (APA, 2013a) has established diagnostic criteria for individuals with Tourette's disorder:

> ***Criterion A.*** In Tourette's disorder, both motor and vocal tics must be present. With persistent (chronic) motor or vocal tic disorder, only motor or vocal tics are present. For provisional tic disorder, motor and/or vocal tics may be present. For other specified or unspecified tic disorders, the movement disorder symptoms are best characterized as atypical in presentation or age at onset (APA, 2013a).

> ***Criterion B.*** There must be a 1-year minimum duration.

> ***Criterion C.*** The onset of tics must occur prior to age 18.

> ***Criterion D.*** Tic symptoms cannot be attributed to physiological effects of a substance or another medical condition.

TREATMENT OPTIONS

There are several treatment modalities that can be used to treat tic disorders, such as behavioral therapies, psychoeducation, and pharmacotherapy. Behavioral therapies consist of relaxation training, psychoanalytic psychotherapy, massed negative practice, habit-reversal training, self-monitoring, biofeedback, and commitment therapy (Verdellen et al., 2011). Psychoeducation is the major form of treatment for tic disorders (Ganos et al., 2016). To understand the nature of tic disorders, psychoeducation is vital to helping patients and families understand the nature of the disorder, neurobiological basis of the condition, and relevant contextual factors, such as stress and fatigue (Verdellen et al., 2011).

- ***Behavioral Therapies.*** This can involve relaxation training, habit-reversal training, exposure-response prevention, contingency management, mindfulness-based approaches, and acceptance and commitment therapy (Verdellen et al. 2011).
- ***Pharmacotherapy.*** Antipsychotics have been used for the treatment of tics for more than 40 years (Goetz et al., 1984; Ross & Moldofsky, 1978). The following antipsychotics have been evaluated for the treatment of tics: Haloperidol, Pimozide, Fluphenazine, Risperidone, Aripiprazole, Tiapride, Sulpiride, Olanzapine, Ziprasidone, Quetiapine, and Ecopipam (Gilbert et al., 2014; Pringsheim et al., 2012; Roessner et al., 2011). In childhood, two different classes of medication are used as a first-line defense in child pharmacotherapy, which consists of adrenergic agonists, antipsychotics, tetrabenazine, topiramate, and potentially baclofen (Ganos et al., 2016). Moreover, dopamine antagonists and typical antipsychotics, such as Aripiprazole and Clonidine, can be used (Ghanizadeh, 2016). Roessner et al. (2011) conducted a survey that examined treatment strategies for tics in individuals with Tourette's syndrome. The results from this study identified Clonidine as the most commonly prescribed form of psychopharmacology agent.

Elimination Disorders

Elimination disorders are the only disorders included in this chapter that are not located within the neurodevelopmental disorders section of the *DSM-5*. There is a separate section labeled "elimination disorders" found after feeding and eating disorders and before sleep-wake disorders. However, the *DSM-5* does state that elimination disorders are usually first diagnosed in childhood or adolescence (APA, 2013a). The *ICD-10* groups elimination disorders within the section labeled "Behavioural and Emotional Disorders with Onset Usually Occurring Childhood and Adolescence" (F90-F98)—the same section that includes hyperkinetic disorders, conduct disorders, separation anxiety disorder, disorders of social functioning (elective mutism, reactive attachment disorder), and tic disorders (just to name a few). Elimination disorders are found under the heading, "Other Emotional and Behavioural Disorders with Onset Usually Occurring in Childhood and Adolescence" (F98; WHO, 1992). There are essentially two kinds of elimination disorders: enuresis and encopresis.

CASE STUDY 3.4 Martin is a 12-year-old boy currently attending Saint Charles middle school. He was able to skip sixth grade and is currently the youngest seventh grader in his class. Whenever he can be of help to his peers, he volunteers to assist them with their coursework, and he also tries to be sociable by joining in conversations that his peers are engaged in. However, Martin is often rejected by his peers and is bullied by them as well.

Every Monday, Wednesday, and Friday for the last 5 months, Martin urinates on himself during his class's lunch period. This causes his peers to not want to be around him, which leads to them calling him names and ostracizing him. Martin does not seem to exhibit any feelings of shame, guilt, or regret when he urinates on himself. However, his teachers report him as being lonely and not fitting in well with the other students. When school officials called Martin's grandmother to report the problem of his frequent urination, she could only offer up, "He does not have these problems at home, but he has been having a hard time since his parents' fatal car accident."

Enuresis (F98.0) (307.6)

Enuresis is the voiding of urine (either involuntarily or intentional) into the bed or clothes. The criteria between the *DSM-5* and the *ICD-10* are relatively similar. Both state that before a diagnosis can be made, the child should at least be 5 years old (both chronologically and mentally). The child must have reached an age where continence is developmentally appropriate. In addition, the voiding of urine should not be the result of the effects of a substance/medication or another medical condition (e.g., seizure disorder, diabetes, structural abnormality of the urinary tract). In general, before considering this diagnosis, all other medical conditions should be ruled out.

Where the *DSM-5* and *ICD-10* differ is the point at which the voiding becomes clinically significant (i.e., the frequency of voiding). The *DSM-5* indicates that the point of clinical significance is voiding at least twice a week for at least 3 consecutive months. The *ICD-10* indicates the point of clinical significance is voiding at least twice a month (for children under 7; for children over 7, it is once per month) for at least 3 consecutive months. Both the *DSM-5* and the *ICD-10* have additional specifiers: nocturnal only (while sleeping), diurnal only (while awake), and nocturnal and diurnal.

Would you diagnose Martin with enuresis?

Encopresis (F98.1) (307.7)

Encopresis is the passage of feces (either involuntarily or intentional) into inappropriate places (e.g., clothing, floor). Like enuresis, the criteria between the *DSM-5* and the *ICD-10* are relatively similar. Both state that before a diagnosis can be made, the child should at least be 4 years old (both chronologically and mentally). In addition, the behavior should not be the result of the effects of a substance/medication (e.g., laxatives) or another medical condition (e.g., chronic diarrhea, spina bifida). Like enuresis, before considering this diagnosis, all other medical conditions should be ruled out.

Where the *DSM-5* and *ICD-10* differ is their duration at which the behavior becomes clinically significant (i.e., how long the behavior has occurred). The *DSM-5* indicates that the point of clinical significance is that there is at least one such event (passage of feces into an inappropriate place) that occurs each month for at least 3 months. The *ICD-10* indicates the point of clinical significance is that there is at least one encopretic event per month for at least 6 months.

Treatment Options

Perhaps one of the first considerations when working with children who meet the criteria for an elimination disorder is whether the behavior is involuntary or intentional. Involuntary events may lead to embarrassment, shame, and/or social rejection, which will possibly present additional concerns that can be addressed through counseling. Intentional events, when the incontinence is clearly deliberate, may coincide with symptoms related to oppositional defiant disorder and conduct disorder (APA, 2013a). Clinicians should consider (and address) other psychological and social factors that may contribute to the behavior.

In terms of options specific to involuntary nocturnal enuresis, clinicians may wish to consider behavioral conditioning using urine alarms (sensors that detect moisture and alert the child to go use the bathroom) or operant conditioning using "dry-bed training" (pairing urine alarms with behavioral strategies, such as frequent waking schedules and having the child change wet bedding; Shepard et al., 2017). For (involuntary) encopresis, biofeedback and "enhanced toilet training" are recommended. Counselors and clinicians will likely need additional resources to use biofeedback, as it involves the use of technology that helps clients observe their own muscular contractions to teach them how to tighten and relax anorectal muscles to improve bowel function. Enhanced toilet training, however, is a behavior modification approach that counselors may attempt to employ. It uses education and training related to breathing techniques and muscle contraction and relaxation to aid defecation. This technique may also incorporate rewards based on successful behavior (Shepard et al., 2017).

Case Study Summary

One of this chapter's case studies reviewed the behaviors of Selena. As you process the story and examine possible diagnostic criteria, take a few minutes to answer the following questions:

1. What would be the correct diagnosis for Selena?

   _____

   _____

2. What are the specific symptoms or criteria that led you to this diagnosis?

   _____

   _____

3. What other possible disorders might you diagnose Selena with and why?

   _____

   _____

4. Briefly discuss what types of treatment may be beneficial for Selena. Could you see using a certain counseling theory and/or medication?

   _____

   _____

Guided Practice Exercises

Scenario 1

Akachi is 10 years old and in the fourth grade. She struggles with making friends and her classroom behavior because of her inability to follow social cues. Akachi tends to use her outside voice, screaming when she is in class receiving instruction from her teacher and when she is redirected or chastised. She will yell at her teacher, "You don't tell me what to do." Her teacher attempts to be patient with Akachi by giving her multiple chances, but at times, Akachi does not properly respond. There was one time where Akachi's teacher was attempting to give the class instructions for their assignment, but Akachi chose to talk over her teacher. This led to Akachi not completing her assignment and being sent out of the classroom for disruptive behavior. These behaviors are not uncommon for Akachi, and the school has been working with her for 3 years now in hopes of shaping up her behavior.

One day during show-and-tell, one of Akachi's peers was sharing a memory behind the necklace his parents had brought him from their trip to Canada, and in the middle of his story, Akachi blurted out her own story about a present she had gotten for Christmas. When Akachi's teacher attempted to reason with her about how the students are to be a set of ears and not a mouth, Akachi went on to say she can't be a set of ears or a mouth. She failed to understand that all her teacher wanted was for her to be quiet and wait her turn to share her story with her classmates.

What would be the correct disorder? What are the specific symptoms or criteria that led you to this diagnosis?

_____

_____

_____

_____

What specific behaviors caused you to diagnose the disorder?

_____

_____

_____

_____

What other possible disorders might you diagnose Akachi with and why?

_____

_____

_____

_____

Scenario 2

James is a 6-year-old who currently attends public school and is enrolled in kindergarten. His mother did not work and kept him at home with his younger brother until enrolling him in kindergarten. He experiences significant social, behavioral, and academic problems each day. Socially, he has difficulty making and keeping friends. He is primarily interested in the game Minecraft, which some of the other kids in his class enjoy but not to extent that James likes to play it. James prefers to play Minecraft alone, and when other kids express their interest in the game, he projects a level of indifference toward them. His life revolves around Minecraft, to the point where his teachers and other children think he is obsessed with it. His book bag, lunchbox, notebook, and clothes are all Minecraft merchandise. He draws Minecraft objects and symbols on his schoolwork and often relates Minecraft facts and trivia in conversation. In terms of conversation, his teachers note that James does not make good eye contact with them or the other children.

James appears to be relatively on grade level, but he has experienced some behavioral issues since starting kindergarten during transition times. He has some anxiety that is displayed when the class transitions between specialists and the classroom teachers—and even when it is time for the things that are fun for most children: lunchtime and playground time. He prefers it when the classroom is quiet and is very evidently not fond of time in the gymnasium with the physical education teacher. The gym tends to reverberate sound, and the children are a bit louder than normal.

What would be the correct disorder? What are the specific symptoms or criteria that led you to this diagnosis?

_____

_____

_____

_____

What specific behaviors caused you to diagnose the disorder?

_____

_____

_____

_____

What other possible disorders might you diagnose James with and why?

_____

_____

_____

_____

Web-Based and Literature-Based Resources

Intellectual Disabilities

The IRIS Resource Center provides module-based learning on a variety of topics, including accommodations, learning strategies, and Individual Education Plans, published by the Peabody College of Education and Human Development at Vanderbilt University: https://iris.peabody.vanderbilt.edu/resources/iris-resource-locator/

Attention Deficit Hyperactivity Disorder

CHADD (Children and Adults with Attention-Deficit/Hyperactivity Disorders) is a national advocacy organization providing web-based resources for adults, children, and their families. They focus on providing evidence-based information and interventions: https://chadd.org/

The Network of Care of Chemung County (New York) provides an overview of attention deficit hyperactivity disorder, including signs and treatment. Of note, they have a link titled Human-Translated Documents and Video to serve multilingual clients: http://chemung.ny.networkofcare.org/mh/nimh/index.aspx?content=signlanguage2&language=signlanguage

Fin, Fur, and Feather Bureau of Investigation provides web-based games to teach school-aged children (K–5) executive functioning and strategies to address a variety of topics, including time management: http://www.fffbi.com/info/academy.html

Autism Spectrum Disorder

The National Alliance on Mental Illness provides resources to explain treatment, prevalence, and means to find support for clients and their families: https://www.nami.org/Learn-More/Mental-Health-Conditions/Related-Conditions/Autism/Support

Autism Speaks provides autism-specific resources for parents, educators, and individuals living with autism: https://www.autismspeaks.org/

Learning and Communication Disorders

Graphic organizers allow students to conceptualize material visually and can be used as an alternative assessment for students with learning differences: http://www.eduplace.com/graphicorganizer/index.jsp

Book Adventure uses varied learning styles and assessment options for reading and addressing test-taking strategies: http://www.bookadventure.com/Home.aspx

Be a Learning Hero offers parents and students a variety of resources, including videos, tips, and experiential activities to address learning: https://bealearninghero.org/

The IRIS Resource Center provides module-based learning on a variety of topics, including accommodations, learning strategies, and Individual Education Plans, published by the Peabody College of Education and Human Development at Vanderbilt University: https://iris.peabody.vanderbilt.edu/resources/iris-resource-locator/

Home Speech Home provides resources for parents and children and adults needing speech therapy, including downloadable tests, word lists, and apps for mobile devices: https://www.home-speech-home.com/

Speech Language provides resources for professionals, including downloadable content for educators, addressing specific sounds (e.g., /s/,/l/,/sh/) and comorbid interventions (e.g., speech development and autism): http://www.speechlanguage-resources.com/

American Speech-Language Hearing Association provides links to apps and links to other online resources, including blogs and recent innovation in the work of speech-language pathologists and audiologists: https://www.asha.org/

The Office of Special Education and Rehabilitative Services is a division of the U.S. Department of Education, and the information provided is designed for birth to age 21 years: https://www2.ed.gov/about/offices/list/osers/osep/index.html?src=mr

Center for Parent Information and Resources provides family-friendly, research-based content, along with webinars on a variety of topics, including language delays, parental advocacy, and best practices: https://www.parentcenterhub.org/

Motor Disorders

CanChild is provided by McMaster University and provides information for parents and schools to find resources related to brain injury, autism, and developmental coordination disorders. Developmental coordination disorder may go unnoticed because clients do not have an identifiable medical or neurological condition to explain their being "clumsy" or their inability to address basic self-care: https://www.canchild.ca/en/discover-canchild

National Ataxia Foundation provides a clearinghouse for information on Ataxia: https://ataxia.org/what-is-ataxia/

Parkinson's Foundation provides information on the signs, movement, and nonmovement symptoms, as well as current research related to Parkinson's diagnosis and prognosis: https://www.parkinson.org/

Elimination Disorders

Created by the Society of Clinical Child and Adolescent Psychology, Effective Child Therapy provides resources for evidence-based therapies, FAQs, and symptoms for a variety of mental health diagnoses, including a tiered approach to addressing nocturnal enuresis and encopresis: https://effectivechildtherapy.org/; https://effectivechildtherapy.org/concerns-symptoms-disorders/disorders/elimination-disorders/

Child Mind Institute provides signs, risk factors, and tips for addressing elimination disorders: https://childmind.org/topics/disorders/elimination-disorders/

References

Alateeqi, N., & Maria, F. J. (2019). Evidence-based treatments of autism spectrum disorder. *Psychiatric Annals, 49*(3), 115–119. http://dx.doi.org.ezproxy.nccu.edu/10.3928/00485713-20190204-01

American Academy of Pediatrics (AAP), Subcommittee on Children and Adolescents with Attention-Deficit/Hyperactivity Disorder. (2019). ADHD: Clinical practice guideline for the diagnosis, evaluation, and treatment of children and adolescents with attention-deficit/hyperactivity disorder. *Pediatrics, 144*(4) e20192528; DOI: 10.1542/peds.2019-2528.

American Association on Intellectual and Developmental Disabilities (AAIDD). (2010). *Intellectual disability: Definition, classification, and systems of supports.*

American Heritage Dictionary of Medicine. (2015). Intellectual disability. *The American heritage dictionary of medicine* (2nd ed.). Houghton Mifflin. http://ezproxy.nccu.edu/login?url=https://search.credoreference.com/content/entry/hmmedicaldict/intellectual_disability/0?institutionId=4295

American Psychiatric Association (APA). (2013a). *Diagnostic and statistical manual of mental disorders* (5th ed.).

American Psychiatric Association (APA). (2013b). *Social (pragmatic) communication disorder.* https://www.psychiatry.org/File%20Library/Psychiatrists/Practice/DSM/APA_DSM-5-Social-Communication-Disorder.pdf

American Psychiatric Association (APA). (2019). *What is ADHD?* https://www.psychiatry.org/patients-families/adhd/what-is-adhd

American Speech-Language Hearing Association. (2015). *Effects of hearing loss audiology on development.* https://www.asha.org/uploadedFiles/AIS-Hearing-Loss-Development-Effects.pdf

American Speech-Language Hearing Association. (2019). *2021 international classification of diseases, tenth revision, clinical modification (ICD-10-CM).* https://www.asha.org/uploadedFiles/ICD-10-Codes-SLP.pdf

Bressert, S. (2019). *Expressive language disorder symptoms.* Psych Central. https://psychcentral.com/disorders/expressive-language-disorder-symptoms/

Callaghan, T., & Sylvester, S. (2019). Autism spectrum disorder, politics, and the generosity of insurance mandates in the united states. *PLoS One, 14*(5). http://dx.doi.org.ezproxy.nccu.edu/10.1371/journal.pone.0217064

Centers for Disease Control and Prevention (CDC). (2018). *What is autism spectrum disorder?* https://www.cdc.gov/ncbddd/autism/facts.html

Centers for Disease Control and Prevention (CDC). (2019). *What are childhood mental disorders?* https://www.cdc.gov/childrensmentalhealth/basics.html

Christiansen, A. (2000). Persisting motor control problems in 11- to 12-year-old boys previously diagnosed with deficits in attention, motor control and perception (DAMP). *Developmental Medicine & Child Neurology, 42*, 4–7. https://doi.org/10.1017/s0012162200000025

Cortiella, C., & Horowitz, S. H. (2014). The state of learning disabilities: Facts, trends, and emerging issues. https://www.ncld.org/wp-content/uploads/2014/11/2014-State-of-LD.pdf

Edelson, S. M. (n.d.). Temple Grandin's 'hug machine'. http://www.autism-help.org/points-grandin-hug-machine.htm

Ferreira, J., Mäkinen, M., & Amorim, K. (2016). Intellectual disability in kindergarten: Possibilities of development through pretend play. *Procedia-Social and Behavioral Sciences, 217*, 487–500. 10.1016/j.sbspro.2016.02.024.

Food and Drug Administration. (2016). *Dealing with ADHD: What You Need to Know.* https://www.fda.gov/consumers/consumer-updates/dealing-adhd-what-you-need-know

Ganos, C., Munchau, A., & Bhatia, K. (2014). The semiology of tics, Tourette's and their association. *Movement Disorder Clinical Practice, 1*, 145–153. https://doi.org/10.1002/mdc3.12043

Ganos, C., Martino, D., & Pringsheim, T. (2016). Tics in the pediatric population: Pragmatic management. *Movement Disorders Clinical Practice, 1*(3), 160–172. https://doi.org/10.1002/mdc3.12428

Ghanizadeh, A. (2016). Twice-weekly aripiprazole for treating children and adolescents with tic disorder, a randomized controlled clinical trial. *Annals of General Psychiatry, 15*(1), 1–8. https://doi.org/10.1186%2Fs12991-016-0112-4

Gilbert, D. L., Budman, C. L., Singer, H., Kurlan, R., & Chipkin, R. E. (2014). A D1 receptor antagonist, ecopipam, for treatment of tics in Tourette syndrome. *Clinical Neuropharmacology, 37*(1), 26–30. https://doi.org/10.1097/WNF.0000000000000017

Goetz, C. G., Tanner, C. M., & Klawans, H. L. (1984). Fluphenazine and multifocal tic disorders. *Arch Neurology, 41*, 271–272.

Grandin, T. (n.d.). *About Temple Grandin.* https://www.templegrandin.com/

Grandin, T. (1992). Calming effects of deep touch pressure in patients with autistic disorder, college students and animals. *Journal of Child and Adolescent Psychopharmacology, 2*, 63–72.

Harris, K. M., Mahone, E. M., & Singer, H. S. (2008). Nonautistic motor stereotypes: Clinical features and longitudinal follow-up. *Pediatric Neurology, 38*, 267–272. https://doi.org/10.1016/j.pediatrneurol.2007.12.008

Harris, S. R., Mickelson, E., & Zwicker, J. G. (2015). Diagnosis and management of developmental coordination disorder. *Canadian Medical Association Journal, 187* (9), 659–665. https://doi.org/10.1503/cmaj.140994

Knight, T., Steeves, T., Day, L., Lowerison, M., Jette, N., & Pringsheim, T. (2012). Prevalence of tic disorders: A systematic review and meta-analysis. *Pediatric Neurology, 47*, 77–90. https://doi.org/10.1016/j.pediatrneurol.2012.05.002

Mackenzie, K. (2018). Stereotypic movement disorders. *Seminars in Pediatric Neurology, 25*, 19–24. https://doi.org/10. 1016/j.spen.2017.12.004

Maguire, G., Yeh, C., & Ito, B. (2012). Overview of the diagnosis and treatment of stuttering. *Journal of Experimental and Clinical Medicine, 4*(2), 92–97.

Mandich, A. D., Polatajko, H. J., & Rodger, S. A. (2003). Rites of passage: Understanding participation of children with developmental coordination disorder. *Human Movement Science, 22*(4–5), 583–595. https://doi.org/10.1016/j.humov.2003.09.011

Marrus, N., & Hall, L. (2017). Intellectual disability and language disorder. *Child and Adolescent Psychiatric Clinics of North America, 26*(3), 539–554. https://doi.org/10.1016/j.chc.2017.03.001

Mayo Foundation for Medical Education and Research. (2019a). *Attention-deficit/hyperactivity disorder (ADHD) in children.* https://www.mayoclinic.org/diseases-conditions/adhd/symptoms-causes/syc-20350889?utm_source=Google&utm_medium=abstract&utm_content=Attention-deficit-hyperactivity-disorder&utm_campaign=Knowledge-panel

Mayo Foundation for Medical Education and Research. (2019b). *Learning disorders: Know the signs, how to help.* https://www.mayoclinic.org/healthy-lifestyle/childrens-health/in-depth/learning-disorders/art-20046105

MentalHealth.net. (2019). Treatment of communication disorders and recommended reading. https://www.mentalhelp.net/disorders-of-childhood/treatment-of-communication-disorders-and-reading/

Miguel, C. F., Clark, K., Terreshko, L., & Ahearn, W. H. (2009). The effects of response interruption and redirection and sertraline on vocal stereotypy. *Journal of Applied Behavioral Analysis, 42*, 883–888. https://doi.org/10.1901/jaba.2009.42-883

Miller, L. T., Polatajko, H. J., Missiuna, C., Mandich, A. D., & Macnab, J. J. (2001). A pilot trial of a cognitive treatment for children with developmental coordination disorder. *Human Movement Science, 20*, 183–210. https://doi.org/10.1016/S0167-9457(01)00034-3

National Academy of Sciences. (2015). *Mental disorders and disabilities among low-income children.* https://www.ncbi.nlm.nih.gov/books/NBK332886/

National Institute on Health (NIH). (2018). *What are the treatments for learning disabilities?* https://www.nichd.nih.gov/health/topics/learning/conditioninfo/treatment

Poulsen, A. A., Ziviani, J. M., M. Cuskelly, M., & Smith, R. (2007). Boys with developmental coordinator disorder: Loneliness and team sports participation. *American Journal of Occupational Therapy, 61*(4), 451–462. https://doi.org/10.5014/ajot.61.4.451

Pringsheim, T., Doja, A., & Gorman, D. (2012). Canadian guidelines for the evidence-based treatment of tic disorders: Pharmacotherapy. *Canadian Journal of Psychiatry, 57*, 133–143. https://doi.org/10.1177%2F070674371205700302

Rasmussen, P., & Gillberg, C. (2000). Natural outcome of ADHD with developmental coordination disorder at age 22 years: A controlled longitudinal, community-based study. *Journal of the American Academy of Child and Adolescent Psychiatry, 39*(11), 1424–1431. https://doi.org/10.1097/00004583-200011000-00017

Ricketts, E. J., Bauer, C. C., Van der Fluit, F., Capriotti, M. R., Espil, F. M., Snorrason, I., Ely, L. J., Walther, M. R., & Woods, D. W. (2013). Behavior therapy for stereotypic movement disorder in typically developing children: A clinical case series. *Cognitive and Behavioral Practice, 20*(4), 544–555. https://doi.org/10.1016/j.cbpra.2013.03.002

Ringdahl, J. E., Andelman, M. S., Kitsukawa, K., Winborn, L. C., Barretto, A., & Wacker, D. P. (2002). Evaluation and treatment of covert stereotypy. *Behavioral Interventions, 17*, 43–49. https://doi.org/10/1002/bin.105.abs

Robinson, S., Woods, M., Cardona, F., & Hedderly, T. (2016). Intense imagery movements (IIM): More to motor stereotypies than meets the eye. *European Journal of Pediatric Neurology, 20*, 61–68. https://doi.org/10.1016/j.ejpn.2015.10.006.

Roessner, V., Plessen, K. J., & Rothenberger, A. (2011). European clinical guidelines for Tourette syndrome and other tic disorders. Part II: Pharmacological treatment. *European Child Adolescent Psychiatry, 20*, 173–196. https://doi.org/10.1007/s00787-011-0165-5

Ross, M. S., & Moldofsky, H. (1978). A comparison of pimozide and haloperidol in the treatment of Gilles de la Tourette's syndrome. *The American Journal of Psychiatry, 135*(5), 585–587. https://doi.org/10.1176/ajp.135.5.585

Shepard, J. A., Poler, J. E., & Grabman, J. H. (2017). Evidence-based psychosocial treatments for pediatric elimination disorders. *Journal of Clinical Child & Adolescent Psychology, 46*(6), https://doi.org/10.1080/153784416.2016.1247356

Simpson, N., Mizen, l. & Cooper, S.A. (2016). Intellectual disabilities. *Medicine, 44* (11), 679–682. https://doi.org/10.1016/j.mpmed.2016.08.008

Singer, H. S. (2011). Stereotypic movement disorders. *Handbook of Clinical Neurology, 100* (63), 19–24. https://doi.org/10.1016/B978-0-444-52014-2.00045-8

Tan, A., Salgado, M., & Fahn, S. (1997). The characterization and outcome of stereotypical movements in nonautistic children. *Movement Disorders Journal, 12,* 47–52. https://doi.org/10.1002/mds.870120109

Taylor, B. A., Hoch, H., & Weissman, M. (2005). The analysis and treatment of vocal stereotypy in child with autism. *Behavioral Interventions, 20,* 239–253. https://doi.org/10.1002/bin.200

U.S. National Library of Medicine. (2019). *Phonological disorder.* https://medlineplus.gov/ency/article/001541.htm

Understood. (2020). *Understanding language disorders.* https://www.understood.org/en/learning-thinking-differences/child-learning-disabilities/communication-disorders/understanding-language-disorders

Van der Linde, B. W., Netten, J. J., Otten, B., Postema, K., Geuze, R. H., & Schoemaker, M. M. (2015). Activities of daily living in children with developmental coordination disorder: Performance, learning, and participation. *Physical Therapy, 95*(11), 1496–14506.

Verdellen, C., van de Griendt, Hartmann, & Murphy, T. (2011). European clinical guidelines for Tourette Syndrome and other tic disorders. Part III: Behavioural and psychosocial interventions. *European Child Adolescent Psychiatry, 20,* 197–207.

Visser, J. (2003). Developmental coordination disorder: A review on subtypes and comorbidities. *Human Movement Science, 22* (4–5), 479–493.

WebMD. (2019). *What is dysgraphia? What should I do if my child has it?* https://www.webmd.com/add-adhd/childhood-adhd/dysgraphia-facts#1

Whiteford, H. A., Degenhardt, L., Rehm, J., Baxter, A. J., Ferrari, A. J., Erskine, H. E., Charlson, F. J., Norman, R. E., Flaxman, A. D., Johns, N., Burstein, R., Murray, C. J. & Vos, T. (2013). Global burden of disease attributable to mental and substance use disorders: Findings from the global burden of disease study 2010. *The Lancet, 382,* 1575–1586.

Willis, C. D. (2014). DSM-5 and neurodevelopmental and other disorders of childhood and adolescence. *Journal of American Academy of Psychiatry and the Law, 42,* 165–172.

World Health Organization (WHO). (1992). *The ICD-10 classification of mental and behavioural disorders: Clinical descriptions and diagnostic guidelines.* Geneva: World Health Organization.

World Health Organization (WHO). (2019). *Autism spectrum disorders.* https://www.who.int/news-room/fact-sheets/detail/autism-spectrum-disorders

Zwicker, J. G., Missiuna, C., Harris, S. R., & Boyd, L. A. (2012). Developmental coordination disorder: A review and update. *European Journal of Paediatric Neurology, 16*(6), 573–581. https://doi.org/10.1016/j.ejpn.2012.05.005

Zwicker, J. G., Harris, S. R., & Klassen, A. F. (2013). Quality of life domains affected in children with developmental coordination disorder: A systematic review. *Child care, health and development, 39*(4), 562–580. https://doi.org/10.1111/j.1365-2214.2012.01379.x

Credits

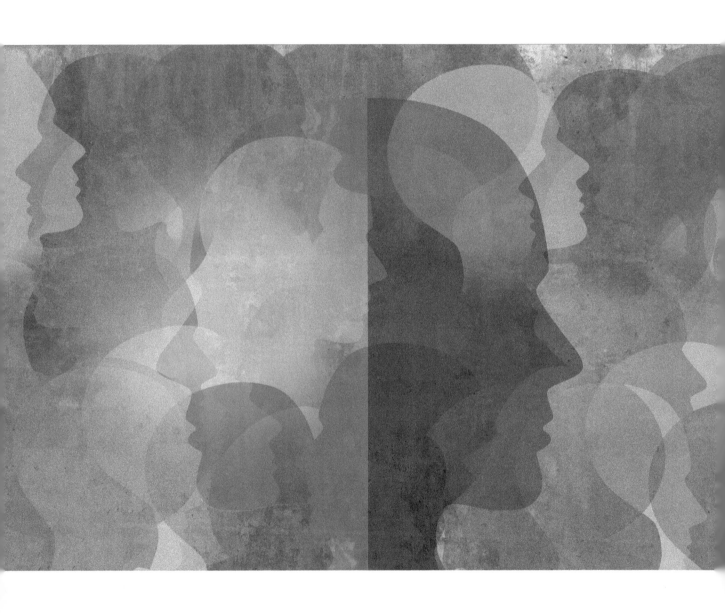

CHAPTER FOUR

SCHIZOPHRENIA AND OTHER PSYCHOTIC DISORDERS

Andy J. Flaherty, David A. Scott, and Michelle Grant Scott

CASE STUDY 4.1 Dietrich, 25, is taken to the hospital by his sister, Anne, and involuntarily admitted. Anne first became concerned about her brother 3 years prior, after their parents' death. Dietrich moved out of the family home to his own apartment following his parents' tragic car accident. When Anne would call or visit, Dietrich would seem "different." His attitude and facial expressions seem very unemotional or flat. She once found him staring at the wall blankly in a rigid position. Anne had no idea how long he had been there, and it took her more than an hour to rouse Dietrich. He never laughed and was not ever excited about anything. He worked at a department store and began to become suspicious of his coworkers. Dietrich told Anne that his coworkers were jealous of him because he had a degree from a community college and was the "boss's favorite employee." He claimed that they used hidden cameras around his register to try to catch him making a mistake. One night he called Anne frantic because he was convinced that one of the coworkers stuck him with a needle and injected a fluid into his body that would allow the Central Intelligence Agency to know his thoughts. He had quit his job, explaining to his boss that he knew about the secret phone tapping and the hidden cameras. Anne drove over to Dietrich's house, but he didn't recognize her and accused her of being a secret government agent. She was finally able to get him into the car and to the hospital.

Did You Know?

- People with schizophrenia are typically portrayed by the media as being prone to violence; however, they are more like to be victims of violence rather than perpetrators.
- Depression is the most prevalent cause of suicide for people suffering from schizophrenia.
- Typically, men between the ages of 16 and 20 will experience schizophrenia for the first time, whereas typically women between the ages of 25 and 30 will experience schizophrenia for the first time.
- Studies have indicated that 25% of those having schizophrenia recover completely, 50% are improved over a 10-year period, and 25% do not improve over time.
- At any given time, there are more people with untreated severe psychiatric illnesses living on America's streets than are receiving care in hospitals.

Overview

The schizophrenia spectrum disorders are characterized and defined by the presence of psychotic symptoms. Much misunderstanding surrounds these disorders, which can lead to underdiagnosis and a significant deal of shame, stigma, and hopelessness surrounding them. However, while they are chronic and/or acute, people can and do recover; however, this is predicated on accurate and effective understanding, diagnosis, and treatment on the part of clinicians. Psychotic symptoms and disorders can be confusing to understand and accurately treat for even seasoned practitioners. With that in mind, this chapter will provide an overview of the schizophrenia spectrum disorder and explore the nature and functioning of a range of psychotic symptoms in addition to the prognosis for these diseases, common treatments, and potential for recovery.

What Do We Mean by the Term "Psychotic"?

In the early editions of the American Psychiatric Association's *Diagnostic and Statistical Manual of Mental Disorders (DSM)*, psychosis was defined broadly as a "gross impairment in reality testing" or the acute "loss of ego boundaries." This definition, which was tied to theory and less to a biological view of psychosis, now seems outdated and challenging for clinicians to understand and apply to their patients.

At present both the American Psychiatric Association (APA, 2013) and the World Health Organization (WHO, 2016) define psychosis in a narrower manner by emphasizing the presence of hallucinations (without insight into their symptomatic nature), delusions, or combination of hallucinations and delusions as the primary indicators of psychosis. Therefore, modern definitions of psychosis still operationalize it as greatly impaired reality testing. However, with the addition of specific symptoms, hallucinations, and delusions, as well as other disorganized thought, speech, and behavior, this provides clear and precise guidelines for understanding what the patient/client is experiencing and how these symptoms are affecting them.

The *DSM-5* and Schizophrenia as a Spectrum of Disorders

Psychotic symptoms common to schizophrenia are evident across several disorders that vary and range in severity and intensity. Therefore, the *DSM-5* (APA, 2013) presents the idea that schizophrenia exists as a part of a continuum of related conditions that share symptoms and causes in common. When viewed as a spectrum of disorders, psychotic disorders can be seen to range between "normal" or typical of the general population at one end (in which no schizophrenia and psychosis is present at all) and severe schizophrenia and extreme mental disorganization at the other end of the scale.

At the mild end of schizophrenia spectrum disorder, several personality disorders are now defined within the *DSM-5* as mild schizophrenia spectrum disorders. Schizoid personality disorder and schizotypal personality disorder sit on the spectrum close to the "normal" or extremely less psychotic side. Like schizophrenia, these are long-term disorders that begin in childhood or early adulthood, which negatively affect people's professional/occupational, social, and family lives. However, while schizoid personality disorder and schizotypal personality disorder share similarities with aspects of schizophrenia, they also differ in significant ways. For instance, people with schizoid personality disorder are "in touch with reality," displaying coherent and clear speech in spite of behaviors and thought patterns that are very atypical from the general population. Likewise, people with schizotypal disorder, in contrast with schizophrenia, are capable of having the insight that thoughts and thinking patterns are disordered.

In the middle of the schizophrenia spectrum disorder are delusional disorder and schizophreniform disorder. While these disorders are more severe than the previously mentioned personality disorders, they feature many more pronounced and intense psychotic symptoms. However, these disorders specifically lack the duration of symptoms that are seen in schizophrenia and schizoaffective disorder.

Schizophrenia and schizoaffective disorder are firmly on the severe end of the spectrum, as these disorders are marked by intense mental disorganization and a pervasive pattern of critical implications to life and social functioning. In addition, these two disorders can be difficult to diagnose, treat, and manage and may require numerous interventions to reach the point at which the disorder goes into remission and recovery begins.

ICD-10 Schizophrenia

Within the *DSM-5*, the diagnostic criteria no longer identify schizophrenia subtypes or the diagnostic divisions based on the acuity of the disorder. Under *DSM-IV*, schizophrenia subtypes were defined and assigned based on the predominant symptoms present at the time that the evaluation was taking place. However, in practice, these subtypes of the disorder often proved unhelpful to clinicians because patients' symptoms and presentation of specific subtypes often changed. Many clinicians reported that some patients moved from one subtype to another and that oftentimes patients present with overlapping subtypes. *ICD-10-CM* eliminated the acuity of schizophrenia as a diagnostic criterion; however, it retains the subtypes of the disorder in contrast to the *DSM-5*.

The *ICD-10* category for schizophrenia (F20) includes the subtypes paranoid, disorganized, catatonic, undifferentiated, residual, and "other."

Schizophrenia Subtypes

- Paranoid
- Disorganized
- Catatonic
- Undifferentiated
- Residual
- Other

Two categories in *ICD-10* that were previously classified under schizophrenia in *ICD-9* are the following:

1. F21—schizotypal disorder, which includes borderline, latent, prepsychotic, prodromal, pseudoneurotic, and pseudopsychopathic schizophrenia, as well as schizotypal personality disorder
2. F25—schizoaffective disorder, which includes bipolar and depressive types

Importantly, while there are significant differences between the *ICD-10* and the *DSM-5*, efforts have been made to improve harmonization between the *DSM* and *ICD* definitions of schizophrenia (Gaebel, 2012; Tandon & Carpenter, 2013). Significantly, although *ICD-11* has not yet been finalized (it is scheduled to be released in 2022), current drafts indicate that all the changes made from *DSM-IV* to *DSM-5* will be included, most notably the deletion of schizophrenia subtypes (Heckers et al., 2010).

Causes of the Schizophrenia Spectrum Disorders

The exact cause of the schizophrenia spectrum disorders is unknown. The best recent research tells us that a combination of factors from across several domains (with some of them overlapping) may contribute to the development of schizophrenia spectrum disorders (Gilmore, 2010).

1. ***Genetic Factors.*** Schizophrenia spectrum disorders tend to have hereditary factors and markers. Yet, this does not mean that if a relative has an illness, then an individual will automatically develop a disorder. However, it does indicate that there is a higher likelihood of a related individual developing the disease. The precise genes that contribute to the development of schizophrenia have yet to be developed, but research is ongoing (Lisman, 2012).

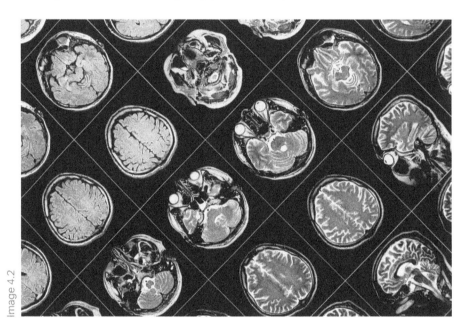

Image 4.2

2. ***Neurological/Brain Chemistry and Structure.*** The function and structure of the brain in people with schizophrenia spectrum disorder conditions may be different and atypical in comparison to the general population in ways that brain science is only beginning to understand. Importantly, brain scans are helping to advance research in this area and providing a full picture of the ways in which neurological factors play a role in the development of schizophrenia spectrum disorders. Sometimes magnetic resonance imaging can be helpful in diagnosing schizophrenia, as typically the imaging shows a smaller total brain volume and enlarged ventricles (Haukvik et al., 2013).

3. ***Environmental Factors.*** Environmental factors may also play a role with some studies indicating that neonatal factors may contribute to the development of schizophrenia spectrum disorders (Dean & Murray, 2005).

4. ***Stress.*** While stress itself does not cause the disorders, stressful events, such as a death of a loved one, divorce, or unemployment, can trigger psychotic symptoms or decompensation of an existing or latent disorder (evident by the worsening of symptoms in those who have a disorder).

5. ***Substance Use.*** Substance use and specifically psychoactive drug use, such as LSD and other hallucinogens, have been linked to the development and the onset of the schizophrenia spectrum disorders (Hambrecht & Hafner, 1996). However, research does not support a link between specific symptoms of schizophrenia and choice of abused drugs (Dixon, 1999).

Schizophrenia

There are significant misunderstandings that surround schizophrenia, and unfortunately, the phrase itself is very commonly overused by the general populace. One effect of the imprecise use of the term is that it causes fear and shame around the disorder, which makes it challenging for professionals to engage people with schizophrenia and other similar mental health challenges. Without early engagement of people with psychotic symptoms, it is difficult to provide early intervention and treatment, which improves the likelihood of someone making a significant recovery, and it can leave patients locked in cycles of stigma, shame, and fear.

The prevalence rate of the disorder is actually much less common than the overuse of the phrase implies. According to the National Institute on Mental Health (NIMH, 2018) studies that use household-based survey samples, clinical diagnostic interviews, and medical records, estimates of the prevalence of schizophrenia and related psychotic disorders in the United States range between 0.25% and 0.64% of the general population.

One frequent and persistent misunderstanding that is important to address about schizophrenia is the idea that it is an indication of multiple or split personalities. Schizophrenia has never referred to the presence of split or multiple personalities, as it is sometimes perceived in the popular imagination, and in reality, schizophrenia has little in common with dissociative identity disorder (the clinical term for multiple personalities), and confusing the two disorders is an unhelpful but sometimes persistent misconception.

Diagnosing Schizophrenia

Even for seasoned clinicians, diagnosing schizophrenia is frequently a complex challenge—a challenge that requires a clinician who can carefully put together diagnostic clues to ensure a complete picture about what the patient is experiencing. Specifically, diagnosing schizophrenia is challenging because other factors not connected to the disorder may contribute to the onset, development, and experience of psychotic symptoms. For instance, drugs like methamphetamines and LSD and other medical factors (other neurological conditions) can cause the onset of schizophrenia-like psychotic symptoms but not the disorder itself.

As many patients are profoundly resistant to the idea that they have a mental health disorder, and because they have such little insight into their symptoms, when they are highly symptomatic, they may believe that, in the fact, nothing is wrong with them. It is important to note that an extreme lack of awareness and insight into their experience with the disorder is a common symptom of people diagnosed with schizophrenia. The effect of this lack of insight is that it considerably complicates treatment and can lead to a worsened prognosis. Therefore, clinicians must carefully and sensitively rule out other factors through gently working with the client over a period of several sessions/weeks before making a diagnosis of schizophrenia.

CLINICIAN'S CORNER 4.1

As a clinician, I am consistently amazed by the extent to which people recover from the schizophrenia spectrum disorders and go on to lead fulfilling and deeply meaningful lives. One of the most remarkable things is that while for many, the symptoms don't completely disappear, they do become manageable. And with a combination of medication and psychosocial supports, their impact can be greatly mitigated. It is important to remember the reality that recovery happens, because when someone is acutely ill with schizophrenia, it can be easy to forget this, especially if the person is having their first psychotic episode. However, in time, and especially with early intervention, people can and do return to a high level of functioning. And with the right supports consistently applied, they go on to lead deeply meaningful and significant lives. The message of the recovery movement is that recovery can and does happen; people are not their diagnoses, and their diagnoses shouldn't be life sentences. It is especially important to remember that as they get older, for many clients, their symptoms will become much less significant and impactful, and it is important to convey with a degree of confidence that things will get better and that the person is not their diagnosis. We must always strive to see the person and not a cluster of symptoms; it is important that we as clinicians see and recognize people first and not their symptoms, however intimidating these may be. Seeing the person has a humanizing effect and helps us to forge connections with our clients that are healing and extremely supportive.

Andy J. Flaherty, MSW

Diagnostic Criteria

There is not a single diagnostic test for schizophrenia; instead, the clinician must evaluate a person's symptoms and the course of their illness and life functioning over at least the previous 6-month period to ensure an accurate diagnosis. It is important to note that many people who eventually receive a diagnosis of schizophrenia will have experienced symptoms for significantly longer than 6 months, in part because of the reasons explained earlier concerning stigma. However, early diagnosis and intervention are very important because research has demonstrated a clear link between early intervention/treatment and greatly improved psychosocial outcomes. To receive a diagnosis of schizophrenia, the individual must have two or more of the following symptoms, with these symptoms persistently occurring in the context of severely reduced functioning:

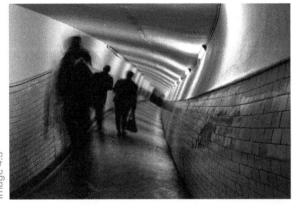

Image 4.3

- Delusions
- Hallucinations
- Disorganized speech
- Disorganized physical behavior or catatonic behavior
- Negative symptoms

As is evident from the diagnostic criteria, schizophrenia involves a range of symptoms that span several domains: the cognitive, the behavioral, and the emotional. In terms of the effect on the individual, the common symptoms of schizophrenia are broken down into three distinct categories: (1) positive symptoms, (2) negative symptoms, and (3) cognitive effects. Positive symptoms are symptoms in which there is the addition of something symptomatic to the individual with the disorder. In contrast, negative symptoms are marked by a deficit or what they take from the person. In addition, it is important to understand that negative symptoms can be somewhat subtle and mimic the symptoms of several other disorders, most notably the mood disorders.

POSITIVE SYMPTOMS

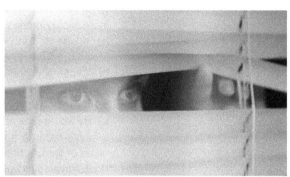
Image 4.4

- *Hallucinations.* These consist of seeing, hearing, or smelling things that are not in reality there. One of the most frequently reported subtypes of hallucinations is hearing voices that are derogatory and threatening.
- *Delusions.* This is a firm belief in ideas or thoughts that are not in fact grounded in reality. Typical examples of delusions include the idea that one is being watched; other delusions are of a persecutory nature and believing oneself to be divine. Significantly, an individual suffering from delusions continues to believe in the legitimacy of these thoughts and ideas even when evidence is presented that comprehensively proves the ideas wrong, meaning they are fixed against contradictory evidence.
- *Thought disorder.* This is characterized by difficulty forming cohesive thoughts and experiencing problems in being understood when attempting to communicate with others. Thought blocking is also a commonly observed symptom in those suffering from schizophrenia in which a person stops talking mid-sentence and may take several seconds to resume the conversation. Likewise, rapidly changing thoughts or creating words that do not exist are other common examples of disordered thinking.
- *Unusual movements.* This can consist of repetitive movements or prolonged episodes of being very still and demonstrating/displaying extreme psychomotor immobility (also known as catatonia). In addition, other unusually slow movements are also frequently observed in people suffering from schizophrenia spectrum disorder.

TRUE LIFE 4.1

John Nash

In the words of the president of Princeton, Christopher L. Eisgruber, "an inspiration to mathematicians, economists and scientists" (Goode, 2015), John Nash is known as one of the greatest thinkers in the realm of mathematics. John Forbes Nash Jr. was born on June 13, 1928, in Bluefield, West Virginia. During his early years, he was classified as socially awkward but did have a small circle of friends. Unfortunately, during one of their experiments, which consisted 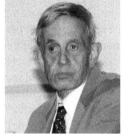 Image 4.5 of making bombs, one of Nash's friends blew himself up (Bell, 2017). During his teen years, he was singled out for his gifted talent in mathematics, and he went on to develop his Nash equilibrium while he studied at Princeton

(continued)

University. He would go on to win two of mathematics' highest honors, the Putnam Competition and the Fields Medal (Goode, 2015).

It was in the 1950s while teaching at Massachusetts Institute of Technology that Nash began to develop symptoms of schizophrenia. His initial symptoms appeared in the form of paranoia and delusions (Goode, 2015). Sometimes, he would disappear for days at a time and return with no explanation of his whereabouts. And in the middle of his lectures, he would make meaningless statements, leaving his students and colleagues frazzled (Bell, 2017). It was Nash's wife who noticed that his conversations became increasingly more strange before she sought the help of a psychiatrist for her husband. John would be admitted into McLean Hospital, part of Harvard Medical, where he would receive a diagnosis of paranoid schizophrenia with grandiose and persecutory delusions (Bell, 2017). The cause ascribed was that of his work and new fatherhood, and a psychoanalyst even suggested it was due to latent homosexuality. After consulting psychiatrists, Nash's family was better able to make sense of his arrest for indecent exposure in a men's bathroom from years prior. This stunt could serve as his possible onset of schizophrenia (Rettner, 2015). During another episode of ill health, Nash traveled to Europe, attempting to convince European governments to grant him refugee status (Bell, 2017). Nash's battle with and recovery from schizophrenia were depicted in the 2001 Oscar-winning film *A Beautiful Mind*.

Despite the many trials encountered by Nash, he had family members and colleagues who were supportive of him and his mental health. His wife divorced him but continued to offer her support by moving him into her home. (They would marry again 38 years later.) John Nash stated he simply decided to return to rationality. "I emerged from irrational thinking, ultimately, without medicine other than the natural hormonal changes of aging" (Goode, 2015). Once he returned to rationality, the Nobel committee awarded John Nash the Nobel Prize in economic sciences. It was this award that transformed Nash from a desolate vandalizing Princeton in scribble to a celebrity. On May 23, 2015, John Nash and his wife were ejected from their car in an accident where they were pronounced dead on arrival.

NEGATIVE SYMPTOMS

- *Lack of Emotions.* This symptom appears to be very similar to a flat affect, as demonstrated within major depressive disorder. A general lack of passion, lack of emotion, lack of interest in life, and lack of joy in previously significant activities may also be prevalent and reported by the client or loved ones. In addition, many individuals with schizophrenia will feel excitement and happiness. However, they are affected by negative symptoms in the sense that the display of their mood (i.e., their affect) is not congruent with their internal experience.
- *Difficulty Maintaining Relationships.* This difficulty is due to a combination of factors, but in particular, a lack of emotions and sometimes a preoccupation with the presence of positive symptoms can make it difficult to attend to relationships. The result of these factors is that they make it easy for individuals with schizophrenia to profoundly disengage from those they care about.

- *Flat Voice.* Evidenced by the client speaking in a dull, flat tone in which inflection or emotion is not present.
- *Difficulty With Caring for Basic Needs.* Because of disorganized thinking, people challenged with schizophrenia display little interest in caring for themselves. This frequently results in decreased personal care and hygiene, as well as a lack of attention to basic health-care needs.

COGNITIVE SYMPTOMS

A range of cognitive symptoms can be present that reflect an impact on overall functioning and affect the completion of activities of daily living. These symptoms include the following:

- *Difficulty Comprehending Information.* This symptom is recognizable as intense confusion about everyday situations or objects.
- *Difficulty in Making Decisions.* This is evidenced by a pronounced difficulty understanding new information and then using this information effectively. This symptom may be referred to as difficulty with "executive functioning."
- *Difficulty in Maintaining Attention.* A general inability to focus or to pay attention.
- *Problems With Memory and Retention of Information.* This symptom can range from chronically misplacing objects to immediately forgetting information as soon as it is learned, with the implication of this symptom being that it seems to be very difficult for those challenged with the disorder to retain information.

Think about our case study of Dietrich. Would Dietrich's symptoms lead you to think about schizophrenia?

Onset and Prevalence of Schizophrenia

Typically, the disorder emerges in the late teens to the early 30s, with the peak onset of the first psychotic episode in the early to mid-20s for men and later 20s for women. While the use of the term is common according to the *DSM-5*, the lifetime prevalence of schizophrenia is approximately 0.3%–0.7% (Saha et al., 2005).

Suicide Risk

Those challenged with schizophrenia are at a significantly elevated risk of suicide, with some 5%–6% of people taking their own lives and about 20% making attempts on more than one occasion (Hor & Taylor, 2010).

The Other Disorders on the Schizophrenia Spectrum

CASE STUDY 4.2 Leonard, 44, is a husband and father of three children. After his last child was born about 10 years earlier, Leonard's wife noticed a marked change in his behavior. He began to withdrawal socially and would go through long bouts of debilitating depression. There would be days where he would not speak, or if he did speak, his speech would not make sense. This resulted in him missing a lot of work. When Leonard returned to work, his boss reprimanded him for missing so much time. Leonard became convinced that his boss and his company were conspiring against him to steal his retirement fund. They were using his social security number to prematurely collect his benefits. Leonard thought that the Federal Bureau of Investigation might be involved as well. These thoughts made Leonard feel worthless and hopeless about the future. One night, Leonard heard a voice calling to him. When Leonard answered, the voice told him how to fix his problems with the retirement fund. If Leonard would collect "codes" from newspapers and television broadcasts and leave those codes in a secret mailbox, then the government would leave him alone.

Schizoaffective Disorder

Schizoaffective disorder is sometimes wrongly thought to be schizophrenia accompanied by major depressive disorder. Because of this, historically, there was much scientific discussion concerning whether schizoaffective disorder is in fact a separate condition from both schizophrenia and depression (Abrams et al., 2008). Yet it is much more complicated than a co-occurrence of these two disorders. Schizoaffective disorder, like schizophrenia, is a complex and chronic mental health condition; it encompasses all the primary symptoms of schizophrenia, such as hallucinations, delusions, and grossly disorganized thinking, along with the symptoms of a mood disorder, such as major depression or bipolar depression. Therefore, scientific consensus is that the disorder is a psychotic condition that is marked by intense disturbances of mood.

SYMPTOMS OF SCHIZOAFFECTIVE DISORDER

The following symptoms are commonly seen in schizoaffective disorder:

- Hallucinations
- Delusions
- Disorganized thinking in which a person may switch very quickly from one topic to another or provide answers that are entirely unrelated to the question
- Depressed mood. If a person has been diagnosed with schizoaffective disorder depressive type, then they will experience feelings of intense sadness, emptiness, feelings of worthlessness, and other symptoms of a depressive disorder (major depressive specifier)
- Manic behavior. If a person has been diagnosed with schizoaffective disorder bipolar type, they will likely experience feelings of euphoria, racing thoughts, increased risky behavior in addition to other symptoms of mania (bipolar specifier)

Like the other psychotic disorders, schizoaffective disorder is also very challenging to precisely diagnose; specifically, because it is not uncommon for psychotic symptoms to be a feature of depression or bipolar disorder. It takes a skilled and experienced clinician to take the required history that will enable a rule out of separate diagnoses.

SCHIZOAFFECTIVE DISORDER DIAGNOSTIC CRITERIA

To be diagnosed with schizoaffective disorder, an individual client must display the following symptoms with the following specifiers:

- A period during which there is a significant mood disorder (either depression or mania) that occurs while symptoms of schizophrenia/psychosis are present.
- Delusions or hallucinations must be present for 2 or more weeks in the absence of a major mood episode.
- Symptoms that meet criteria for a significant mood disorder are present for most of the total duration of the illness.
- Symptoms are not better explained by drug use, a medication reaction, or some other medical condition.

CASE STUDY 4.3 Geoffrey, 32, is a husband and a father of two. He works as a mechanic at a local body shop. In the last 2 months, his behavior has drastically changed. First, he begins to suspect that the government is spying on his behavior. In response, he changes his route to work each day to throw off anyone following him. He has purchased disposable cell phones for himself and his wife to be able to be sure that their phones are not tapped and has taken his family to his sister's house for several nights because he did not believe their house to be safe. One night, a man named Richard meets him outside his back door and offers to help his family. If Geoffrey will decode messages from the government written in magazines and then drop his analysis in a special mailbox, his family will be safe. Geoffrey's wife, Marie, hears him talking outside. When she walks out, it appears that Geoffrey is having a conversation with thin air. When she asks him about it, he is convinced there is another person with them. Geoffrey spends large amounts of time standing in a rigid position and is unresponsive to his family.

Schizophreniform Disorder

Schizophreniform disorder represents the halfway point on the schizophrenia spectrum disorder between brief psychotic disorder and schizophrenia. This condition is defined by the presence of two or more psychotic and related symptoms (delusions, hallucinations, disorganized speech, and abnormal psychomotor behavior, such as grossly disorganized or catatonic speech), with at least one of these symptoms being delusions, hallucinations, or disorganized speech (Gubi et al., 2014). Schizophreniform disorder symptoms must last for at least 1 month but less than 6 months. Schizophreniform disorder is differentiated from schizophrenia by the amount of time that the individual has been experiencing the disorder; therefore, in some instances schizophreniform disorder is used as a precursor diagnosis before a diagnosis of schizophrenia is given, if 6 months have not elapsed since the onset of the symptoms.

Delusional Disorder

Delusional disorder is clearly distinguishable from schizophrenia because it consists of the presence of delusions without any of the other psychotic symptoms of schizophrenia. Clients with delusional disorder only exhibit delusional thinking; their other cognitive faculties remain intact; therefore, people can live with this condition with significantly less impairment than the other schizophrenia spectrum disorders. Interesting delusions demonstrated in this condition follow similar themes, and they can be divided into two categories and then into several subtypes. The two categories are nonbizarre and bizarre.

Nonbizarre. The content of these delusions involves situations that could occur in reality—for example, being followed, poisoned, infected, loved at a distance, or deceived by one's spouse or lover. Clinicians must carefully assess the validity of clients claims as sometimes what is delusional upon first hearing seems somewhat plausible.

Bizarre. The content of these delusions features impossible situations (i.e., such as having one's thoughts controlled by aliens). Typically, these types of delusions are much more noticeable than the nonbizarre and are more quickly identified by clinicians.

DELUSIONAL SUBTYPES

Delusional disorder can be further broken down into several different subtypes based on the primary theme and content of the delusions.

The various thematic specifiers of delusional disorder include the following:

- *Erotomaniac.* This is a belief that another person, typically significant, famous, or influential, is in love with the person with the delusion (patient). Therefore, the person with the delusion may attempt to contact the romantic object, and unfortunately, highly obsessive and stalking behavior may follow.
- *Grandiose.* The primary feature of this delusion is an overinflated sense of worth, power, personal capabilities, and talent. Oftentimes, people with this delusion may believe that they have made a great or unique discovery or are an undiscovered talent or that their true identity is known only to them.
- *Jealous.* The main feature of this delusion is the belief that the sufferer's spouse or partner is unfaithful and is engaged in a sexual relationship with another person. In particular, male clients may be especially tormented by the thought that they are being cuckolded.

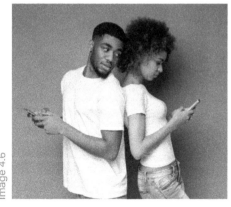

Image 4.6

  - *Persecutory.* The main feature of this delusion is that the patient is being mistreated, being spied on, or that someone or some entity is planning to harm them. Frequently, people with this type of delusion come into contact with legal authorities as they make repeated complaints about how they are being treated.

  - *Nihilistic.* The main feature of this delusion is the belief that the self, or a part of the self, has died or has somehow ceased to exist. This delusion can also present as the conviction that nothing in fact exists. Intense guilt over things that the person is not responsible for and could not have caused may also accompany this delusion.

  - *Somatic.* In this delusion, the sufferer has the belief that they have a serious medical problem or a physical defect.

  - *Mixed.* This delusion features a combination of the various aforementioned specifiers.

DELUSIONS OF REFERENCE

Delusions of reference are frequently seen in people challenged with delusional disorder (and other schizophrenia spectrum disorders). These delusions manifest as the belief that everything that is happening is somehow connected to the individual suffering from the delusion regardless of the theme of the delusion. Oftentimes, for people presenting with this symptom, it can seem as if they are the center of the universe and everything revolves around them. For instance, they may believe that all people are talking about them, and they are the focal point of attention from others. In people with these types of symptoms, seemingly random and everyday events are perceived as being interconnected, forming a giant conspiracy at which the individual is at the center.

Brief Psychotic Disorder

A diagnosis of brief psychotic disorder is marked by the presence of delusions, halluci-nations, disorganized speech, or other grossly disorganized behavior (such as catatonia). These symptoms must not be better explained by another mental disorder, substance use disorder, or medical condition with symptoms lasting at least 1 day but less than 1 month, with eventual full return to functioning as before the symptoms. The important metric in determining if someone has delusional disorder is the duration of time the symptoms have been present. When assessing and considering brief psychotic disorder, the symptoms last more than 1 day and but remit by 1 month (Tandon et al., 2013).

Other Psychotic Disorders

CASE STUDY 4.4 Shufen, 20, is pursuing an art degree at a local community col-lege. She presents to the clinic with her mother. Six months ago, Shufen moved out of the family home into an apartment. After not hearing from Shufen for several weeks, her mom became worried. Her mom found Shufen alone in her apartment with a num-ber of Ouija® boards and other equipment for talking to the deceased. Shufen has always been more of a "loner" and states that she does not fit in with the others at her school. She does not live with a roommate, nor does she want to live with anyone. Since she was in high school, Shufen has been obsessed with communicating with the dead. She is convinced that she is a medium and often tries to use a Ouija board to talk with the dead. Shufen says she has never audibly heard voices of the dead, but they have "given her signs." Shufen speaks to the therapist with no hint of emotion on her face. She dresses only in black, and her long fingernails are also painted black. She is constantly tapping her nails against something or filing them loudly.

Schizotypal Personality Disorder

Schizotypal personality disorder is at the mild end of the schizophre-nia spectrum of disorders. The common features of this disorder are impairment and reduced capacity for social functioning and interper-sonal relationships. These relational deficits are often accompanied by unusual perceptual experiences (illusions) and cognitive distortions (such as paranoia, odd beliefs, magical thinking, and obsessions that are held with delusional conviction).

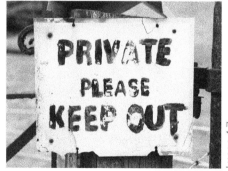

Image 4.7

A diagnosis of schizotypal personality disorder typically includes five or more of the following signs and symptoms:

- The patient lacks close friends and relationships outside of their immediate family

- Persistent incorrect and inaccurate interpretation of events
- Highly eccentric and unusual thinking, beliefs, and mannerisms
- Peculiar dress and wearing mismatched clothes that are inappropriate for the social setting
- The belief that one has special powers and intense superstitions
- Unusual perceptions, such as sensing an absent person's presence or experiencing illusions and visions
- Persistent and excessive social anxiety
- Peculiar styles of speech, unusual speech patterns, rambling, and lack coherence in conversation
- Suspicious or paranoid thoughts and questions about the loyalty of others
- Flat affect and inappropriate emotional responses

Some of the symptoms of schizotypal personality disorder, such as intense social anxiety and interest in solitary pursuits, may be first observable during the teenage years. For youth with schizotypal personality disorder, some of the indicators are being socially challenged, challenged with poor school performance, and experiencing difficulties with making friends and close social relationships.

Schizotypal Personality Disorder Versus Schizophrenia

Without extensive knowledge of the differences between the two disorders, schizotypal personality disorder can easily be confused with schizophrenia. However, there are several important differences that differentiate the two disorders. Most notably, while people with schizotypal personality disorder may experience brief psychotic episodes in which delusions or hallucinations are present, these episodes are not as frequent, prolonged, or intense as is the case with the diagnosis of schizophrenia proper.

Treatment Options

A standard group of treatments is typically used for various disorders within the schizophrenia spectrum disorders. While all the treatments listed next are helpful in addressing many of the symptoms of schizophrenia spectrum disorder, it is important to note that in terms of chronic and persistent mental health challenges, "recovery" is multidimensional and can look different from one client to the next. Specifically, recovery in mental illness does not require a complete remission of symptoms, as for many clients with schizophrenia spectrum disorder, complete remission of symptoms will not happen. However, "recovery" means facilitating and supporting the client as they work toward their goals for an active and fulfilling social life with meaningful relationships and employment opportunities while effectively managing symptoms. A broader "recovery movement" within the mental health arena has worked over the past 4 decades to provide people with chronic and persistent mental health challenges with the unshakable hope that recovery is multifaceted, that life can be meaningful, and that recovery can be facilitated through numerous supports and treatments.

Medications

Various medications are used to treat schizophrenia and its related disorders on the spectrum. However, antipsychotics are usually the first choice for prescribing physicians when trying to reduce the effect of psychotic symptoms. Antipsychotic medications manage the symptoms of schizophrenia but do not "cure" the disease. It usually takes several weeks for antipsychotics to begin to take full effect. In addition, it is common for a patient to have to try a variety of medications, including antidepressants and antianxiety medications, to identify the right blend of drugs to manage as many of the symptoms as possible. In practice, this means that it may take some time before the proper dosage and combination of medications are identified. Once the most optimal dosages have been established, it is vital that the individual does not stop taking their medication without lengthy consultation with their doctor and psychiatrist.

Talk Therapy

Psychotherapy can be used to help an individual manage their day-to-day symptoms of their schizophrenia spectrum disorder. It is also helpful in educating people to identify signs that relapse and reoccurrence of symptoms are imminent. However, talk therapy will not resolve the symptoms, yet developing greater insight into their symptoms can lead to an individual patient learning to manage their own mental health recovery and wellness with more confidence and self-determination. The ability to identify their symptoms and to have increased insight into the course of their symptoms will provide patients with greater mastery over them. In addition, social skills training, group and family therapy, and vocational rehabilitation services are all helpful for those individuals who require additional support around activities of daily living.

Electroconvulsive Therapy (ECT)

ECT is typically now only used in cases of very severe depression and bipolar disorder that are resistant to treatment, but it can in some cases be useful for schizophrenia. Therefore, ECT is sometimes used as a last resort treatment when other treatments no longer have the desired effect.

Inpatient Care

When the symptoms of schizophrenia become extremely severe or life-threatening to the individual or anyone else then inpatient mental health treatment is the optimal and most secure option for treatment to take place. However, it is important to note that it can be distressing and even intensely traumatizing to be placed in a hospital; this is especially true if the hospitalization occurs against the person's will. Yet oftentimes, hospitalization is the best option to ensure that people are stabilized as soon as possible and that recovery can begin again.

Assertive Community Treatment (ACT)

ACT is a treatment model for people with chronic and persistent mental health challenges, such as those included on the schizophrenia spectrum disorder. This treatment model is community based, and the individual is served by a mobile mental health treatment team. The treatment team is multidisciplinary and designed to provide the individual with comprehensive treatment, psychiatric care, rehabilitation, and support. Persons served by ACT often have multisystemic problems ranging across several domains, such as substance use, homelessness, criminal justice system involvement, and frequent hospitalization. ACT team members work with clients in their homes and other community settings; these clients are those who typically have not been well served by traditionally less intensive services.

Clubhouses

The clubhouse model has proved to be helpful for people with persistent and serious mental health challenges, such as schizophrenia spectrum disorder. Clubhouses are community-based drop-in centers for people with persistent and chronic mental health challenges. Membership in a club is open to anybody with a serious mental illness and participation is strictly voluntary. The purpose of clubhouses is to strengthen members' sense of community and integration into the wider society. Programs in clubhouses take a strengths-based approach, and staff members support clients as they take advantage of opportunities to experience education, social support, and meaningful work and employment. Clubhouses are democratic and have a decentralized and empowerment approach to supporting individuals; this allows people with chronic mental health challenges to develop a sense of advocacy and agency concerning their opportunities for socialization and recovery support.

Case Study Summary

One of this chapter's case studies reviewed the symptoms of Dietrich. As you process the story and examine possible diagnostic criteria, take a few minutes to answer the following questions:

1. What would be the correct diagnosis for Dietrich?

   _____
   _____

2. What are the specific symptoms or criteria that led you to this diagnosis?

   _____
   _____

3. What other possible disorders might you diagnose Dietrich with and why?

   _____
   _____

4. Briefly discuss what types of treatment may be beneficial for Dietrich. Could you see using a certain counseling theory and/or medication?

   _____
   _____

5. What kinds of support can be offered for the caregiver?

   _____
   _____

Guided Practice Exercises

Scenario 1

Kaylee, 23, believes adamantly that she is a reincarnation of Gandhi. This started around the time she was 18 and just graduating from high school. Her family started noticing changes in Kaylee's behavior at this time. She would go mute for hours or even days. Then she would tell her family that she had seen a great vision of "what is to come." She confided to her mom that she is actually Gandhi, and her identity has not been discovered yet. Kaylee claims to hear the voice of the "almighty." Once, when Kaylee was at the market, she became irrationally irritated with another customer. Kaylee ordered the customer to bow down to her and revere her. When the customer did not obey, Kaylee became irritable and lost touch with reality. She babbled incoherently until one of the other customers called the police.

What would be the correct disorder? What are the specific symptoms or criteria that led you to this diagnosis?

What specific behaviors caused you to diagnose the disorder?

What other possible disorders might you diagnose Kaylee with and why?

What are the most common types of hallucinations?

There is a huge amount of schizophrenia within the homeless populations in big cities. Why do you think that is?

Scenario 2

Zhang, 30, is a single mother of two girls who lives primarily on disability benefits. Her friend, Sally, becomes concerned after talking to one of Zhang's daughters one day. It seems that Zhang has an irregular sleep pattern. She will spend weeks not sleeping and be extremely social and bubbly during this time. She will claim that a man has appeared in the house and tells her that she is one of the smartest people in the world. She will have long conversations with this man whom her daughters cannot see. Zhang claims to be the lost great-great-granddaughter of Galileo. She must work on a new theory of angular momentum or physics will derail in the future. After weeks of work, Zhang will be depressed and unable to get out of bed. During this time, the man appears to her and tells her that she is worthless and has no future. Sally is thinking about calling children's services for the safety of Zhang's two daughters. It is clear when Sally talks to Zhang that she no longer recognizes reality and is unable to take care of her children because of her unbalanced mental state.

What would be the correct disorder? What are the specific symptoms or criteria that led you to this diagnosis?

_____
_____
_____

What specific behaviors caused you to diagnose the disorder?

_____
_____
_____

What other possible disorders might you diagnose Zhang with and why?

_____
_____
_____

Describe the similarities and differences between schizoaffective disorder and schizophrenia.

_____
_____
_____

What would it feel like to see and hear things that do not actually exist? Explain.

_____
_____
_____

Scenario 3

Megha, 19, is an Indian exchange student at a large public university. Her roommate, Suzanne, takes her to the hospital because in the last month, she has "lost her grip on reality." Megha tells the nurse, "The clock will strike 12. The clock will. ... Then the owl will tell it to control the gears. Gears move and go. The gears will control my mind and then the owl will have it. The owl always has ham." Suzanne explains that a few months ago, Megha acted like a typical college student. She would study during the week and socialize on weekends with her friends. About a month ago, Megha began to suspect that someone called the "owl" was spying on her. Apparently, the owl is a creature that Megha believes to be extraterrestrial. Megha explained to Suzanne that the owl would often talk to her at night when she was trying to sleep. Megha began to speak incoherently about the owl (as she did to the nurse) and stopped going to classes because she was so disturbed by the owl's threats.

What would be the correct disorder? What are the specific symptoms or criteria that led you to this diagnosis?

_____
_____
_____

What specific behaviors caused you to diagnose the disorder?

_____
_____
_____

What other possible disorders might you diagnose Megha with and why?

_____
_____
_____

Scenario 4

Braxton, 28, is a third-year medical student. According to his girlfriend, Kristen, his behavior has become odd in the last few months. Braxton has spent a lot of time watching the national news and writing vigorous notes in a journal. He claims that the Nigerians are sending messages meant for him through CBS and CNN. If Braxton is to help free child soldiers, he must jot down the messages and decipher the codes. Although Braxton is still able to keep up his schoolwork, he is spending increasing amounts of time decoding the messages. His sleeping pattern has not changed, and he has not experienced any auditory or visual hallucinations. Kristen is worried that if his behavior does not change, he may need to drop out of school.

What would be the correct disorder? What are the specific symptoms or criteria that led you to this diagnosis?

_____
_____
_____

What specific behaviors caused you to diagnose the disorder?

_____
_____
_____

What other possible disorders might you diagnose Braxton with and why?

_____
_____
_____

Explain what referential delusions are and give an example.

_____
_____
_____

Scenario 5

Carson, 55, is employed as a freelance author. He comes to the clinic at the request of his wife, Edna. When asked why he is there, he explains that his wife does not understand his fascination with aliens. He confides that aliens are currently selecting individuals to take to the new planet. Carson has rigged his and Edna's house to protect against the attack. He has attached new wires and satellite dishes to different parts of the house to deter the signals. He has also erected a storm shelter with water, canned food, flashlights, radios, and blankets. Carson dresses in an aluminum jogging suit because he is convinced it will best protect him in space if the aliens select him. Although Carson obsesses over aliens, he is still able to carry out his work as a writer. His maternal grandfather and two of his uncles had/have schizophrenia. Besides his wife, he does not have any friends and tends to "keep to himself." He claims to be uncomfortable in any social situation. During the interview, Carson continues to tilt his head back and forth several times.

What would be the correct disorder? What are the specific symptoms or criteria that led you to this diagnosis?

_____
_____
_____

What specific behaviors caused you to diagnose the disorder?

_____
_____
_____

What other possible disorders might you diagnose Braxton with and why?

_____
_____
_____

Differentiate between schizophrenia and schizotypal personality disorder.

_____
_____
_____

Web-Based and Literature-Based Resources

Recovery After an Initial Schizophrenia Episode (RAISE): https://www.nimh.nih.gov/health/topics/schizophrenia/raise/raise-resources-for-patients-and-families.shtml

Schizophrenia and Related Disorders Alliance of America: https://sardaa.org

National Alliance on Mental Illness—Schizophrenia: https://www.nami.org/Learn-More/Mental-Health-Conditions/Schizophrenia/Support

Support groups for Schizophrenia: www.Schizophrenia.com

References

Abrams, D. J., Rojas, D. C., & Arciniegas, D. B. (2008). Is schizoaffective disorder a distinct categorical diagnosis? A critical review of the literature. *Neuropsychiatric Disease Treatment*, 4(6), 1089–1109.

American Psychiatric Association (APA). (2013). *Diagnostic and statistical manual of mental disorders* (5th ed.).

Bell, D. (2017). *John Nash*. Living with Schizophrenia. https://www.livingwithschizophreniauk.org/john-nash/

Dean, K., & Murray, R. M. (2005). Environmental risk factors for psychosis. *Dialogues in Clinical Neuroscience*, 7(1), 69.

Gaebel, W. (2012). The status of psychotic disorders in ICD-11. *Schizophrenia Bulletin*, 38, 895–898.

Gilmore, J. H. (2010). Understanding what causes schizophrenia: A developmental perspective. *American Journal of Psychiatry*, 167, 8–10. https:doi.org/10.1176/appi.ajp.2009.09111588

Goode, E. (2015, May 24). John F. Nash Jr., math genius defined by a 'beautiful mind,' dies at 86. *New York Times*. https://www.nytimes.com/2015/05/25/science/john-nash-a-beautiful-mind-subject-and-nobel-winner-dies-at-86.html?_r=0

Gubi, A. A., McDonnell, C., & Bocanegra, J. O. (2014). Changes to DSM-5 schizophrenia diagnosis. *Communique*, 43(4), 1–23.

Hambrecht, M., & Häfner, H. (1996). Substance abuse and the onset of schizophrenia. *Biological Psychiatry*, 40(11), 1155–1163.

Hor, K., & Taylor, M. (2010). Suicide and schizophrenia: a systematic review of rates and risk factors. *Journal of psychopharmacology (Oxford, England)*, 24(4), 81–90. https://doi.org/10.1177/1359786810385490

Haukvik, U. K., Hartberg, C. B., & Agartz, I. (2013). Schizophrenia-what does structural MRI show? *Tidsskrift for den Norske laegeforening: Tidsskrift for praktisk medicin, ny raekke*, 133(8), 850–853.

Heckers, S., Tandon, R., & Bustillo, J. (2010). Catatonia in the DSM. Shall we move or not? *Schizophrenia Bulletin*, 36, 205–207.

National Institute of Mental Health. (2018). *Schizophrenia. https://www.nimh.nih.gov/health/statistics/schizophrenia.shtml*

Rettner, R. (2015, June 2). How '*Beautiful Mind*' mathematician John Nash's schizophrenia 'disappeared'. Live Science. https://www.livescience.com/51058-schizophrenia-recovery-john-nash.html

Tandon, R., Gaebel, W., Barch, D. M., Bustillo, J., Gur, R. E., Heckers, S., Malaspina, D., Owen, M. J., Schultz, S., Tsuang, M. & Van Os, J. (2013). Definition and description of schizophrenia in the *DSM-5*. *Schizophrenia Research*, 150(1), 3–10.

Tandon, R., Carpenter, W. T. (2013). Psychotic disorders in DSM-5. *Die Psychiatrie 10*, 5–9.

Saha, S., Chant, D., Welham, J., & McGrath, J. (2005). A systematic review of the prevalence of schizophrenia. *PLoS Med*, 2(5), e141.

World Health Organization (WHO). (2016). *International statistical classification of diseases and related health problems, 10th revision (ICD-10)*.

Credits

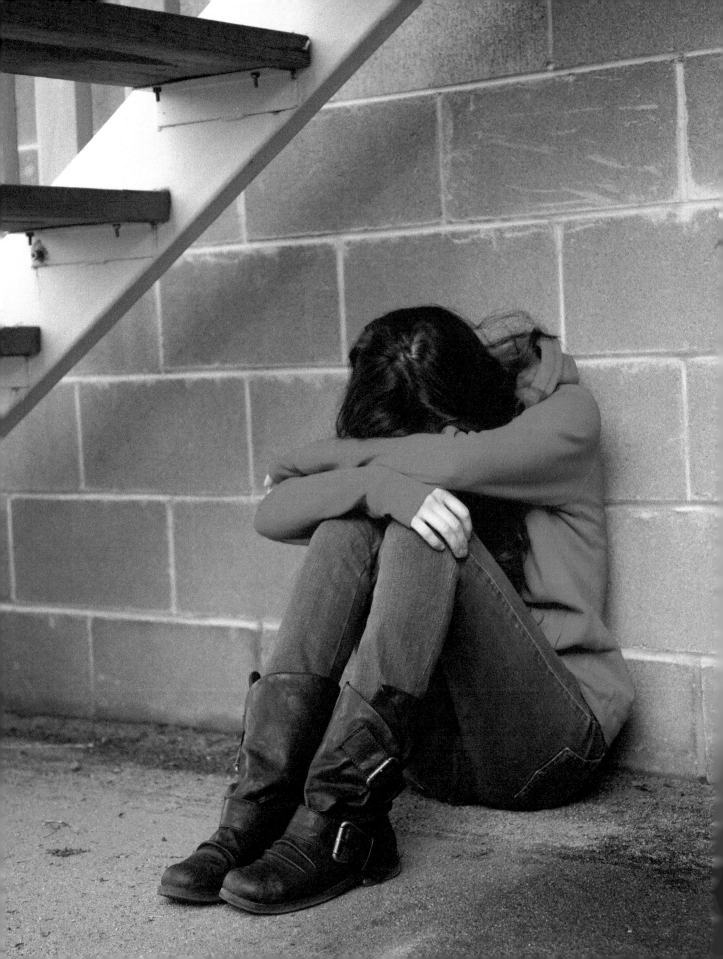

CHAPTER FIVE

MOOD DISORDERS

David A. Scott and Michelle Grant Scott

CASE STUDY 5.1 Kwan is a 30-year-old Asian American male admitted to the emergency room by his wife for reporting to her that he "just felt like killing myself" a week prior. Kwan had been to his primary physician complaining of headaches, insomnia, and lower back pain that he had been experiencing for a little over a month. The doctor could not find medical reasoning and referred Kwan to mental health services to which Kwan declined.

Kwan has lived in the United States his whole life, but his parents are from Korea. He reports that there is a rumor that his great-grandfather died by suicide, but he is never talked about within the family. There are no other known diagnoses. Kwan has no prior mental health diagnoses but reports times in college where he felt fleeting feelings of depression. He reports that he consistently feels "hopeless" for the majority of his days for the past month. He does not see a future for himself with his family or his occupation. He strongly believes that he is burdening his family and that killing himself would help them in the long run.

He can no longer bring himself to engage in golf, kayaking, or reading, which he used to enjoy deeply. His wife reports that he was once very actively engaged with his family, his work, and his leisure activities, but since he began having somatic symptoms a month prior, this has not been the case. Although he reports that he is not active, Kwan is surprisingly fatigued at the end of each day. Because of his exhaustion, he is sleeping much longer hours and feels that sometimes he "cannot get out of bed." When he does wake up and go to work, he has a difficult time concentrating on his assigned tasks. He is easily distracted by the idea of suicide and finds himself obsessing about ending his life. This is affecting his occupation severely, and he has already been written up once for missing work. Kwan self-reports that he does not have any current alcohol or drug use but that he would binge drink in college.

Did You Know?

- Depression affects an estimated 350 million people worldwide.
- Mood disorders rank in the top 10 of reasons for disability with about 6.7% of adults in the United States experiencing a major depressive disorder (NIMH, 2015).
- Japan's definition of a mood disorder is *kokoro no kaze*, which means "the soul catching a cold." And one of the first selective serotonin reuptake inhibitors (SSRIs) was not sold in Japan until the late 1990s (Landers, 2002).
- There were more than 800,000 deaths by suicide in 2012 worldwide.

Overview

At some point in our lives, most of us experience feelings of sadness, low energy levels, and changes in our sleeping and eating patterns. Many of us have also said, "*I'm just feeling depressed today*," without really understanding the true meaning of depression and how it can affect a person's life. Having a diagnosed depressive disorder is more than being sad, blue, or grieving. It can be a debilitating disorder that affects children, adolescents, and adults. In 2012, it was estimated that around 350 million people worldwide were affected by depression (Marcus et al., 2012). Depression does not discriminate between male and female, cultural background, or race. The study and treatment of depression continues to be one of the major issues in mental health, and there has been an explosion in pharmacological treatment options.

Depression is certainly not the only type of mood disorder. In this chapter, we will explore mood disorders, including major depressive disorder, bipolar disorder I and II, and other related affective disorders. The *Diagnostic and Statistical Manual of Mental Disorders, 5th Edition* (*DSM-5*) moved bipolar disorders into a separate category from depressive disorders, while the *International Statistical Classification of Diseases* (*ICD-10*) kept all of these disorders within their mood (affective) disorders category. The disorders covered in this chapter are not exhaustive but a coverage of the most common mood disorders. Table 5.1 provides a brief comparison of mood disorders in the *ICD-10* and *DSM-5* to give you a quick view of some of the most prevalent disorders discussed in this chapter.

TABLE 5.1 *ICD-DSM* Comparison

ICD-10 **CODES** Mood disorders (F30-F39)	*DSM-5* **CODES** Depressive disorders
Manic episode (**F30**) Symptoms could include increased energy, less need for sleep, out of character behavior, possible delusions	**Moved out of depressive disorders into a separate chapter for bipolar and other similar disorders**
Bipolar affective disorder (**F31**) Symptoms could include a vacillation between elevated mood and lowered mood and below normal levels of energy	**Moved out of depressive disorders to a separate chapter for bipolar and other similar disorders**
Depressive episode (**F32**) Symptoms could include lower than normal mood, energy, and self-esteem. Loss of interest in normal activities, appetite, and libido	**Major depressive disorder** (**296.xx**) Symptoms could include lower than normal mood, energy, and self-esteem. Loss of interest in normal activities, appetite, and libido
Recurrent depressive disorder (**F33**) Symptoms could include repeated bouts of depression without episodes of mania or hypomania	**Not included in** *DSM-5*
Persistent mood disorders (**F34**) Symptoms could include episodes of mood disturbances that do not qualify for bipolar or depressive disorder. Include cyclothymia and dysthymia	**Disruptive mood dysregulation disorder** (**296.99**) Symptoms could include extreme temper outbursts that are not consistent with the situation **Persistent depressive disorder** (**300.4**) Symptoms could include a depressed mood that is more chronic than major depressive disorder (at least 2 years) but does not meet the full criteria for major depressive disorder. Only includes dysthymia

Other mood disorders (F38)	**Other Specified Depressive Disorder (311)**
Any mood disturbance that does not meet the criteria for the mood disorders listed earlier	Any mood disturbance that does not meet the criteria for the mood disorders listed earlier
Premenstrual tension syndrome	**Premenstrual dysphoric disorder (625.4)**
*In ICD-10 Chapter XIV, "Diseases of the Genitourinary System"	Symptoms include severe symptoms of premenstrual syndrome that affect daily living

Note: Adapted from ICD-10 (WHO, 2016) and DSM-5 (APA, 2013)

Depressive Disorders

Depressive disorders are the disorders typically consisting of significant changes in a person's mood and activity. The episodes can be mild, moderate, or severe and can be only one episode or multiple (recurring) episodes. Around 80% of those who experience an episode of depression will go on to experience multiple episodes.

Depressive disorders include the following:

- Major depressive disorder
- Disruptive mood dysregulation disorder
- Persistent mood disorder/dysthymic disorder
- Premenstrual dysphoric disorder

Major Depressive Disorder (F32.2) (296.xx)

The most commonly diagnosed of the depressive disorders is major depressive disorder (MDD). It is one of the most prevalent mental disorders in the United States, occurring in between 6.7% and 9% of adults each year; the amount of people who have experienced the condition at some point in their lives is 16.6%. In U.S. children (4–11 years old), 3.3% are diagnosed yearly. Women are thought to be twice as likely to be diagnosed (Marcus et al., 2012), and adults age 59 and under are twice as likely to be diagnosed with major depressive disorder as adults 60 and older. Diagnoses of major depressive disorder are also found to be more prevalent in people with a family history of the disorder. Research indicates, however, that causes may stem from a combination of genetics, environmental, biological, and psychological factors. The average age of onset is 32 years old, but it can occur in children, adults, and the elderly.

Box 5.2 Is It Grief or Depression?

At some point in our lives, we all have experienced or will experience the loss of a loved one. When we do experience this loss, we will typically have symptoms associated with grief and bereavement. Examining grief, we can see that some of the symptoms are similar to those associated with depression. Typical symptoms of grief and bereavement include the following:

- Sadness
- Lower levels of energy

- Guilt
- Hard time concentrating
- Feeling alone

Mental health professionals are quick to point out that grief and bereavement are not the same as clinical depression. Grief is a natural response to a loss in a person's life. Although there is not a definitive point (or specific amount of time) at which grief could progress into depression, there are *red flags* that may warrant an evaluation by a mental health professional. The diagnosis of major depressive disorder only comes into play when these thoughts and feelings are pervasive and persistent and create an inability to perform daily tasks.

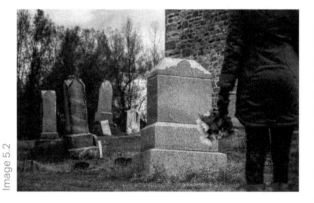

Image 5.2

To be diagnosed with major depressive disorder, a person will have had at least one depressive episode (see Table 5.2) with minimum duration of 2 weeks in which five or more symptoms are experienced. As seen in Table 5.2, major depressive disorder can interfere with a person's ability to concentrate, sleep and eat regularly, complete tasks, find joy in activities, and be hopeful.

Think about our case study of Kwan. Is Kwan exhibiting some of these symptoms?

Some people with major depressive disorder may have recurring thoughts of death and dying and may attempt self-harm. Later in the chapter, we will discuss how this relates to suicide rates. The good news is, with intervention, major depressive disorder is treatable (National Institute of Mental Health [NIMH], 2015) and manageable.

TABLE 5.2 Depressive Episode

Symptoms can include the following:
• Lowering of mood. Varies little from day to day
• Reduction of energy and concentration
• Decrease in activity and marked tiredness
• Reduced capacity for enjoyment
• Loss of interest and pleasurable feelings, including loss of libido
• Disturbed sleep (waking hours before usual time) and loss of appetite
• Reduced self-esteem and self-confidence
• Thoughts of guilt or worthlessness
Depressive episodes can be categorized as follows:
• Mild (two or three symptoms)
• Moderate (four or more symptoms with difficulty completing daily tasks)
• Severe (several symptoms that are marked and possible suicidal ideation)

Note: Adapted by World Health Organization (WHO, 2016). ICD-10

Disruptive Mood Dysregulation Disorder (F34.8) (296.99)

One of the newer and more controversial disorders in the *DSM-5* is disruptive mood dysregulation disorder. Disruptive mood dysregulation disorder (DMDD) was not a diagnosis in previous *DSM* editions. The *ICD-10* includes this disorder under F34.8 (other persistent mood [affective] disorders). One of the reasons disruptive mood dysregulation disorder was created was to address the concerns of practitioners who noticed that children and adolescents were being misdiagnosed with bipolar disorders (Gotlib & LeMoult, 2014). This misdiagnosis has led to children and adolescents being prescribed medications that are inappropriate and possibly harmful if they truly do not have bipolar disorder (Leibenluft, 2011). Behaviors in children and adolescents with this disorder are typically as follows:

- Severe outbursts (up to three or more times per week)
- Irritability more often than not during the day
- Reactions that are larger than expected for the situation

These behaviors would need to be present for more than a year, and the child would need to be at least 6 years old. The behaviors would also need to not meet the symptomology of bipolar disorder, conduct disorder, or oppositional defiant disorder. These behaviors are also persistent and do not include a manic or hypomanic episode (i.e., bipolar disorder).

Dysthymic Disorder/Persistent Depressive Disorder (F34.1)(300.4)

The chronic version of major depressive episode is called dysthymic disorder (*ICD-10*), or persistent depressive disorder, as referred to in the *DSM-5*. People diagnosed with this disorder must have less severe symptoms than those of major depressive disorder, which last for more than 2 years (1 year for adolescents).

Depressive symptoms can also last for several years if left untreated. Would this apply to Kwan?

The prevalence rate of adults in the United States who are diagnosed with dysthymic disorder is 1.5%, with the average age of onset being 31 years old (Kessler et al., 2005). Many times, clients with this disorder will describe their mood as feeling less happy than in the past, low energy levels, and an overall feeling of sadness. Since it is chronic in nature, many people with dysthymic disorder will struggle with daily functioning even more than those diagnosed with major depressive disorder and may have trouble with eating, sleeping, and maintaining high levels of energy for any period of time (Klein et al., 2000). This chronic level of depression can also severely affect relationships and a person's career by hindering their ability to complete daily tasks at home and required tasks at work.

Premenstrual Dysphoric Disorder (N94.3) (625.4)

Readers may be familiar with the term premenstrual syndrome (PMS), referring to typical symptoms occurring a week to 10 days prior to a female's monthly menstrual cycle. During the premenstrual period, women may experience typical premenstrual syndrome symptoms, such as fatigue, irritability, abdominal bloating or cramping, and mild anxiety, among others. With premenstrual syndrome, symptoms may be uncomfortable but do not typically interrupt a woman's level of functioning or cause significant distress.

Premenstrual dysphoric disorder, however, encompasses increased severity of these symptoms, especially with mood changes. Women who experience significant social and relational problems, along with intense behavioral and biological symptoms, during the premenstrual time period may be diagnosed with premenstrual dysphoric disorder. This is a newer disorder found in the *DSM-5*. In addition to significant mood changes, women with premenstrual dysphoric disorder may have intense bouts of anxiety, irritability, poor concentration, fatigue, and physical symptoms, such as abdominal bloating, body aches, and sleep disturbances. Typically, the symptoms lessen dramatically after the menstruation period begins but occur during most cycles within a year's time.

Because differentiating premenstrual dysphoric disorder from premenstrual syndrome can sometimes be difficult, having the client document mood changes and symptoms can be helpful in both diagnosing and in planning treatment. A few such journaling tools are presented next:

- Calendar of premenstrual experiences
- Daily record of severity of problems
- Prospective record of the severity of menstruation

Specific causes of premenstrual dysphoric disorder are not known, but research (Huo et al., 2007) indicates there is a biological component to the disorder, specifically effecting serotonin transmission. For this reason, one front-line treatment option is antidepressants, specifically selective serotonin reuptake inhibitors (SSRIs). There are a variety of other treatment options, some of which are herbal supplements, increasing sleep quality, aerobic exercise, nutrition monitoring, reducing caffeine and sugar, and cognitive behavioral therapy.

Postpartum Depression (Depressive Disorder Specifier)

Although many women experience mild mood changes referred to as *baby blues* (periodic sad, negative mood) during the 1–2 weeks after giving birth, the symptoms of postpartum depression are more severe. This is not an official disorder appearing in the *ICD-10* or *DSM-5* but a specifier for depressive disorders. It is worthy of focus, however, since research indicates that up to 15% of birthing mothers are estimated to have symptoms of postpartum depression (Cohen et al., 2010). The symptoms can occur anytime from 1 week to approximately 1 year after giving birth.

Postpartum depression can include the following symptoms: severe sadness, low energy, anxiety, irritability, difficulty sleeping, excessive guilt, and thoughts of death or harming self or others. There may also be symptoms related to the care of the baby, as the mother may fear harming the child, fear being alone with the baby, have excessive worry about the baby's care, or difficulty bonding with the infant.

Most at risk are mothers under the age of 20 and those who have been previously diagnosed with depression, a mood disorder, or anxiety disorder. Sleep deprivation may be a major factor in a woman experiencing postpartum symptoms. Treatment options such as antidepressants and talk therapy have been found to successfully lessen symptoms. It is important to note, however, that research suggests women who experienced postpartum depression after one pregnancy are up to 50% more likely to have depressive symptoms after subsequent births (Hirst & Moutier, 2010). Several well-known celebrities have struggled with postpartum depression, including Gwyneth Paltrow, Courteney Cox, and Marie Osmond (CBS News, 2016). Famous actress, Brooke Shields (2006) even wrote a bestselling memoir detailing her struggles with postpartum depression.

CLINICIAN'S CORNER 5.1

Mood Disorders

As a clinician for more than 20 years, I've learned so much from clients battling depression. One thing I have learned is how powerful *knowledge* can be in the fight. Clients with depression, and those who love them, often thirst for information on how to understand it, manage it, and prevent it from coming back. They can learn, for example, how getting daily sunlight, even small amounts of exercise, and adequate sleep really can make a difference in how they feel. Arming them with information about how to make long-term lifestyle changes empowers them and helps lessen feelings of hopelessness. If you are treating someone with depression or a mood disorder, I encourage you to give them a takeaway item during each session, such as written reminders of their goals, websites, or apps you recommend; hotline numbers; or other resources. Finally, I encourage you to give them *hope*! There is hope in hearing that we now have empirically proven treatments for depression. People *do* thrive with and overcome depression and mood disorders.

Michelle Grant Scott, MSW, LISW-CP(S)

Treatment Options

The good news concerning depression and other mood disorders is that we are currently getting better at diagnosing and treating these disorders than at any other point in history. The bad news is the majority of individuals with depression do not seek treatment or do not have access to treatment. With a focus on treating the individual by addressing their needs from a biopsychosocial approach, clinicians can work in a collaborative manner with other health-care providers to provide the most effective treatment for mood disorders. As with any treatment option, it is critical that the client works closely with their mental health professional(s) to determine the best course of action for their treatment. The following is a more in-depth look at treatment from the biological, psychological, social, and integrative approaches.

Would any of these options work for Kwan?

BIOLOGICAL

Knowing the client's medical history and encouraging them to have an updated physical examination will help clinicians take a holistic approach to treatment. For example, medical issues such as diabetes, overactive or underactive thyroid (for females), sleep disorders, and other issues can contribute to mood problems and may be easily treated by a physician.

Our ability to explore regions of the brain continues to expand at a very fast pace. Brain imaging machines such as magnetic resonance imaging, computed axial tomography scan, and functional magnetic resonance imaging can provide researchers with even more in-depth exploration of the brain and the possible locations in the brain that are responsible for depression. Most research suggests that the limbic system, hypothalamus, hippocampus, amygdala, and anterior cingulate gyrus all play a role in depression within the brain. Depression can also be a cause of stress on the brain. This stress can lead to atrophy and diminished nerve connectivity, which could lead to negative physiological changes (i.e., heart and organ problems), high levels of cortisol, lowered immunity, and a myriad of medical problems (Frodi et al., 2008).

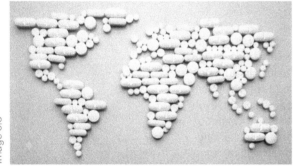

Image 5.3

Biologically speaking, we know that depression runs in families. We also know that depression can occur in a person with no family history of a mood disorder. A meta-analysis conducted by Sullivan, Neale, and Kendler (2000) suggested that the heritability of major depressive disorder is between 31% and 42%. Having this information is critical for discussing the possible development of depression in clients who have a family history of the disorder.

We are familiar with the association of mood disorders and neurotransmitters, such as serotonin levels in the brain. Norepinephrine and dopamine are also considered possible factors related to depression. We are now also in a proliferation period of treating depression with medications, mainly SSRIs and serotonin-norepinephrine reuptake inhibitors (SNRIs). Table 5.3 provides a list of some of the most widely used SSRIs and SNRIs on the market today. While this list is not exhaustive, and there will undoubtedly be more and more psychotropic medications in use over the next decade (as we uncover more information through research), it is critical that mental health professionals have a working knowledge of medications that many of their clients will be using in treatment.

TABLE 5.3 SSRIs and SNRIs Used to Treat Mood Disorders

GENERIC NAME	BRAND NAME	TYPICAL DOSE
SSRIs		
Fluoxetine	Prozac	20–80mg/day
Sertraline	Zoloft	50–200mg/day
Paroxetine	Paxil	20–50mg/day
Citalopram	Celexa	10–60
Escitalopram	Lexapro	5–20mg/day
SNRIs		
Mirtazepine	Remeron	15–45mg/day
Venlafaxine	Effexor	50–300mg/day

Buproprion	Wellbutrin	75–450mg/day
Duloxetine	Cymbalta	20–60mg/day
Nefazodone	Serzone	100–500mg/day

The psychotropic medications listed in Table 5.3 help in the treatment of depression by blocking the reuptake of either serotonin (SSRI) or norepinephrine (SNRI). This blockage is believed to turn on and off receptors that play a role in producing the symptoms of depression.

Another biological treatment is exercise. Considered both a biological and behavioral treatment, exercise has empirical support from numerous studies (Craft & Perna, 2004), indicating how people who engage in exercise can have a long-lasting reduction in depressive symptoms. The reasons why exercise is beneficial in treating depression are varied, but we do know there are measurable changes in the brain during and after exercise that play a role in its effectiveness. Part of a mind-body movement in the treatment of depression includes examining how the body can naturally combat depression. Included in the web-based resources is the link to a TedxTalk by Dr. Charles Raison discussing one interesting option.

PSYCHOLOGICAL

Mental health professionals are now well equipped with various forms of evidence-based psychotherapy to treat mood disorders. The key to deciding on which therapy to use will depend on your training, the client's specific needs, and the use of a treatment that has empirical support for its use in treating depression. The World Health Organization (WHO, 2015) conducted a large-scale, meta-analysis examining the effectiveness of different types of psychotherapy for depressive disorders. Their study found the following types of psychotherapy to be effective modes of treatment for moderate to severe depression:

1. Cognitive behavioral therapy
2. Interpersonal therapy
3. Behavioral activation therapy

The study also supported group therapy and the possible use of web-based mental health services (with a trained mental health professional) for those without access to services in their communities.

Box 5.3 Alternative Treatment for Depression

Another interesting form of treatment for depression is focusing on how treating a mother's depression can actually affect their child's depression without treating the child directly. Researchers found that children's levels of depressive symptoms lowered when the parent's levels of depressive symptoms decreased (Garber et al., 2011). The parents were treated using cognitive behavioral therapy and/or psychotropic medications. The children did not receive treatment for depression, only the parents. Pilowsky et al. (2008) followed a group of mothers and their children for a year after treatment and found a decrease in the children's psychiatric symptoms and the mothers' depression. This direct association between a parent's depressive symptoms and their child's depression may have an effect on how we provide treatment in communities in the near future.

SOCIAL

Sullivan et al. (2014) in the large-scale, meta-analysis mentioned the importance of environmental influences and how they are specific to each individual. People who have gone through the same exact experiences are affected differently; some individuals walk away from the experience with little to no disturbance, while others are deeply affected and struggle to cope with the experience. Social factors that could contribute to mood disorders include military conflicts, neglect, social isolation, political unrest, socioeconomic factors, social or gender inequality, oppression, and environmental disturbances. Social factors that can play roles as protective factors include connectedness to family members and others in the community, a safe environment, access to care (medical and mental), and access to quality education.

Image 5.4

Any social factors for Kwan?

INTEGRATIVE APPROACH

There are multiple integrative approaches to treating depression and mood disorders, which sometimes include both Eastern and Western medicine approaches. The idea that people feel healthier when the mind, body, and spirit are in harmony is not a new concept, but we now have more empirical evidence to support the effectiveness of such integrative approaches. As reported by Segal et al. (2012), the mindfulness-based cognitive therapy approach combines cognitive techniques with meditation and other thought awareness components. This approach is reported to have as much effectiveness in treating depression as medication does (Segal et al., 2012). Other approaches, such as Reiki, yoga, and breathing techniques have been found to effectively reduce depressive symptoms in some clients. Furthermore, research conducted by Boelens et al. (2012) found clients with depression who engaged in daily prayer had less depressive symptoms up to 1 year later. Thus clinicians may encourage clients to explore their spirituality, however it is defined by the client, and offer an integrative approach to treatment.

Bipolar Disorders (F31.x) (296.xx)

CASE STUDY 5.2 Vanessa, 33, is described by most of her friends as mercurial. They will not see Vanessa for weeks at a time, and then suddenly Vanessa will show up more energetic than ever and unable to stop talking. She works at a local insurance agency and has an apartment with her longtime partner, Phillip. Police took Vanessa into custody a few days ago for sleeping with multiple underage boys. She also drained her own savings account, along with the savings of her parents, claiming that she is going to start "the best bakery in the world." She spent the money on a storefront, machines, and baking mixes. Her parents recount that Vanessa has not slept for days but that, several weeks ago, she seemed extremely distraught and depressed. They do not understand what has changed.

The bipolar disorders, previously referred to as *manic depression*, are disorders of the brain, which include major changes in mood and behavior beyond what is typical for the affected individual. Manic (or hypomanic) episodes of elevated or intensely joyful mood, increased energy level, and possible agitation separate these disorders from the depressive disorders. The manic episode may alternate with depressive episodes, but a bipolar disorder *can* be diagnosed without the presence of a depressive episode. Bipolar disorders may also co-occur with substance abuse and anxiety disorders. Do you see Vanessa or Ingrid (see Case Study 5.3) exhibiting any of these symptoms? Bipolar disorders include bipolar I, bipolar II, cyclothymic disorder, and bipolar not otherwise specified. The information later in this section will help clinicians differentiate between the varying types. Table 5.4 provides a brief description of the various episodes related to bipolar disorders. Are Vanessa and Ingrid experiencing any of these episodes?

TABLE 5.4 Episodes of Bipolar Disorder

Manic Episode. Characteristics of a manic episode include elevated or irritable mood, along with increased energy that is not typical for the client and decreased need for sleep. Many times, mania may cause extreme excitement about events, flight of ideas, and even engaging in atypical risky behaviors (spending sprees, out of control gambling, uninhibited sexual encounters).

Hypomanic Episode. A milder increase in mood, energy, and participation in activities. Friends and family members may see an increase in talking and being social and a decrease in the need for sleep. Since hypomania affects the client less than a full manic episode, there may not be as dramatic a change observed in behavior.

Depressive Episode. Characteristics include a loss of energy, disturbed sleep, changes in appetite, loss of interest in activities, possible agitation, and/or thoughts of death.

Mixed Episode. Mixed episodes can include both manic and depressive symptoms.

Source: ICD-10 (WHO, 2016).

Prevalence and Causes of Bipolar Disorders

In an 11-nation study, researchers found the prevalence rates for bipolar disorders are 2.4% worldwide and 4.4% in the United States (Merikangas et al., 2011). The United States reported the highest percentage of bipolar diagnoses in the study. Just as with depressive disorders, most research suggests the causes of bipolar disorders can be genetically based and possibly environmentally influenced. Dr. Francis McMohan and colleague's research highlights a centralized genetic location within the brain that could be an indicator for both depressive and bipolar disorders (McMahon et al., 2010). Regarding environmental factors, it appears that clients with high levels of life stressors are at higher risk for symptom expression and development. Further research will be needed in this area to help determine the true causes and possible prevention of bipolar disorder.

As you may have discussed in class, heard from the media, or witnessed firsthand, there has been a major increase in youth diagnosed with bipolar disorder. One of the reasons for the creation of the disruptive mood dysregulation disorder, as discussed earlier, was this rapid increase in adolescents and children being diagnosed with bipolar disorder. Moreno et al. (2007) reported that there was a *40-fold* increase in children and adolescents being diagnosed with bipolar disorder over a 10-year span. The study went on to discuss that more than 90% of youth who were diagnosed with bipolar disorders were prescribed a psychotropic medication as part of their treatment. There remains controversy around the diagnosis of bipolar disorder in youth and the true causes. The media attention to the disorders in recent years is thought to have a possible effect on the overdiagnosis of youth.

Bipolar I

The National Institute of Mental Health (NIMH, 2015) describes bipolar I as a disorder of the brain that includes major changes in emotions or mood. Specific to bipolar I is the presence of a manic or mixed episodes that can last more than 7 days or a manic episode that would require hospitalization because of the severity level. The manic episodes can be categorized as mild, moderate, or severe. Bipolar I may also include mild or moderate depressive episodes that can last at least 2 weeks. In addition, bipolar I may include grandiosity (heightened sense of self-confidence) and psychosis, which is seen less in other bipolar disorders. An individual with this disorder may exhibit exaggerated or risky behavior that could be more easily noticeable than in other bipolar disorders.

CASE STUDY 5.3 Ingrid, 60, is a retired French freelance writer and editor. She moved to the United States with her partner, Amelia, following their retirement. They both present to the clinic claiming relationship issues. Ingrid seems extremely sociable and tells the counselor all about her favorite places in France and her job as a writer. Amelia cuts her off to explain that Ingrid is self-centered and does not pitch in around the house. She will go for weeks without being able to get out of bed simply because she is sad. Amelia finds this preposterous. Then Ingrid becomes extremely sociable and bubbly. During these times, she hardly sleeps and goes out to bars with her friends as if she were in her 20s. Amelia is feed up with 30 years or so of dealing with Ingrid's up and downs.

Bipolar II

Bipolar II is also a disorder characterized by major changes in emotions or mood. It differs from bipolar I, however, in that the individual will have at least one occurrence of a depressive episode and at least one occurrence of a hypomanic episode. Typically, bipolar II symptoms may present as milder than those of bipolar I. The individual's hypomanic episode would not meet the full criteria of a full manic episode and would be shorter in duration than a manic episode. The hypomanic episode will last only 4 days, whereas the manic episode will last at least 7 days. Clinicians should take note, however, that a person with bipolar II may experience more risk of suicidality than a person with bipolar I since the likelihood of a major depressive episode is more likely with bipolar II. In the event that an individual has bipolar symptoms that do not meet fit criteria for another bipolar disorder, bipolar not otherwise specified may be considered. Do you think Ingrid would be considered bipolar I or II?

Cyclothymic Disorder

This disorder is considered less severe but more chronic than the other bipolar disorders. People diagnosed with cyclothymic disorder may have multiple hypomanic episodes, as well as depressive episodes for at least 2 years (1 year time span for adolescents or children). There are frequent mood swings, episodes of high (mania) or low (depressions) energy lasting from a few days up to a few weeks, with no more than 2 months symptom-free. The symptoms are significant but do not meet the full criteria for a manic episode or for major depressive disorder. Cyclothymic disorder can occur early in life and is more frequent in people who have a family history for bipolar disorder or other mood disorders. Could Vanessa be diagnosed with cyclothymic disorder? The National Institute of Health (2014) reports that cyclothymic disorder affects men and women equally. It is estimated that less than half of those with cyclothymic disorder will develop symptoms of bipolar disorder. Effective treatment for this disorder, similar to bipolar disorder, can include medications, such as mood stabilizers and antidepressants, psychotherapy, or a combination (Kessler et al., 2005). As we conclude the discussion on the bipolar disorders, Table 5.5 provides a brief comparison of the bipolar disorders and cyclothymia.

TABLE 5.5 Comparison of Bipolar Disorders and Cyclothymic Disorder

BIPOLAR I	BIPOLAR II	CYCLOTHYMIA *
Presence of one or more manic episodes	Presence of one or more hypomanic episodes	Presence of more than one period of hypomanic symptoms
Presence of depressive episodes are *possible*	Presence of one or more major depressive episodes	Presence of more than one period of mild depressive symptoms
Acute episodes, Symptom length of time varies	Acute episodes, symptom length of time varies	Symptom length of time at least 2 years duration (1 year in children)
Moderate risk for suicidality	Highest risk for suicidality	Less risk for suicidality
		May develop bipolar I or II

Hypomanic and depressive symptoms of cyclothymic disorder do not fully meet the criteria for a hypomanic or depressive episode.

Treatment Options

Treatment of bipolar disorder typically involves both mental health therapy and a course of treatment with psychopharmacological medications. In 2001, the National Institute of Mental Health began the largest-scale research program ever to evaluate bipolar disorders (Systematic Treatment Enhancement Program for Bipolar Disorder). Multiple studies resulted from these clinical trials. One study by Miklowitz et al. (2007)

found that patients who were prescribed medications for their bipolar disorder had longer lasting positive results if they were also involved in intensive mental health psychotherapy. The researchers provided intensive therapy on a weekly and biweekly schedule for 9 months. The three therapies used were family-focused, interpersonal and social rhythm, and cognitive behavioral.

For years, the medication of choice to treat bipolar was lithium. While lithium was considered a groundbreaking medication in the treatment of bipolar, it does have its drawbacks. Because of lithium's narrow therapeutic window (normal dose is close to a toxic dose) and the fact that clients must routinely have their blood levels checked, many clients found the side effects (i.e., nausea, diarrhea, weight gain) to be problematic. Would you feel comfortable referring Vanessa and Ingrid for a medication evaluation? Prescribing physicians are now using various medications in different combinations to treat bipolar disorder, including antipsychotics, benzodiazepines, and mood stabilizers (see Table 5.6). Some of the non-lithium medications used to treat bipolar include various forms of carbamazepine, lamictal, and valproate.

TABLE 5.6 Medications Used to Treat Bipolar

TYPE	COMMON NAMES
Antipsychotics	Abilify
	Latuda
	Risperdal
	Seroquel
Mood Stabilizers	Lithium
	Depakote
	Lamictal
	Symbyax
Antianxiety	Benzodiazepines (i.e., Ativan, Xanax, Valium)

TRUE LIFE 5.1

Vincent van Gogh

We all know of the famous artist Vincent van Gogh and some of his most popular works of art. There is a popular consensus that he struggled with mental illness throughout his life. His condition reflects both medical and psychological underpinnings, and diagnoses span from epilepsy to bipolar disorder and many in between (Blumer, 2002).

Based on asymmetry in van Gogh's facial features, it is suspected that he had suffered from early brain injury (most likely during birth). This may have contributed to his self-described passion and emotional intensity (Blumer, 2002). These qualities led to a tumultuous love life. Van Gogh was

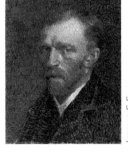

Image 5.5

rejected at the age of 16 by his first crush, sending him into a deep depression. His next love interest was his recently widowed cousin, Kee. She was disgusted by his infatuation and rejected van Gogh, which lead to another episode of depression. Van Gogh's mental problems did not seem to be a major issue until he was living in Paris with his brother, Theo.

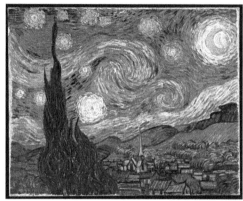

Image 5.6

During this time (1886–1888), van Gogh experienced symptoms such as sudden outbursts of terror, paralyzing stomach pain, involuntary hand movements, and amnesia (Biography.com, 2015). He would stay up arguing with his brother for most of the night. Theo described van Gogh as seeming like two different persons in one body. When van Gogh moved to Southern France in 1888, his mental stability was further shaken. In his letters, van Gogh described his inner state during this time as a "storm within him" (Blumer, 2002, p. 520). He characterized bipolar symptoms, describing periods of ecstasy and enthusiasm toward his work, with contrasting periods of debilitating anxiety and depression (Blumer, 2002).

Theo conversed daily with van Gogh through letters and became concerned about his brother's lonely and depressed state. Theo convinced Paul Gauguin (future famous impressionist painter) to join van Gogh in Arles, France. Like most of van Gogh's relationships, his relationship with Gauguin was fraught with emotions and arguments. Gauguin left after only visiting for 2 months (Biography.com, 2015). His departure was the seeming precipitating event for the most famous story about van Gogh. Paul left the house after van Gogh had thrown alcohol in his face. Van Gogh followed him out with a razor blade in his hand. Van Gogh eventually was deterred from hurting Gauguin and returned home. He proceeded to cut off his own ear and went to a brothel to give the ear to his favorite prostitute, Rachel. He evidenced signs of a psychotic break, including hallucinations and delusions (Blumer, 2002).

Eventually, van Gogh voluntarily checked into an asylum for a year. Van Gogh had made a number of suicide attempts during his life. On several occasions, he drank turpentine or paint in an attempt to die but was never successful until July 27, 1890. This is when van Gogh went out to paint as usual but took a gun with him and shot himself in the chest. He did not die immediately but passed on a few days later with Theo at his side. Although his exact diagnoses are debated, it is clear that van Gogh had both a brilliant and tortured mind (Blumer, 2002).

Suicide

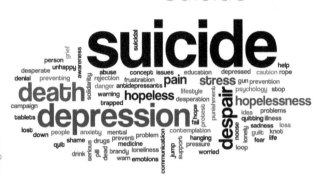

Image 5.7

Typically, suicide is most associated with the category of mood (affective) disorders. Suicide is not a specific diagnosis, but suicidal ideation is listed as a possible symptom of several mood disorders. The World Health Organization (WHO, 2014) reports that there were more than 800,000 suicide deaths in 2012 worldwide; it is the second-highest cause of death for 15- to 29-year-olds. The Centers for Disease Control and Prevention (CDC), National Vital Statistic Reports by Kochanek et al. (2019) stated the number of deaths by suicide in the United States in 2017 was more than 47,173 with an average of 129 per day. The study also reports that more than 10 million adults in the United States reported having suicidal thoughts in 2017. Suicide can affect loved ones, friends, and family members, as well as the community.

Colleges and universities are also struggling with the rise in suicidal ideation and attempts. The Center for Collegiate Mental Health (2015) reported that over the past 5 years, the number of students who reported that they had seriously considered suicide jumped from 25% to 31%. There were a reported 1,100 deaths by suicide on college campuses in 2011 (American College Health Association, 2012).

Another alarming population with growing suicide rates is United States' veterans. The most recent U.S. Department of Veteran Affairs (Kemp & Bossarte, 2012) reports reveal that the number of suicides by veterans (which was typically lower than the general population) has now almost doubled. The report suggested that, in 2010, 22 veterans died from suicide each day. Kang et al. (2015) also reported that veterans have a much higher risk of suicide (41%–61% higher) but that deployment to a war zone was not necessarily associated with this higher risk.

Risk factors for suicide and suicidal ideation can vary from one person to the next. The Centers for Disease Control and Prevention (2015) provides a list of risk factors, with a caveat that these are not necessarily direct causes.

- Physical illness (acute or chronic)
- Family history of suicide
- Lack of access to mental health services
- Easy access to lethal methods
- History of alcohol or substance abuse
- History of childhood abuse or neglect
- Cultural and religious beliefs (culture or religion believes that suicide is a noble resolution)
- History of mental disorders, particularly depression
- Isolation and feelings of hopelessness
- Loss of job, relationship, or finances

Suicide does not have to be viewed as a problem with no answers. There are many organizations around the world that are working to combat the issues related to suicide and provide outreach and help for those contemplating suicide. Information about agencies that are working in the field of suicide are located at the end of this chapter in the "Web-Based and Literature-Based Resources" section. The World Health Organization (WHO, 2014) and the U.S. Public Health Service (1999) have provided information on protective factors and ways to prevent suicide:

- Establish early identification methods so that people can receive adequate services. This includes incorporating suicide prevention as a core issue in health-care services
- Providing family and community support (i.e., follow-up care, supporting those affected by a suicide, and fighting the stigma of suicide and mental health)
- Collaboration between health-care providers. Relationships must be developed between medical and mental health professionals
- Continuing to examine and use evidence-based treatments for mental health and substance abuse disorders

---

Would you feel comfortable talking with Kwan about his suicidal ideation?

Case Study Summary

One of this chapter's case studies reviewed the behaviors of Kwan. As you process the story and examine possible diagnostic criteria, take a few minutes to answer the following questions:

1. What would be the correct diagnosis for Kwan?

2. What are the specific symptoms or criteria that led you to this diagnosis?

3. What other possible disorders might you diagnose Kwan with and why?

4. Briefly discuss what types of treatment may be beneficial for Kwan. Could you see using a certain counseling theory and/or medication?

Guided Practice Exercises

Scenario 1

Mr. Smith was a middle-aged White male living in an apartment complex with his wife. One night, a maintenance worker for the complex observed Mr. Smith working on his car in the parking lot at 2 a.m. After several complaints were filed to the complex management, it was discovered that Mr. Smith was spending all hours of every night working on his car in the parking lot. Complaints were filed because he had started playing music loudly over his car speakers while working. One complex resident was greatly disturbed when she returned home from a night shift at 4 a.m. to view Mr. Smith standing in the parking lot completely naked.

When spoken to, Mr. Smith responded energetically and enthusiastically. His speech was racing, and his thought process was tangential. One resident, unaware of Mr. Smith's recently strange behavior, engaged Mr. Smith in conversation; Mr. Smith then became agitated when the person tried to remove himself from the conversation to tend to other things. Mr. Smith exhibited feelings of grandiosity and confronted the person for walking away from him and not listening to his "important" thoughts.

After about a week of Mr. Smith exhibiting this behavior, a member of the complex management team viewed him driving home one day in a brand-new car. That night, Mr. Smith spent the entire night "working" on the new car. When management called Mr. Smith's wife to gain some insight into Mr. Smith's behavior, she informed them that she had been locking herself in their bedroom at night because he had been coming in and stealing her things while she was asleep. Mrs. Smith reported that her husband refused to be seen by a doctor and kept stating that he was fine and enjoyed his "new energy." She stated that Mr. Smith was not a heavy drinker (maybe a glass of wine with a meal) and had never used illegal drugs in his life. Mrs. Smith did comment that she remembered his uncle behaved in similar ways years ago before he was treated at the local mental health center. She could not remember what the uncle was diagnosed with at the time.

What would be the correct disorder? What are the specific symptoms or criteria that led you to this diagnosis?

_____
_____
_____
_____

What specific behaviors caused you to diagnose the disorder?

_____
_____
_____
_____

What other possible disorders might you diagnose Mr. Smith with and why?

_____
_____
_____
_____

Scenario 2

Tracy was a missionary for her church in Costa Rica for about 8 months when she started feeling depressed. She would have very negative thoughts, and no matter how hard she tried, she could not feel happy. She attributed her mood to the stressful nature of the mission, the difficulty of learning Spanish, and adjusting to a new culture. The depressive symptoms lasted for a few months, and then one day she woke up with a significant amount of energy. After that, she could not sleep for several days. She would lie down and try to fall asleep but was unable to. After a few days, she fell into the depressive state again.

Suicidal thoughts became a common occurrence. Tracy could not grasp why she had these thoughts since she considered her life to be great. Thoughts of her family and how much she knew they loved her kept her from committing suicide. She went through two more cycles of the extreme high-energy days to the long low-energy months. Finally, one of her mission leaders noticed that something was off. She talked with Tracy and learned all that Tracy had been experiencing over the past several months. Tracy was flown home to the United States where she saw a clinical mental health counselor and a psychiatrist. They noted a family history of a mood disorder in her grandfather and an aunt.

What would be the correct disorder? What are the specific symptoms or criteria that led you to this diagnosis?

_____
_____
_____
_____

What specific behaviors caused you to diagnose the disorder?

_____
_____
_____
_____

What other possible disorders might you diagnose Tracy with and why?

_____
_____
_____
_____

Web-Based and Literature-Based Resources

American Association of Suicidology: http://www.suicidology.org/ncpys

International Association for Suicide Prevention: http://www.iasp.info/resources/Crisis_Centres/

National Alliance on Mental Illness (Depression): https://www.nami.org/Learn-More/Mental-Health-Conditions/Depression

National Suicide Prevention Lifeline: www.suicidepreventionlifeline.org, 1-800-273-8255

Raison, C. (2013). *Rethinking how we understand and treat depression: Charles Raison at TEDxTucsonSalon.* http://tedxtalks.ted.com/video/Rethinking-How-We-Understand-an;search%3ARethinking%20How%20We%20Understand%20and%20Treat%20Depression

Systematic Treatment Enhancement Program for Bipolar Disorder: https://www.clinicaltrials.gov/ct/show/NCT00012558?order=1

References

American College Health Association. (2012). *American College Health Association–national college health assessment II: Reference group executive summary fall 2011.*

American Psychiatric Association (APA). (2013). *Diagnostic and statistical manual of mental disorders* (5th ed.).

Biography.com Editors. (2015). *Vincent van Gogh.* Biography.com. http://www. biography.com/people/vincent-van-gogh-9515695

Blumer, D. (2002). The illness of Vincent van Gogh. *American Journal of Psychiatry, 159*(4), 519–526.

Boelens, P. A., Reeves, R. R., Replogle, W. H., & Koenig, H. G. (2012). The effect of prayer on depression and anxiety: Maintenance of positive influence one year after prayer intervention. *International Journal of Psychiatry in Medicine, 43*(1), 85–98. https:doi.org/10.2190/PM.43.1.f

CBS News. (2016). *10 celebrities who battled postpartum depression.* http://www.cbsnews.com/pictures/10-celebrities-who-battled-postpartum-depression/6/

Center for Collegiate Mental Health. (2015, January). *2014 annual report* (Publication No. STA 15-30).

Centers for Disease Control and Prevention. (2015). *Preventing Suicide. https://www.cdc.gov/violenceprevention/suicide/fastfact.html*

Cohen, L. S., Wang, B., Nonacs, R., Viguera, A. C., Lemon, E. L., & Freeman, M. P. (2010). Treatment of mood disorders during pregnancy and postpartum. *Psychiatric Clinics of North America, 33*(2), 273–293. https:doi.org/10.1016/j.psc.2010.02.001

Craft, L. L., & Perna, F. M. (2004). The benefits of exercise for the clinically depressed. *Primary Care Companion to the Journal of Clinical Psychiatry, 6*(3), 104–111.

Frodl, T. S., Koutsouleris, N., Bottlender, R., Born, C., Jäger, M., Scupin, I., Reiser, M., Möller, H. J., & Meisenzahl, E. M. (2008). Depression-related variation in brain morphology over 3 years: Effects of stress?. *Archives of General Psychiatry, 65*(10), 1156–1165. https://doi.o

Garber, J., Ciesla, J. A., McCauley, E., Diamond, G., & Schloredt, K. A. (2011). Remission of depression in parents: Links to healthy functioning in their children. *Child Development, 82*(1), 226–243. http://doi.org/10.1111/j.1467-8624.2010.01552.x

Gotlib, I. H., & LeMoult, J. (2014). The 'ins' and 'outs' of the depressive disorders section of *DSM-5. Clinical Psychology: Science And Practice, 21*(3), 193–207. https:doi.org/10.1111/cpsp.12072

Hirst, K. P., & Moutier, C. Y. (2010). Postpartum major depression. *American Family Physician, 82*(8), 926–933

Huo, L., Straub, R. E., Schmidt, P. J., Shi, K., Vakkalanka, R., Weinberger, D. R., & Rubinow, D. R. (2007). Risk for premenstrual dysphoric disorder is associated with genetic variation in ESR1, the estrogen receptor alpha gene. *Biological Psychiatry, 62* (8), 925–933. https:doi.org/10.1016/j.biopsych.2006.12.019

Kang, H. K., Bullman, T. A., Smolenski, D. J., Skopp, N. A., Gahm, G. A., & Reger, M. A. (2015). Suicide risk among 1.3 million veterans who were on active duty during the Iraq and Afghanistan wars. *Annals of Epidemiology, 25* (2), 96–100.

Kemp, J. & Bossarte, R. (2012). *Suicide data report, 2012.* Department of Veterans Affairs.

Kessler, R. C., Berglund, P. A., Demler, O., Jin, R., & Walters, E. E. (2005). Lifetime prevalence and age-of-onset distributions of *DSM-IV* disorders in the national comorbidity survey replication (NCS-R). *Archives of General Psychiatry, 62*(6), 593–602.

Klein, D. N., Schwartz, J. E., Rose, S., & Leader, J. B. (2000). Five-year course and outcome of dysthymic disorder: A prospective, naturalistic follow-up study. *American Journal of Psychiatry, 157*, 931–939.

Kochanek, K. D., Murphy, S. L., Xu, J., & Arias, E. (2019). *Deaths: Final data for 2017.* U.S. Department of Health and Human Services. Centers for Disease Control and Prevention. https://www.cdc.gov/nchs/data/nvsr/nvsr68/nvsr68_09-508.pdf

Landers, P. (2002, October). Drug companies push Japan to change view of depression. *Wall Street Journal.* http://www.globalaging.org/health/world/japandepression.htm

Leibenluft, E. (2011). Severe mood dysregulation, irritability, and the diagnostic boundaries of bipolar in youths. *American Journal of Psychiatry, 168*, 129–142. https:doi.org/10.1176/appi.ajp.2010.10050766

Marcus, M., Yasamy, M. T., Ommeren, M. V., Chisholm, D., & Saxena, S. (2012). *Depression: A global public health concern.* World Health Organization Department of Mental Health and Substance Abuse. http://www.who.int/mental_health/management/depression/who_paper_depression_wfmh_2012.pdf

McMahon, F. J., Akula, N., Schulze, T. G., Muglia, P., Tozzi, F., Detera-Wadleigh, S. D., Steele, C. J., Breuer, R., Strohmaier, J., Wendland, J. R., Mattheisen, M., Mühleisen, T. W., Maier, W., Nöthen, M. M., Cichon, S., Farmer, A., Vincent, J. B., Holsboer, F., Preisig, M., Rietschel, M. (2010). Bipolar Disorder Genome Study (BiGS) Consortium. Meta-analysis of genome-wide association data identifies a risk locus for major mood disorders on 3p21.1. *Nature genetics, 42*(2), 128–131. https://doi.org/10.1038/ng.523

Merikangas, K. R., Jin, R., He, J. P., Kessler, R. C., Lee, S., Sampson, N. A., Viana, M. C., Andrade, L. H., Hu, C., Karam, E. G., Ladea, M., Medina-Mora, M. E., Ono, Y., Posada-Villa, J., Sagar, R., Wells, J. E., & Zarkov, Z. (2011). Prevalence and correlates of bipolar spectrum disorder in the world mental health survey initiative. *Archives of General Psychiatry, 68*(3), 241–251. https://doi.org/10.1001/archgenpsychiatry.2011.12

Miklowitz, D. J., Otto, M. W., Frank, E., Reilly-Harrington, N. A., Wisniewski, S. R., Kogan, J. N., Nierenberg, A. A., Calabrese, J. R., Marangell, L. B., Gyulai, L., Araga, M., Gonzalez, J. M., Shirley, E. R., Thase, M. E., & Sachs, G. S. (2007). Psychosocial treatments for bipolar depression: A 1-year randomized trial from the Systematic Treatment Enhancement Program. *Archives of General Psychiatry, 64*(4), 419–426. https://doi.org/10.1001/archpsyc.64.4.419

Moreno, C., Laje, G., Blanco, C., Jiang, H., Schmidt, A. B., & Olfson, M. (2007). National trends in the outpatient diagnosis and treatment of bipolar disorder in youth. *Archives of General Psychiatry, 64*(9), 1032–1039. https:doi.org/10.1001/archpsyc.64.9.1032

National Institute of Health (NIH). (2014). *Cyclothymic disorder.* https://www.nlm.nih.gov/medlineplus/ency/article/001550.htm

National Institute of Mental Health (NIMH). (2015). *Health & education database.* http://www.nimh.nih.gov/health/index.shtml

Pilowsky, D. J., Wickramaratne, P., Talati, A., Tang, M., Hughes, C. W., Garber, J., Malloy, E., King, C., Cerda, G., Sood, A. B., Alpert, J. E., Trivedi, M. H., Fava, M., Rush, A. J., Wisniewski, S., & Weissman, M. M. (2008). Children of depressed mothers 1 year after the initiation of maternal treatment: Findings from the STAR*D-Child Study. *The American Journal of Psychiatry, 165*(9), 1136–1147. https://doi.org/10.1176/appi.ajp.2008.07081286

Segal, Z. V., Williams, J. M. G., & Teasdale, J. T. (2012). *Mindfulness-based cognitive therapy for depression* (2nd ed.). Guilford Press.

Shields, B. (2006). *Down came the rain: My journey through postpartum depression.* Hyperion.

Sullivan, P. F., Neale, M. C., & Kendler, K. S. (2000). Genetic epidemiology of major depression: Review and meta-analysis. *American Journal of Psychiatry, 157* (10), 1552–1562.

U.S. Public Health Service. (1999). *The surgeon general's call to action to prevent suicide.* US Department of Health and Human Services.

World Health Organization. (2014). *Preventing suicide: A global perspective.* http://apps.who.int/iris/bitstream/10665/131056/1/9789241564779_eng.pdf?ua=1&ua=1

World Health Organization. (2015). *Comparative effectiveness of different formats of psychological treatments for depressive disorder.* http://www.who.int/mental_health/mhgap/evidence/resource/depression_q8.pdf

World Health Organization (WHO). (2016). *International statistical classification of diseases and related health problems, 10th revision (ICD-10).*

Credits

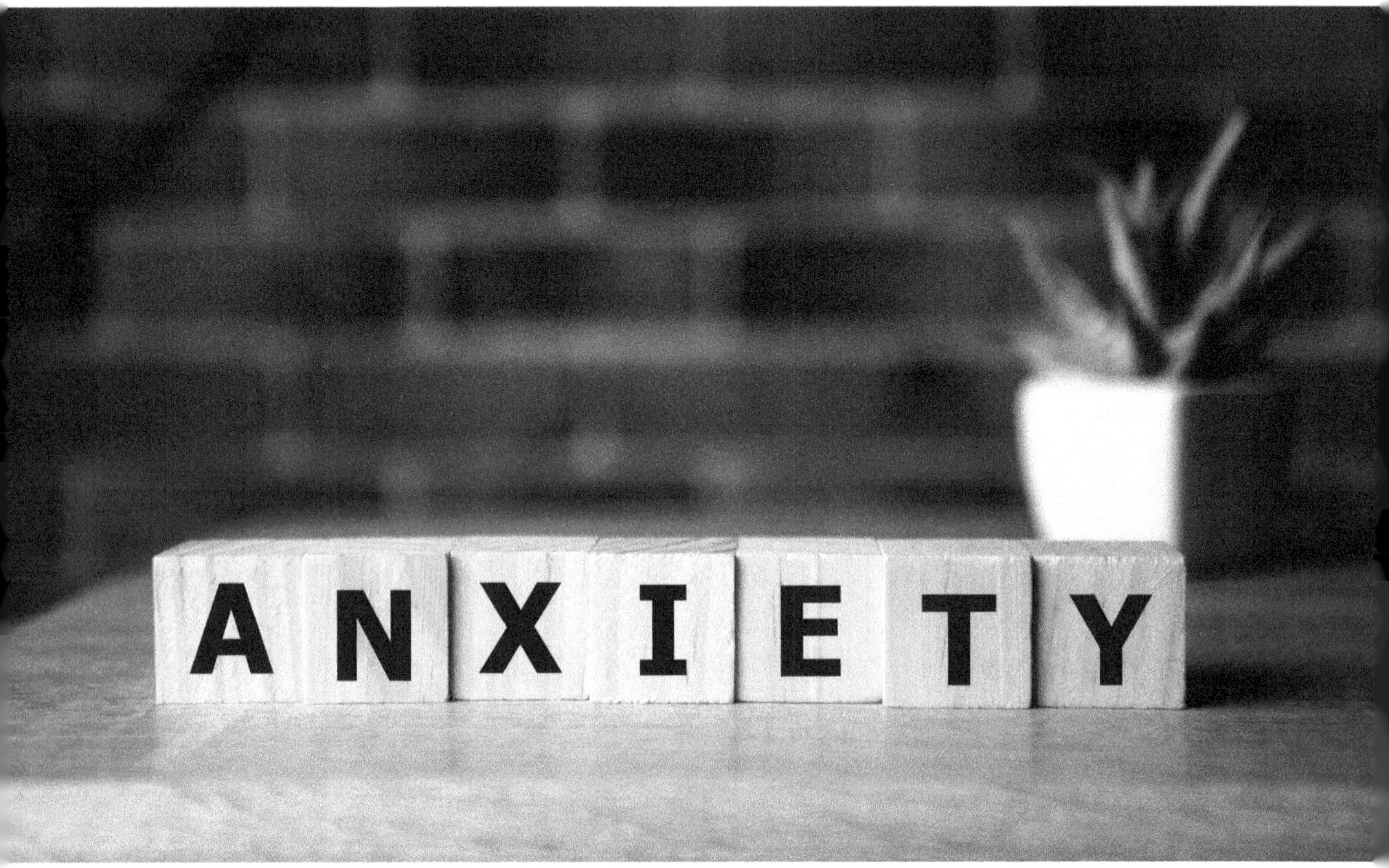
ANXIETY

CHAPTER SIX

ANXIETY DISORDERS

Michelle Grant Scott and David A. Scott

CASE STUDY 6.1 Sean, 23, still lives at home with his parents. He considered going to college after high school but knew that the pressure of living with a stranger and being surrounded by others in a classroom would be too much to take. He knows that his fear of interacting with others is irrational but accepts that it is unchangeable. Sean never had a big friend group in high school. In fact, he only had one close friend, Dave, whom Sean would only hang out with occasionally outside of school. The thing Sean liked the most about Dave was that he was comfortable with silence. Sean hates talking to others because he knows that he will say something stupid and be ashamed and embarrassed. He is thankful for his parents. They talked to school administrators throughout his schooling about his "shyness," which allowed him many times to write papers instead of speaking in front of the class. They always answer the phone and door and do not make Sean go to social or family events. Sean now works a night-shift job at a factory in town. It is a role that requires him only to interact with a small number of coworkers. Sean wants to have friends and especially a girlfriend but cannot bear the anxiety of asking a girl out. The only way Sean can go out to a club with his friends is if he drinks several beers beforehand. Usually, by that time, he is so drunk that he can't get the words out. He did once try to ask Tina, a friend, out when he was sober, but he was so nervous that he quickly blurted out his question, and she did not understand him.

Did You Know?

- Around 40 million people in the United States suffer with issues related to anxiety (Anxiety and Depression Association of America [ADAA], 2016a).
- Of the world's elderly population, 3.8% are affected by anxiety disorders (World Health Organization, 2016b).
- There are hundreds and hundreds of specific phobias: from ablutophobia (fear of washing) to zemmiphobia (fear of the great mole rat).

Overview

We all have and need some level of anxiety in our lives. Experiencing some anxiety about life events, such as passing an exam, getting a job, or even getting married, is typical and motivates us to prepare for success. Some typical symptoms of anxiety are sweaty palms, change in heartbeat (often more rapid), worrisome thoughts, and restlessness. For most, coping with those symptoms and anxiety-producing events may be uncomfortable at times, but it is manageable. It is normal to experience temporary anxiety when faced with a challenging situation or decision. However, if the anxiety does not go away or worsens, this could be a sign of an anxiety disorder. Anxiety affects one in five Americans each year (National Institute of Health [NIH], 2016a). Research suggests that anxiety disorders are the most common mental health problems for both adults and children (Kessler et al., 2005).

But for those 264 million people in the world (WHO, 2017; Table 6.1) living with an anxiety disorder, managing unwanted thoughts and other anxiety symptoms is more complicated and can interfere with daily functioning and lessen a person's quality of life. These feelings can last 6 months or more and increase the risk of other medical issues, including heart disease, diabetes, substance abuse, and depression (NIH, 2016a). In addition, symptoms may be more intense and include physical symptoms, such as shortness of breath and dizziness, which can mimic symptoms of physiological conditions. Anxiety disorders often accompany other conditions, including depression and obsessive-compulsive disorder. Overactive thyroid or low blood sugar are some of the physical conditions that can mimic the symptoms of or worsen an existing anxiety disorder (NIMH, 2016). Thus it is important for clinicians to not only develop a knowledge base of anxiety disorders but also to know when to refer clients for medical evaluations to rule out physical illness.

TABLE 6.1 Global Cases of Anxiety Disorders

Southeast Asia Region	**60.05 million** (23%)
Region of the Americas	**57.22 million** (21%)
Western Pacific Region	**54.08 million** (20%)
European Region	**36.17 million** (14%)
Eastern Mediterranean Region	**31.36 million** (12%)
African Region	**25.91 million** (10%)

Note: Adapted from World Health Organization (WHO, 2017).

According to the Anxiety and Depression Association of America (ADAA, 2016b), anxiety disorders are the most commonly diagnosed mental disorders in the United States. More than six million people are thought to suffer from generalized anxiety disorder. Other anxiety disorders include specific phobias, panic disorder and agoraphobia, social anxiety disorder, separation anxiety disorder, selective mutism, and others. Approximately one in three children or adolescents suffer from an anxiety disorder at some point. A majority of children outgrow their anxiety disorders. However, many anxiety disorders in adults began in childhood. Since around half of diagnosable mental health disorders begin by age 14, the National Institute of Health is funding a study of 200 teens ages 14–15 with and without anxiety or depression. The aim of this study is to use detailed magnetic resonance imaging to determine neurological causes for anxiety disorders (NIH, 2016a). Obsessive-compulsive disorder is also anxiety-based but has been moved to its own section in the *Diagnostic and Statistical Manual of Mental Disorders, 5th Edition (DSM-5)*. This chapter covers symptoms of these anxiety disorders, comparisons between disorders, and some effective treatment options.

Generalized Anxiety Disorder (F41.1) (300.02)

Generalized anxiety disorder in an interesting disorder in that there is not necessarily a specific issue the client is worried about. Clients present with a general, overarching worry about everyday situations or things. Many times generalized anxiety disorder (GAD) can be long lasting (6 months or longer), and the client acknowledges that there is no specific reason for them to worry about an issue.

Typical symptoms for both adolescents and adults consist of the following (NIH, 2016b; WHO, 2016a):

- Worrying about their health and the health of their family
- Not being able to control their worrying
- Worrying about their school or job performance
- Have trouble relaxing

Clients can also have the following physical symptoms:

- Headaches and muscle aches
- Issues with their sleep (falling and/or staying asleep)
- Feeling light-headed and out of breath
- Sweating
- Trembling

While there is not a specific cause for generalized anxiety disorder, several factors, such as a family history of anxiety, changes in the brain, childhood abuse, or environmental stressors, may contribute to the development of generalized anxiety disorder. Early research of generalized anxiety disorder suggests that there are changes in the inferior frontal and medial orbitofrontal cortices in adults (Rauch et al., 1997), but more research is needed to clear up the exact causes of generalized anxiety disorder. As with most mental health issues, you may want to refer your client to a physician to rule out any physical problems (i.e., heart and/or thyroid problems) that may be causing the anxiety.

Think about our case study of Sean. Is Sean exhibiting some of these symptoms?

Treatment Options

Treatment options for generalized anxiety disorder include both psychotherapy and medication. Cognitive behavioral therapy (CBT) seems to be one of the most popular forms of psychotherapy treatment for generalized anxiety disorder (Andrews et al., 2016; NIH, 2016a). Typical medications used to treat generalized anxiety disorder include Buspirone, selective serotonin reuptake inhibitors (SSRIs; Prozac and Paxil), serotonin-norepinephrine reuptake inhibitors (Cymbalta and Effexor), anticonvulsants (Lyrica), and benzodiazepines (Ativan and Halcion). Zoberi and Pollard (2010) suggested that benzodiazepines not be used as a long-term treatment option because of possible medication dependence. Daily exercise, meditation, and changes in routines may also help in reducing generalized anxiety disorder symptoms.

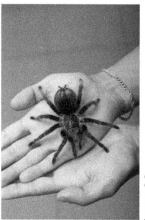

Image 6.2

CASE STUDY 6.2 Allie, 18, used to think she wanted to become a nurse. During a junior high shadowing program, she followed a physician for a day and observed different medical procedures and protocols. At the end of the day, the physician examined a cut on a patient's leg. As the physician probed the cut, it began to bleed. Suddenly, Allie became light-headed, and all she remembers next is waking up with a cold pack on her head in the waiting room. During subsequent encounters with blood, Allie has had similar reactions. It has become such an issue that Allie has quit the track team for fear of seeing a runner fall and scrape their knee. She can only watch certain television shows and read certain books and magazines for fear of a reference to blood. Allie's biology teacher requires a dissection of a pig for a passing grade. She told Allie's mom that she may fail the course because of the pervasive fear of passing out. Allie's mother brings Allie to the clinic one day after school. As Allie talks about her fear of blood, the counselor recognizes how much of Allie's life is organized around the fear of encountering blood and passing out.

Specific Phobia (F40.2) (300.xx)

One of the more unique anxiety disorders is specific phobia. The *International Statistical Classification of Diseases (ICD-10)* also includes the term specific (isolated) phobias in their description. Specific phobia is an extremely intense fear and avoidance of a specific object or situation. Typically, the person realizes that the fears are irrational but are still unable to control their thoughts. This fear can also materialize when they are just thinking about the object or situation. If one can think of it, there probably is a named phobia for it. A quick internet search for lists of phobias will generate several hundred phobias—all with a specific identifier. Table 6.2 provides a small sample of specific phobias. Specific phobias are generally grouped together in one of the following areas:

- Animal phobias
- Environment phobias
- Injury phobias
- Specific situation phobias
- Other phobias

TABLE 6.2 Specific Phobias

Ablutophobia	Fear of washing or bathing
Arachibutyrophobia	Fear of peanut butter sticking to the roof of the mouth
Coulrophobia	Fear of clowns
Pentheraphobia	Fear of mother-in-law
Triskaidekaphobia	Fear of the number 13

While there is not an exact cause for specific phobias, Linares et al.'s (2012) meta-analysis found that there is activation in several parts of the brain (amygdala, prefrontal, and orbitofrontal cortexes) in those who have been diagnosed with a specific phobia. Treatment consists of CBT, relaxation techniques, medications, and exposure therapy (ADAA, 2016b). With little conclusive research on what medications actually work with specific phobias, the majority of the time, clients will be prescribed an SSRI or antianxiety medication (i.e., Ativan).

CLINICIAN'S CORNER 6.1

Anxiety Disorders

Before diagnosing a client with an anxiety disorder, I recommend that clinicians complete their usual thorough assessment with added emphasis on the client's medical history, substance consumption, and daily lifestyle habits. Because anxiety symptoms may be manifested physically (shortness of breath, stomach upset, trembling, headache, dizziness), it is of the utmost importance to also rule out physical illness first. Sometimes a vitamin deficiency, thyroid or hormone irregularities, or cardiac problems can be mistaken for or related to anxiety symptoms. For example, I met with a young adult male client who presented with symptoms similar to panic attacks. After much discussion, we found the cause of his symptoms directly related to his changes in caffeine intake. Changing his daily habit from four cups of coffee per day back to one decreased his symptoms so much that he did not meet the criteria for an anxiety disorder. Another client, who was a middle-aged female, spent much time with physicians and spent money as she sought a medical diagnosis for her symptoms of dizziness, restlessness, and heart palpitations. After multiple medical providers agreed there was no physical illness causing the symptoms, she pursued CBT and nutrition changes to successfully treat her anxiety. Finally, clinicians are encouraged to include a spiritual component in all assessments, especially with an anxious client who worries often. Encouraging clients to seek spiritual solace, however they define it, has benefited many clients in my practice.

Michelle Grant Scott, MSW, LISW-CP(S)

Social Anxiety Disorder (F40.1) (300.23)

Social anxiety disorder (SAD) is the third most common mental health disorder in the United States (Doehrmann et al., 2013). It is a very common type of anxiety, occurring in about 15 million American adults (NIH, 2016a). Sometimes referred to as social phobia, social anxiety disorder clients have an extreme fear of social situations in which they *expect* to feel embarrassed, rejected, or judged.

Would this apply to Sean?

The *ICD-10* suggests that this fear of scrutiny can lead clients to avoid many social situations and also be associated with low self-esteem. The *DSM-5* notes that for social anxiety to be diagnosed in children, the anxiety needs to be in peer settings and not just with adults. People with social anxiety disorder may present with the following and other symptoms (NIMH, 2016; WHO, 2016a):

- Afraid of other people judging them
- Avoiding places where there are other people
- Physical complaints (nausea, blushing, hand tremors)
- Problems making and maintaining friendships

CASE STUDY 6.3 Drew, 8, shifts uncomfortably in the waiting room and stays close to his parents. After walking into your office with his parents, he does not respond to your greeting. His parents explain that Drew's increasing anxiety around his peers prompted them to come to a session. Drew hides or throws away invitations to birthday parties from other children. The teacher and guidance counselor both have shown concern for Drew. During free time, he sits alone in a corner with a puzzle. If another classmate asks him to play, he does not respond. The teacher has tried calling on Drew in class, but he does not answer. Typically, he looks down at his desk shamefully. After aptitude testing the previous year, Drew's teacher was shocked because he scored higher than most of his classmates.

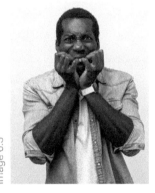

Image 6.3

Treatment options for social anxiety disorder are similar to the treatment of other anxiety disorders. Clinicians do need to understand that clients diagnosed with social anxiety disorder may not be willing to participate in group counseling because of the nature of their symptomology. Many times, the treatment clients receive will be based on their service provider and not on individualized treatment. Doehrmann et al. (2013) suggested that newer brain imaging techniques (functional magnetic resonance imaging), focusing on the occipitotemporal region, can help predict the optimal treatment for clients diagnosed with social anxiety disorder. The research reported that the patients who responded more to the images of faces (and not scenes), responded better to CBT (exposure therapy, social skills training). If medications are used, they are usually SSRIs, benzodiazepines, and even beta-blockers.

Panic Disorder (F41.0) (300.01)

Panic disorder is diagnosed when a person experiences sudden bouts of intense discomfort and anxiety, known as panic attacks (NIMH, 2016). As noted in the *DSM-5*, a person having a panic attack may experience heart palpitations, trembling, shortness of breath, dizziness, a tingling sensation, perspiration, abdominal and/or chest discomfort, and intense fear (APA, 2013). Most panic attacks last a few minutes or more but the person experiencing them may fear the symptoms will never cease. Sometimes the fear can include concerns of passing out, losing control of behavior, or even dying (APA, 2013).

According to the *ICD-10*, some typical symptoms of panic disorder are experiencing the following for at least 1 month after a panic attack:

- Recurrent and sudden periods of intense fear or panic attacks
- Strong desire to avoid locations and situations where panic attacks have happened or could potentially occur
- Unhealthy or maladaptive responses to the fear of having a panic attack

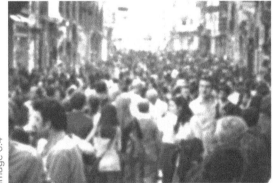

Image 6.4

As with most anxiety disorders, panic disorder can bring great distress and concern to those living with the symptoms. Because some symptoms may mimic those of cardiac or other physiological problems, clinicians should encourage clients to seek a thorough medical evaluation to rule out such possible physiological illnesses or effects of a substance before completing a treatment plan.

Although each plan should be based on the needs of the individual, treatment of panic disorder can be similar to those of other anxiety disorders. Treatment may include any combination of psychotherapy, medication, and behavioral or exposure therapy. As noted with other anxiety disorders, CBT is effective in assisting clients in correcting faulty, irrational thought patterns. Medication such as SSRIs, beta-blockers, and benzodiazepines may also be prescribed to reduce symptoms. Healthy exercise and nutrition habits, along with relaxation and breathing training, can be effective in treating panic disorder.

Agoraphobia (F40.0) (300.22)

In previous versions of the *DSM*, agoraphobia was a subcategory of panic disorder. The *DSM-5* now lists agoraphobia within anxiety disorders but as a separate disorder (clients can also be diagnosed with both panic disorder and agoraphobia). The *ICD-10* lists agoraphobia within the phobic anxiety disorders but with its own code (F40.0). The *ICD-10* and *DSM-5* include the following diagnostic symptoms:

1. Fear of crowds and public spaces
2. Fear of public transportation
3. Fear of leaving or being outside of the home

When asked, many people will say that they do not prefer to be in large crowds or overcrowded elevators. People with agoraphobia have marked increases in anxiety and panic when *even thinking* about the situations presented earlier, so much so that they will refuse to leave their homes and can have negative outcomes for their quality of life (unable to travel outside of their safety zones, unable to leave home to go to work, etc.). These symptoms need to last at least 6 months and have a higher than normal effect on daily living. Agoraphobia affects women more than men.

TRUE LIFE 6.1

Paula Deen

Paula Deen is best known for her decade-long popularity on Food Network with shows featuring her southern-style cooking. Deen has a classic "American Dream" story going from having $200 after her divorce in 1989 and starting a small catering business to becoming a Food Network celebrity. What is lesser known about Deen is her life-long struggle with panic attacks and agoraphobia. Deen began her struggle with anxiety and panic at the age of 23. At that time, both of her parents had passed away (Moskin, 2007). Deen told Oprah in an interview that she struggled with agoraphobia for 20 years. Deen described agoraphobia as "pure unadulterated hell" (Salata, 2012).

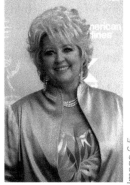

Image 6.5

Deen started her home catering business because it was something that she could do without leaving the house, and it was a distraction from her many problems. "Some days I could get to the supermarket, but I could never go too far inside," Ms. Deen said. "I learned to cook with the ingredients they kept close to the door." She consulted her pastor for help, and his response was that she was a "spoiled brat." She did not want to go to a psychiatrist at the time because of the stigma still surrounding treatment (Moskin, 2007).

After Paula and her first husband divorced in 1989, Paula saw a TV show naming agoraphobia as her illness. She claimed that this and her success and eventual television offer were what "saved her from agoraphobia" (Moskin, 2007). Deen was involved in controversy in 2013 when she made inappropriate racial comments during a deposition for a lawsuit. As a result, the Food Network did not renew her contract. In an interview with Nancy O'Dell, Dean commented about the controversy: "My darkest moment was when I had to face the fact that I had hurt people." She went on to say, "It got bad. I went on a 20-year ride with agoraphobia, from the time I was 20 to the time I was 40. I knew that if I was not careful, that I could slip right back into that." Deen has since debuted on a new television network, as well as written a new cookbook (Oshmyansky, 2014).

There are effective treatment options for agoraphobia. CBT, exposure therapy, flooding techniques, and relaxation training are some of the common treatment options for agoraphobia. Typical medications used in treatment consist of SSRIs and benzodiazepines. The main issue is how to administer the treatment options if the person is afraid to leave their home. With the advances in online mental health services, people diagnosed with agoraphobia (who can't leave their homes) now have alternative ways to receive treatment. The online mental health services could be used early on in the treatment and then possible transition to face-to-face counseling for the remainder of the treatment sessions.

Separation Anxiety Disorder

Dropping off a young child on the first day of school or childcare can be challenging. We have probably all observed the child that really did not want to leave their parent and became extremely emotional when their parent left the room. Most of the time, those reactions are short-lived, and a child will find eventually find a comfortable way to separate to attend childcare or school.

While some anxiety and emotions are common in children, those diagnosed with separation anxiety disorder are significantly distressed to the point of interfering with daily routines, and it continues into adolescence. Separation anxiety disorder is considered one of the most commonly diagnosed anxiety disorders in children (Ehrenreich et al., 2008; Herren et al., 2013). The *ICD-10* and *DSM-5* describe several symptoms of separation anxiety disorder, including the following:

- Excessive anxiety when anticipating or separated from the attachment family member
- Experience is different from normal anxiety when it is severe and beyond the normal age period
- Associated with problems in social functioning
- Can include persistent worry about losing the attached family member because of injury, illness, or death
- Refusing to be alone or without the family member
- Somatic symptoms can include nausea, headaches, and nightmares (Last, 1991)

The *DSM-5* removed the age of onset requirements for separation anxiety disorder, thus allowing for the examination of separation anxiety disorder in adults. Adult separation anxiety disorder describes a person whose symptoms did not start in childhood but in adulthood. Symptoms must be present for at least 6 months in adults and 4 weeks in children. Adults will experience intense fears (interfere with their daily routines) that their attachment figure could be harmed (Pini et al., 2010) or when they are separated from their attachment figure. More research in this area is needed, but early studies have suggested that there is a relatively high rate of comorbidity with mood disorders (Shear et al., 2006) and may have been thought of as panic disorder (or other disorders) in the past (Rochester & Baldwin, 2015). Currently, there is not a clear form of treatment for adult separation anxiety.

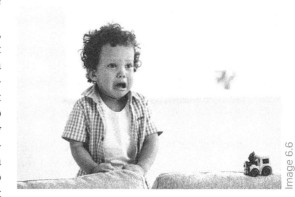

There is a clear need to expand the research on effective, evidence-based treatment for separation anxiety (Vaughan et al., 2016). Some of the current treatment options for separation anxiety disorder include CBT (exposure therapy and relaxation training) and the involvement of the family in treatment (Ehrenreich et al., 2008). Family involvement is critical to help the child and educate the parent(s) on how to effectively work with their child to alleviate their anxiety. When medication is needed to help, a combination of CBT and SSRIs can be effective. Benzodiazepines are currently not approved to treat children with separation anxiety disorder (Vaughan et al., 2016).

Selective Mutism (F94.0) (313.23)

Selective mutism, also known as elective mutism (WHO, 2016b), is a somewhat rare disorder involving emotionally related speaking behavior, including episodes when a verbal person does not speak in specific situations. Selective mutism is more frequent in girls than boys and typically occurs between 2 and 5 years old but could occur at any age. Researchers also suggest that selective mutism rates are higher in children whose parents also had selective mutism (Remschmidt et al., 2001). Comorbidity includes other anxiety disorders and even oppositional defiant disorder. According to the *ICD-10* and *DSM-5*, the duration of symptoms is at least 1 month and can include the following:

- Ongoing lack of speaking in some settings where speaking is an expectation (workplace, classroom), while engaging in speaking in other settings.
- The behavior and symptoms interfere with the person's performance in educational, occupational, or social settings.
- The lack of speaking is not related to language barriers of the spoken language, a communication disorder, or other mental disorder.
- Usually involves social anxiety, resistance, or withdrawal.

Effective treatment options continue to be limited, as evidence-based treatments for selective mutism are scarce. Researchers have suggested that selective mutism-focused CBT has shown promise as a treatment option (Lang et al., 2016). Medications such as SSRIs and monamine oxidase (MAO) inhibitors have been used, but currently, there are limited studies supporting a specific psychopharmacological approach for selective mutism.

Wrap Up

Researchers have identified risk factors for developing an anxiety disorder. Shyness in childhood could be an indicator that a person will develop an anxiety disorder. Having limited economic resources, being divorced, or the death of a spouse also puts a person at higher risk. Elevated afternoon cortisol levels in the saliva can be a predictor. Those with a parent or other close biological relative with an anxiety or other mental disorder are more likely to develop one (NIMH, 2016). However, no specific gene linked to anxiety disorder has been identified. Although social anxiety occurs equally in women and men, other forms of anxiety disorder are more common in women (NIH, 2016a).

Treatment for anxiety disorders include psychotherapy, medication, or a combination of the two (NIH, 2016a). CBT is often used to treat anxiety disorders. It teaches people to change the way they react to stressful or fearful situations. CBT also instructs people in social skills (NIMH, 2016). Initial research has uncovered similar neural patterns in adults who responded well to CBT. This information may lead to better predictions of treatment than just a clinician's assessment (NIH, 2016a). Exposure therapy is an alternative to CBT. In exposure therapy, people are taught relaxation techniques and address the underlying fear that causes their anxiety disorders. Stress management techniques or meditation can teach people with anxiety disorders to calm themselves and complement the effects of psychotherapy. Also, support groups and family members are often helpful for those with anxiety disorders. Caffeine, cold medicine, and illicit drugs should be avoided, as they can exasperate symptoms of anxiety. The types of medications usually used to treat the symptoms of anxiety disorders include antidepressants, antianxiety drugs, and beta-blockers (NIMH, 2016).

Case Study Summary

One of this chapter's case studies reviewed the behaviors of Sean. As you process the story and examine possible diagnostic criteria, take a few minutes to answer the following questions:

1. What would be the correct diagnosis for Sean?
    _____
    _____

2. What are the specific symptoms or criteria that led you to this diagnosis?
    _____
    _____

3. What other possible disorders might you diagnose Sean with and why?
    _____
    _____

4. Briefly discuss what types of treatment may be beneficial for Sean. Could you see using a certain counseling theory and/or medication?
    _____
    _____

5. How do you think introversion versus extraversion plays into social phobia? Are those with social phobia displaying extreme introversion? Defend your position after reading about Carl Jung's opinion on introversion and extraversion.

_____

_____

6. You've been working with Sean for about a year, and he has made a lot of progress. He is thankful for your help and brings you tickets to the next college football game as a thank you present. Do you accept or decline, and what do you tell Sean? Defend your position using the ethics code.

_____

_____

Guided Practice Exercises

Scenario 1

Christian is a 54-year-old business owner with a wife and four children. He presents at the clinic following a physician referral. He went to the doctor to address his depression, difficulty sleeping, and muscle tightness. Despite ample finances and familial support, he is convinced that it is only a matter a time before something disastrous happens. It is a challenge to pinpoint the source of Christian's worries. Not only is he concerned about his marriage, but he is also worried about his health, his business, and his children. Christian states three times during the first session that he is terrified of his wife leaving him. When questioned further, the counselor finds that he has been married for 23 years, and his wife has never threatened to leave. Still, Christian asserts that it will inevitably happen soon. Christian runs a computer accessory store downtown that has been in business for more than 30 years. He fervently believes he will be the owner to ruin it. Several times, employees have quit because Christian told them that the store's future is bleak. Yet the financial reports of the store show no sign of deterioration. Christian's eldest daughter (19 years old) recently moved out because of her dad's perpetual worry that she would become involved with drugs and ruin her life. She has had no previous drug history.

What would be the correct disorder? What are the specific symptoms or criteria that led you to this diagnosis?

_____

_____

_____

_____

What specific behaviors caused you to diagnose the disorder?

_____

_____

_____

_____

What other possible disorders might you diagnose Christian with and why?

_____

_____

_____

_____

Scenario 2

Trish, a 20-year-old college student, comes to the university counseling center looking bleak. She is consumed by her worries about failing out of school. This is her second time trying to complete a degree at Rink University. The first time Trish quit 2 weeks into the year because "she knew that she couldn't do it." When questioned about her grades during high school and community college, Trish responds that she mostly received A's and B's. The counselor soon finds that school is not the only concern on Trish's mind; she also worries that she is not socially competent, that her parents are disappointed in her, and that her religious beliefs are not strong enough.

What would be the correct disorder? What are the specific symptoms or criteria that led you to this diagnosis?

_____

_____

_____

_____

What specific behaviors caused you to diagnose the disorder?

_____

_____

_____

_____

What other possible disorders might you diagnose Trish with and why?

_____

_____

_____

_____

You are friends with Trish, and she confides that she is worrying about a lot of things. What is your reaction? What advice would you give Trish?

_____

_____

_____

_____

What distinguishes a person having generalized anxiety disorder from just being a "worrier"? Explain.

_____

_____

_____

_____

Your fellow counselor, Chad, has a client with generalized anxiety disorder. He has shared that his client's insurance will not pay for Chad's care unless his client has a "serious mental health condition." Chad thinks that he is going to diagnose the client with a more serious condition to get more sessions approved. Do you agree with Chad? Use the code of ethics to back up your argument.

_____

_____

_____

_____

Scenario 3

Jasmine, 44, will never forget her first panic attack. She was a 20-year-old college student and went with her boyfriend, Miguel, to a local Indian restaurant. During the course of the spicy meal, she suddenly couldn't breathe. She sunk to the floor with the sensation of choking, a racing heart, and trouble breathing. Miguel called an ambulance, and she was rushed to the hospital. The doctors never found any physical cause for her illness. For the next 22 years, her life has changed, but her attacks have been much the same. Jasmine is now the secretary at a local dentist's office and is married with three children. Once or twice a year, Jasmine will have an attack. She will usually be out in a public place and suddenly become gripped with dizziness, an inability to breathe, excessive sweating, a racing heart, and a seeming "detachment from her body." This has happened in the grocery store, at the bus station, while driving her car, and in the park with her kids. The attacks happen in a variety of locations, and she is unsure of any triggers for the attacks. Jasmine has successfully been able to go back to the grocery, the park, and even Indian restaurants, but she is still gripped by the terror that her next attack will end her life. Although she has not suffered major occupational or social problems as a result of the attacks, Jasmine still constantly worries about the next attack.

What would be the correct disorder? What are the specific symptoms or criteria that led you to this diagnosis?

_____

_____

_____

_____

What specific behaviors caused you to diagnose the disorder?

_____

_____

_____

_____

What other possible disorders might you diagnose Jasmine with and why?

_____

_____

_____

_____

Web-Based and Literature-Based Resources

Anxiety Disorders Association of America: www.adaa.org

Mental Health America (anxiety section): http://www.mentalhealthamerica.net/ conditions/anxiety-disorders

References

American Psychiatric Association (APA). (2013). *Diagnostic and statistical manual of mental disorders* (5th ed.).

Andrews, G., Mahoney, A. J., Hobbs, M. J., & Genderson, M. R. (2016). *Treatment of generalized anxiety disorder: Therapist guides and patient manual.* Oxford University Press.

Anxiety and Depression Association of America (ADAA). (2016a). *Understand the facts.* https://www.adaa.org/understanding-anxiety

Anxiety and Depression Association of America (ADAA). (2016b). *Specific phobias.* Retrieved from: https://www.adaa.org/sites/default/files/July%2015%20Phobias_adaa.pdf

Doehrmann, O., Ghosh, S. S., Polli, F. E., Reynolds, G. O., Horn, F., Keshavan, A., Triantafyllou, C., Saygin, Z. M., Whitfield-Gabrieli, S., Hofmann, S. G., Pollack, M., & Gabrieli, J. D. (2013). Predicting treatment response in social anxiety disorder from functional magnetic resonance imaging. *JAMA Psychiatry, 70*, 87–97.

Ehrenreich, J. T., Santucci, L. C., & Weiner, C. L. (2008). Separation anxiety disorder in youth: Phenomenology, assessment, and treatment. *Psicologia Conductual, 16*(3), 389–412. https://doi.org/10.1901/jaba.2008.16-389

Herren, C., In-Albon, T., & Schneider, S. (2013). Beliefs regarding child anxiety and parenting competence in parents of children with separation anxiety disorder. *Journal of Behavior Therapy and Experimental Psychiatry, 44*, 53–60.

Kessler, R. C., Chiu, W. T., Demler O, & Walters E. E. (2005). Prevalence, severity, and comorbidity of twelve-month *DSM-IV* disorders in the national comorbidity survey replication (NCS-R). *Archives of General Psychiatry, 62*(6), 617–627.

Lang, C., Nir, Z., Gothelf, A., Domachevsky, S., Ginton, L., Kushnir, J., & Gothelf, D. (2016). The outcome of children with selective mutism following cognitive behavioral intervention: A follow-up study. *European Journal of Pediatrics, 175*, 481–487. https://doi.org/10.1007/s00431-015-2651-0

Last, C. G. (1991). Somatic complaints in anxiety disordered children. *Journal of Anxiety Disorders, 5*, 125–138.

Linares, I. M., Trzesniak, C., Chagas, M. N., Hallak, J. C., Nardi, A. E., & Crippa, J. S. (2012). Neuroimaging in specific phobia disorder: A systematic review of the literature. *Revista Brasileira De Psiquiatria, 34*(1), 101–111. https://doi.org/10.1016/S1516-4446(12)70017-X

Moskin, J. (2007, February 28). From phobia to fame: A southern cook's memoir. *New York Times.* http://www.nytimes.com/2007/02/28/dining/28deen.html?fta=y&_r=1&

National Institutes of Health (NIH). (2016a). Understanding anxiety disorders: When panic, fear, and worries overwhelm. *NIH News in Health.* Retrieved September 28, 2016, from https://newsinhealth.nih.gov/issue/Mar2016/Feature1

National Institute of Health (NIH). (2016b). *Generalized anxiety disorder: When worry gets out of control.* NIH publication NO. QF 16-4677. https://www.nimh.nih.gov/health/publications/generalized-anxiety-disorder-gad/index.shtml

National Institute of Mental Health (NIMH). (2016, March). *Anxiety disorders.* https://www.nimh.nih.gov/health/topics/anxiety-disorders/index.shtml

Oshmyansky, R. (2014, September 23). Exclusive: Paula Deen struggled with agoraphobia fears after racial slur scandal. *Entertainment Tonight Online.* http://www.etonline.com/news/151490_paula_deen_struggled_with_agoraphobia/

Pini, S., Abelli, M., Shear, K. M., Cardini, A., Lari, L., Gesi, C., Muti, M., Calugi, S., Galderisi, S., Troisi, A., Bertolino, A., & Cassano, G. B. (2010). Frequency and clinical correlates of adult separation anxiety in a sample of 508 outpatients with mood and anxiety disorders. *Acta Psychiatrica Scandinavica, 122*(1), 40–46.

Rauch, S. L., Savage, C. R., Alpert, N. M., Fischman, A. J., & Jenike, M. A. (1997). The functional neuroanatomy of anxiety: A study of three disorders using positron emission tomography and symptom provocation. *Biological Psychiatry, 42*, 446–452.

Remschmidt, H., Poller, M., Herpertz-Dahlmann, B., Hennighausen, K., & Gutenbrunner, C. (2001). A follow-up study of 45 patients with elective mutism. *European Archives of Psychiatry and Clinical Neuroscience, 251,* 284–296.

Rochester, J., & Baldwin, D. S. (2015). Adult separation anxiety disorder: Accepted but little understood. *Human Psychopharmacology, 30*(1), 1–3. https://doi.org/10.1002/hup.2452

Salata, S. (2012, March 4). Paula Deen's fear of death and struggle with agoraphobia [TV series episode]. *Oprah's Next Chapter.* Oprah Winfrey Network. http://www.oprah.com/own-oprahs-next-chapter/Paula-Deens-Fear-of-Death-and-Struggle-with-Agoraphobia-Video

Shear, K., Jin, R., Ruscio, A. M., Walters, E. E, Kessler, R. C. (2006). Prevalence and correlates of estimated DSM-IV child and adult separation anxiety disorder in the national comorbidity survey replication. *American Journal of Psychiatry, 163,* 1074–1083.

Vaughan, J., Coddington, J. A., Ahmed, A. H., & Ertel, M. (2016). Separation anxiety disorder in school-age children: What health care providers should know. *Journal of Pediatric Healthcare, 31*(4), 433–440. https://doi.org/10.1016/j.pedhc.2016.11.003

World Health Organization. (2016a). *International statistical classification of diseases and related health problems, 10th revision (ICD-10).*

World Health Organization (WHO). (2016b). *Mental health and older adults. Fact sheet.* http://www.who.int/mediacentre/factsheets/fs381/en/

World Health Organization (WHO). (2017). *Depression and other common mental disorders: Global health estimates.*

Zoberi, K., & Pollard, C. A. (2010). Treating anxiety without SSRIs. *Journal of Family Practice, 59*(3), 148–154.

Credits

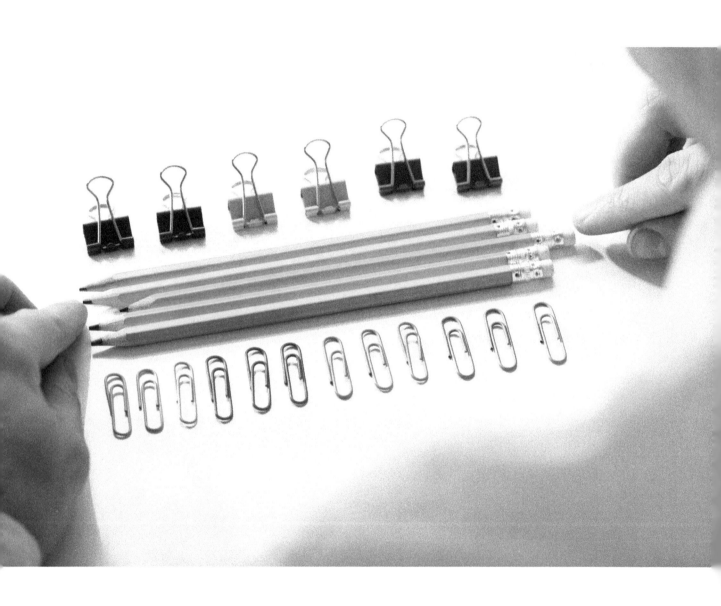

CHAPTER SEVEN

OBSESSIVE-COMPULSIVE DISORDER AND RELATED DISORDERS

Michelle Grant Scott and David A. Scott

CASE STUDY 7.1 Tyrell, 53, is haunted by thoughts of uncleanliness. In fact, most of his days are spent performing ritualistic cleaning behaviors. His hands are red and swollen from spending 2–3 hours a day scrubbing them. He will also take multiple showers each day and meticulously wipe down all surfaces in the house with disinfectant wipes. He is married and has two children. In the kitchen, he buys and keeps separate food from the rest of the family, afraid that another family member could contaminate it. When faced with not being able to perform his rituals or share his "clean" food, Tyrell goes into a panic. In fact, to keep up the rituals, he had to quit his job about 10 years ago and now his wife supports the family. This gives him time to clean both himself and the house. Tyrell refuses to go to hospitals, funerals, or nursing homes because of his fear of obtaining a disease or sickness from one of these places.

Overview

Obsessive-compulsive disorder (OCD) is often portrayed as a personality trait seen in film, the news, and other media sources, such as social networking sites. Individuals who struggle with obsessive-compulsive disorder may be described as having "perfectionistic" tendencies or a "type A" personality. Others may think of someone who is overly concerned about germs. We may even causally say, "I'm *so* OCD" to describe our behavior of being picky. Because of the normalization of the acronym for obsessive-compulsive disorder, some fail to recognize the true meaning of the disorder and the severity it can involve. In this chapter, we hope to assist the reader in understanding just that, along with briefly reviewing related disorders.

Research shows and individual testimonies reveal the covert distress obsessive-compulsive disorder and related disorders bring. For obsessive-compulsive disorder, a commonality, and diagnostic criterion, is a person experiencing distress in multiple settings, with variations of the two main symptoms: obsessions and compulsions.

There are several disorders listed in the *Diagnostic and Statistical Manual of Mental Disorders, 5th Edition* (*DSM-5*) related to obsessive-compulsive disorder. As noted, here we will discuss the psychopathology behind obsessive-compulsive disorder, body dysmorphic disorder, hoarding disorder, trichotillomania, and excoriation. The *DSM-5* lists obsessive-compulsive disorder and related disorders in their own category and

Did You Know?

- Some common obsessive-compulsive disorder (OCD) obsessions are not only related to germs and maintaining order but also fear of sudden crisis and unintended violence. Mental images such as unwanted sexual acts or harming others may occur as well. Often, people with obsessive-compulsive disorder fear they will act on these intrusive thoughts and cause harm (as depicted in their images).

- When hoarding involves large volumes of possessions or unsanitary items, it can result in home safety hazards. In some states, fire and emergency responders have created task forces to assist families affected by hoarding.

- There are hair salons throughout the United States designed specifically to assist individuals suffering from trichotillomania. Wigs with human hair and spaces providing privacy are features found in some of these specialized salons.

- Many celebrities and famous persons have publicly reported having obsessive-compulsive disorder or related disorders. See Howie Mandel's story as one example.

- According to the National Institute of Mental Health, children who exhibit sudden, new, or exacerbated obsessive-compulsive disorder symptoms after having a streptococcal infection could be suffering from pediatric autoimmune neuropsychiatric disorders associated with streptococcal infections. This is primarily found in children and young teens and rarely in adults (2020).

chapter, while the *International Statistical Classification of Diseases (ICD-10)* lists obsessive-compulsive disorder and related disorders under the neurotic, stress-related, and somatoform disorders category.

TRUE LIFE 6.1

Howie Mandel

Howie Mandel—Obsessive-Compulsive Disorder

Most people know Howie Mandel as a host of television shows such as *Deal or No Deal* and *America's Got Talent.* Mandel is also an actor and a comedian. He is one of only a handful of celebrities to be open about his struggle with obsessive-compulsive disorder. He was born in Canada in 1955 and had a fear of germs from a young age. Mandel would refuse to tie his shoes, not because he did not know how but because they were dirty (Haddad et al., 2009). Mandel had a talent for humor, but that took the shape of becoming the class clown.

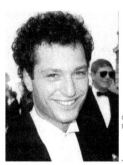

Image 7.2

His behavior led to three expulsions from different high schools. He eventually got his general equivalency diploma instead of attending traditional high school. His first career was as a carpet salesman. However, he tried out for a comedy show in Los Angeles and ended up impressing a producer and getting hired. Much of his early career was spent as a comedian (Biography.com, 2015).

Mandel became known from his appearances on *The Tonight Show with Johnny Carson.* He also had a short-lived talk show. Mandel admits that he kept a bucket of Purell hand sanitizer under his desk during the talk show because he had to shake hands with guests. Mandel was going to give up on his television career when he got the offer for *Deal or No Deal.* He turned it down because he thought it was insulting. But his wife of more than 30 years convinced Mandel to try it out. Little did he know that he would get the most recognition from that role (Haddad et al., 2009).

In 2009, Mandel went public about his obsessive-compulsive disorder with a humorous autobiography entitled *Here's the Deal: Don't Touch Me.* One of his trademarks on *Deal or No Deal* is fist bumping contestants. Few people know that this is due to a fear of germ contamination. In an interview with ABC, Mandel said that an open hand is like a "petri dish of germs" to him. Contestants are told prior to the show not to shake Mandel's hand if they are chosen to play. Mandel's makeup artists have to buy new sponges and applicators every day or Howie will refuse to let them touch him. Mandel also avoids handrails at all costs and tries not to touch doorknobs. Raising children (of which he has three) was a nightmare. Mandel was horrified when the children would crawl on the floor. He would not let many people touch the children without washing their hands. Even his bald head is intentional because it makes him feel cleaner (Haddad et al., 2009).

Mandel has gotten both therapy and medication for his condition. He is becoming an advocate for mental health, even speaking in Washington on behalf of those struggling with mental health issues. "You know, in the middle of a workday, wherever you work in America, if you got up and say, 'I'm gonna go see my dentist,' nobody would even flinch," Mandel said. "But if you got up in the middle of the day and said, 'You know what, I gotta go, I'm having a little issue. I've gotta go to my psychiatrist. I'll be back in an hour.' I think that people would—'Did he just say he's going to the psychiatrist?' ... There's a stigma" (Haddad et al., 2009). Despite his obsessive-compulsive disorder, Mandel has done well professionally and continues to travel extensively to perform at comedy clubs. He braves hotel rooms because performing is what he loves to do (Haddad et al., 2009).

Obsessive-Compulsive Disorder and Related Disorders

Obsessive-compulsive disorder and related disorders share similar symptoms known as obsessions and compulsions. *Typically,* **obsessions** are thoughts, impulses, or images that occur repeatedly and are out of the person's control. **Compulsions** can be repetitive thoughts or behaviors a person uses to try to reduce or stop their obsessions. A compulsion may be a coping response to an obsession one experiences. Depending on the person, however, there may be various combinations of symptoms (presence of obsessions, absence of compulsions, vice versa, both). These symptoms can be observed in other related disorders but are characterized as cognitive preoccupations followed by repetitive behaviors. Individuals with these disorders often feel powerless, and the symptoms tend to worsen over time.

Obsessive-compulsive disorder and related disorders include those listed in Box 7.2.

Box 7.2 Obsessive-Compulsive Disorder Disorders

- Obsessive-compulsive disorder
- Body dysmorphic disorder
- Hoarding disorder
- Trichotillomania
- Excoriation disorder

CASE STUDY 7.2 Angelica, 34, lives alone in a Chicago suburb. She often fears for her safety, despite an absence of threats. She cannot remember a time when she was not tortured with thoughts of being attacked or mugged. To go to bed at night, Angelica needs to check each of the locks on the house seven times and switch the lights on and off nine times. She was almost fired from her job last week because she went out to the parking lot multiple times to check that her car was locked during her workday. Before stepping into bed, she needs to take four steps backward and two steps forward and will often repeat the routine "to be safe." She believes that these rituals are the only things that keep her thoughts at bay and keep her safe.

Questions

- Many people will say, "Sorry I'm a little OCD" in everyday life. Differentiate between what these people may be implying and what those clinically diagnosed with obsessive-compulsive disorder experience.
- Obsessive-compulsive disorder can manifest itself in different ways. For example, one person may spend hours cleaning the house each day, while another may be haunted by inappropriate thoughts and ritualistic responses to those thoughts. How can two seemingly opposite situations both exemplify obsessive-compulsive disorder?

Obsessive-Compulsive Disorder (F42) (300.3)

In 2008, it was estimated that one in 100 adults and one in 200 children in the United States were struggling with symptoms of obsessive-compulsive disorder (Ruscio et al., 2010). Thus it is estimated that there are approximately 20 high school–aged kids per public school who struggle with obsessive-compulsive disorder symptoms (March & Benton, 2007). Although more males are affected by the disorder during childhood, there appear to be higher numbers of females with obsessive-compulsive disorder in adulthood. The World Health Organization also ranks obsessive-compulsive disorder as one of the "most debilitating conditions" as it relates to symptom severity (Veale et al., 2014). Other risk factors of obsessive-compulsive disorder sufferers include poor life quality, difficulty living independently (Veale et al., 2014), and higher suicide risks (Angelakis et al., 2015). These statistics show the severity and magnitude of symptoms that can occur in sufferers of obsessive-compulsive disorder.

The *ICD-10* indicates that the diagnosis of obsessive-compulsive disorder is based on an individual experiencing obsessions (irrational thoughts/ruminations), compulsions (compensatory/repetitive behavior), or both. These symptoms must be time-consuming and take more than 1 hour a day to complete. Symptoms must cause significant distress or impairment in daily activities, such as social engagements or work or interfere with a variety of task completions. A list of common obsessions and compulsions are listed in Table 7.1. These symptoms should not be attributed to substance use or other medical conditions (WHO, 2016).

Consider the case study of Tyrell. Is Tyrell exhibiting some of these symptoms? If so, which ones?

TABLE 7.1 List of Some Common Obsessions and Compulsions

OBSESSIONS	COMPULSIONS
Having things symmetrical	Arranging things in a precise way
Wanting things in perfect order	Compulsive counting
Fear of germs or contamination	Excessive cleaning
Unwanted thoughts of causing harm to self or others, safety fears	Excessive handwashing
	Repeatedly checking on things (i.e., if oven is off, if door is locked, child is safe)

Source: National Institute of Mental Health (2020)

Body Dysmorphic Disorder (F45.22) (300.7)

CASE STUDY 7.3 Liam, 34, rarely leaves the house without a hat because of his concern with his hair. He believes that his hair has been the cause of many of his breakups and a reason he does not have a better job. Despite changing the style and color multiple times, it never seems to satisfy Liam. He always has to have a comb and will comb his hair more than 10 times each day in an effort to make it look "less hideous." Liam does not feel much anxiety about hanging out with friends or with women but is anxious that they will reject him after noticing his hair. This has greatly influenced his social life because he feels he can only hang out when it is acceptable to wear a hat. He has been invited to church by one of his close friends and would love to go to a service but fears he would be judged for wearing a hat in a religious environment.

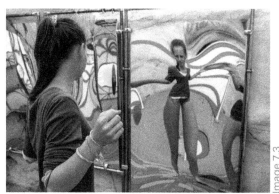

Image 7.3

According to the American Psychiatric Association (2013), about one in 50 people in the general population are affected by body dysmorphic disorder (BDD). The *ICD-10* describes this disorder as the persistent preoccupation with a person's appearance as being abnormal when most would consider the person's appearance normal or commonplace. An individual's preoccupation with their perceived flaws may last hours or days, causing them to experience great distress. A person may often exhibit compulsive behaviors, such as mirror checking, and as a result, they find it difficult to make it to work or even socially related functions in a timely manner.

Because of the severe cognitive impairment body dysmorphic disorder can cause an individual, suicidality rates have shown to be high in this population. According to a study done in Germany, individuals diagnosed with body dysmorphic disorder had significantly more reports of cosmetics surgeries (15.6%) and higher rates of suicide ideation (31%) and attempts (22.2%) compared to controls (Buhlmann et al., 2010). This may not be singularly attributed to this population's self-scrutiny over their perceived flaws but also potentially to the persistent invalidation and judgment they may receive from their support systems. Individuals with body dysmorphic disorder exhibit very rigid thinking and poor insight (Hartmann & Buhlmann, 2017), so others consistently telling these individuals what they see isn't real or rational can result in social isolation and a damaged sense of self.

The onset of this disorder occurs in adolescence (Hartmann & Buhlmann, 2017). With the great emphasis on body image in contemporary culture, this leads clinicians and researchers to ponder the etiological underpinnings of body dysmorphic disorder when it comes to the influence of our environment. More research is indicated to further understand how the development of body dysmorphic disorder may be influenced by a person's access to images on the internet and social media sites.

According to the *ICD-10*, the criteria for diagnosing someone with body dysmorphic disorder would include preoccupations with one or more perceived defects or flaws in physical appearance and the strong desire to perform repetitive behavior or mental acts in response to the physical concerns. Symptoms must cause significant distress or impairment in daily activities, such as social engagements or work. These symptoms are not better explained by concerns with body fat or any eating-related disorders (WHO, 2016).

CASE STUDY 7.4 Emmett, 45, keeps and collects a large number of possessions in his home. He began doing this after tragedy struck in his life. Emmett's wife and his two daughters died in a bus accident 10 years ago. Following the traumatic event, Emmett was unable to throw away or give away any of their possessions. In fact, he

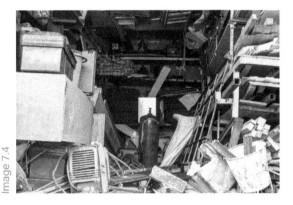

began keeping everything that reminded him of his wife or daughters. His living room is full of toys, news clippings, coloring books, and hairbrushes. There is one small pathway to get from the bedroom to the kitchen. The old rooms of his daughters' are too full for anyone to go into them. Emmett's best friend, Dave, expresses concern that Emmett is not coping well with his loss years ago. Dave notices Emmett misses work periodically and does not eat regularly because of the state of his kitchen. Finally, the health department threatens to condemn Emmett's house if he does not clean it. The thought of throwing anything away to Emmett is like forgetting his wife and little girls; it is unbearable. Dave finally convinces Emmett to go to the mental health clinic to see a therapist.

Image 7.4

Hoarding Disorder (F42) (300.3)

Approximately 2% to 6% of adults (Pertusa et al., 2010) and 2% percent of adolescents (Ivanov et al., 2013) are diagnosed with hoarding disorder. Symptoms can begin emerging in individuals as early as 11 years of age. Diagnosed individuals, however, tend to be older, single, and unemployed compared to their undiagnosed counterparts (Nordsletten et al., 2013). Hoarding behavior was previously considered a symptom of obsessive-compulsive disorder but with the development of updated diagnostic criteria, hoarding disorder was given its own *DSM-5* diagnosis code (2013).

Hoarding disorder involves much more than an individual's desire to collect things or keep some items of sentimental value. A person diagnosed with hoarding disorder shows persistent difficulty in discarding items of little value, experiences significant distress related to parting with such items, and strongly feels the need to save the items. Hoarding disorder involves difficulty parting with possessions but may also involve accumulating more items than is considered safe or tolerable for a clean, functional living or working space. According to the *DSM-5*, these items may be newspapers or magazines, books, or clothing but could be any items that the individual feels must be saved (2013). The symptoms are not better accounted for by a medical diagnosis, substance use disorder, or other disorder.

Would this apply to Tyrell?

CASE STUDY 7.5 Stella, 24, is extremely self-conscious about the way she looks. She has several bald spots on her head and little arm hair. Her hairdresser, Steven, has done the best he can to style her hair to hide the bald spots, but her hair keeps getting thinner each time she sees him. Stella confides in Steven that she has an undying desire to pull out her hair. She will feel sad once she has large bald spots on her head after she pulls each piece out, but she is unable to stop. Stella describes it as an "itch-like" sensation. Stella is a bank teller and takes night classes at a community college. After her 3-hour class, she will often try to hide a small pile of hair that has built up as she pulls her hair out strand by strand. She once plucked all of her eyebrow hair out and had to stencil them in for a month.

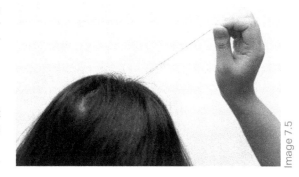

Image 7.5

Questions

- Do you think most people with trichotillomania pull out their hair unconsciously, knowingly, or both? What leads you to your answer?
- Describe some of the stress a person living with trichotillomania faces because of the hair-pulling behavior.

Trichotillomania (F63.3) (312.39)

Trichotillomania is estimated to affect 0.5% to 2% of the population in the United States, where it is more common in females than males: 4:1 (Grant et al., 2016). This disorder is characterized by the compulsive desire and habitual behavior of pulling out one's own hair. The result is hair loss and sometimes bald spots (WHO, 2016). The hair pulled can be on one's head, face (brows, eyelashes, beard), arms, or other body parts. The disorder is also characterized by unsuccessful attempts to stop the behavior. Some triggers for hair pulling are thought to be emotional distress and times of distraction, during which a person may be hair pulling without realizing the severity until later when they look in a mirror (Grant et al., 2012).

Trichotillomania can be associated with secondary complications, such as low self-esteem and shame, especially when hair loss causes unwanted appearance changes, such as bald spots. It is estimated that 5% to 20% of individuals with trichotillomania eat the hair they pull, a behavior referred to as *trichophagia*. Eating the pulled hair can lead to gastrointestinal issues and, in extreme cases, require medical and surgical intervention (Grant et al., 2016). Despite a person's desire to break the cycle, changing this compulsive behavior can be a lengthy and intensive process (Grant et al., 2016).

CASE STUDY 7.6 Leo, 14, presents to the clinic with scars and scratches all over his face. For the last 3 years, he has had the persistent urge to scratch his face. He verbalizes that sometimes he does not realize that he has been scratching until his face is bleeding. His mother reports that they've "tried everything" to get him to stop, but nothing has helped. Leo says that scratching makes him feel calmer, especially after stressful situations. The worst time he scratched was after receiving a low grade on an algebra test. Leo scratched scabs and healthy skin on his face that night, causing it to bleed while he slept. His mother reportedly cried when she saw him the following morning. His mother reports increased "moodiness" in Leo and irritability since the scratching began.

Questions

* Discuss what additional questions you would ask Leo and his mother about his situation.
* What are some physical and emotional consequences of engaging in this behavior? Discuss treatment options for Leo.

Excoriation Disorder (F42.4) (L98.1)

According to Dr. Jon Grant, approximately 1.4% to more than 5% of the people in the United States have excoriation disorder (also known dermotillimania), with a usual onset in adolescence (2012). The majority of persons seeking treatment for excoriation disorder are female. The *ICD-10* describes excoriation disorder as involving the habitual behavior of skin picking, which can result in skin abrasions (WHO, 2016). Criteria for the disorder also include the desire or effort to stop the skin-picking behavior, and the behavior is not attributable to another physical or mental health disorder (APA, 2013). Skin picking can take various forms, including pulling off scabs of healing wounds to scratching or tearing skin with fingernails. Secondary physical damage can occur depending on the severity, including skin lesions, infections, or scaring of the skin (Odlaug & Grant, 2008). Furthermore, excoriation disorder can cause shame and embarrassment when it affects one's physical appearance and may add to or cause much psychological distress (Grant et al., 2012). Persons with existing skin problems, such as eczema, are at higher risk of developing excoriation disorder. Triggers for skin picking or pulling vary but can be related to feelings of stress or

---

CLINICIAN'S CORNER 7.1

When working with clients living with obsessive-compulsive disorder and related disorders, I have heard many say they are embarrassed or feel shame about their symptoms. Many have sat across from me and explained how it feels to be perceived by others as needy or selfish, saying, "I wish I could just stop." Time-consuming compulsive behaviors (checking, hoarding, even scratching) can all have an effect on those who love the client. Some relationships struggle if a loved one perceives demands are being made of him or her. Some examples are if a loved one is asked not to sit on the family furniture after being out of the home, is asked to wait often on a chronically late client, or is requested to provide frequent reassurance to offset the client's intrusive thoughts. Taking some time to help clients understand how and why obsessive-compulsive disorder behaviors affect others while offering resources and possible solutions can help empower clients toward change. Meeting with loved ones of a person with obsessive-compulsive disorder can also prove powerful, improve relationship quality, and often result in a team approach to the client's treatment.

Michelle Grant Scott, MSW, LISW-CP(S)

anger, along with engaging in the behavior during times of distraction or boredom (Odlaug et al., 2011). One treatment specific to skin picking is called habit reversal training. With this therapy, clients learn to be more aware of their tendencies while learning healthier behaviors to replace the skin-picking behavior (Grant et al., 2012). Other types of treatment for obsessive-compulsive disorder and related disorders will be shared later in this chapter.

Treatment Options

Treatment options for obsessive-compulsive disorder and related disorders are often derived from the biopsychosocial model, emphasizing a holistic approach by addressing individuals' complex biological, psychological, and social aspects (Borrell-Carrió et al., 2004). Psychotherapy can help clients address cognitive issues, learn relaxation and breathing techniques, and create a treatment plan. Talk therapy best suited for these disorders often includes some form of cognitive behavioral therapy (CBT), which has proven effective in treating faulty thoughts and increasing desensitization responses (Borrell-Carrió et al, 2004).

For treating obsessive-compulsive disorder symptoms, variations of CBT, along with exposure response prevention therapy (ERP therapy) may be used with clients. With ERP, clients are gradually and purposefully exposed to their obsessions (or fears) and assisted with developing a healthier coping response. By doing so, clients gradually learn to tolerate exposure to their obsessions without relying on a compulsion or ritual for coping (Grant et al., 2016). Flooding, also referred to as in vivo exposure, is a behavioral technique used to expose clients more quickly to obsessions while also giving them support in coping with related feelings. For example, a client who obsesses over germs or contamination might participate in touching dreaded items, such as trash or a restroom doorknob during a flooding session. Both ERP and flooding requires guidance by a trained clinician to avoid causing harm to the client.

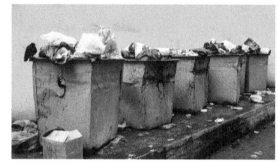

Image 7.6

In addition to varieties of talk therapy, the use of selective serotonin reuptake inhibitors (SSRIs; such as Prozac, Zoloft, and Luvox), along with antipsychotics, have been found effective in treating obsessive-compulsive disorder and related disorders (Veale et al., 2014). Because SSRIs may take several weeks to months to provide relief of obsessive-compulsive disorder related symptoms, a combination approach of talk therapy and medication is further supported to provide symptom relief.

While these treatments continue to be viable options for most, a percentage of clients with severe cases of obsessive-compulsive disorder and related disorders may continue to experience chronic symptoms. For this treatment-resistant population, emerging research suggests there are client benefits from the use of ablation surgery and deep brain stimulation (also used for movement disorders) as treatment options (Tierney et al., 2013). The Food and Drug Administration also approved transcranial magnetic stimulation in 2018 as a treatment option for obsessive-compulsive disorder in adults. This procedure involves stimulating nerve cells in the brain and is considered a noninvasive treatment (NIMH, 2020). More research on these techniques is indicated to ensure that they are viable and effective treatments for clients with obsessive-compulsive disorder.

Case Study Summary

One of this chapter's case studies reviewed the behaviors of Tyrell. As you process the story and examine possible diagnostic criteria, take a few minutes to answer the following questions:

1. What would be the correct diagnosis for Tyrell?

    _____

    _____

2. What are the specific symptoms or criteria that led you to this diagnosis?

    _____

    _____

3. What other possible disorders might you diagnose Tyrell with and why?

    _____

    _____

4. Briefly discuss what types of treatment may be beneficial for Tyrell. Could you see using a certain counseling theory and/or medication?

    _____

    _____

Guided Practice Exercises

Scenario 1

Scarlett, 23, describes herself as a "monster." Despite being a well-liked and attractive young woman, she is consumed by her belief that her nose is atypically large and unsightly. While the clinician does not notice any deficiency, Scarlett is convinced that all anyone can see is her nose. Scarlett has expended a great amount of money on surgeries to correct her nose. Thus far, she has had three surgeries and is considering suing her latest plastic surgeon because of her unhappiness with his job. Scarlett has begun to miss work quite frequently and rarely spends time with friends anymore because of her extreme discomfort with her appearance. She looks at her nose in the mirror frequently during the day. The time she feels most comfortable is when there is dim lighting or it is dark, thus shielding sight of her nose.

What would be the correct disorder? What are the specific symptoms or criteria that led you to this diagnosis?

_____

_____

_____

_____

What specific behaviors caused you to diagnose the disorder?

_____

_____

_____

_____

What other possible disorders might you diagnose Scarlett with and why?

_____

_____

_____

_____

Scenario 2

Charlotte, 73, seeks services at the insistence of her daughter, Camille. Camille claims that Charlotte is barely able to get around her home because of the mass amounts of possessions Charlotte is unable to throw away. The health department has lodged several complaints against Charlotte and noted that she must deal with the rotting food and trash disposal issues in her kitchen, or her house may be condemned. When one looks at Charlotte's house, one sees piles of trash and unusable items. In her kitchen alone, there are bottles and cans, pots, half-opened containers of food, and old fast-food bags. Other rooms are equally packed with a variety of items. To Charlotte, the possessions are meaningful, and it feels unbearable to lose them. She cannot remember a time when she did not hold on to possessions. Charlotte remembers hiding old newspapers and candy wrappers from her mom as a child. She has not had anyone over to the house in years because of its unsanitary state. Although she expresses a want for more social interaction, she has few friends. Charlotte declines treatment because of her age and fear of having to throw away loved possessions.

What would be the correct disorder? What are the specific symptoms or criteria that led you to this diagnosis?

_____

_____

_____

_____

What specific behaviors caused you to diagnose the disorder?

_____

_____

_____

_____

What other possible disorders might you diagnose Charlotte with and why?

_____

_____

_____

_____

Web-Based and Literature-Based Resources

International OCD Foundation: https://iocdf.org/about-ocd/

The TLC Foundation: https://www.bfrb.org/learn-about-bfrbs/trichotillomania

The Center for Anxiety and OCD: https://www.caocd.com

Intrusive Thoughts Project: https://www.intrusivethoughts.org

References

American Psychiatric Association. (2013). *Diagnostic and statistical manual of mental disorders* (5th ed.).

Angelakis, I., Gooding, P., Tarrier, N., & Panagioti, M. (2015). Suicidality in obsessive compulsive disorder (OCD): A systematic review and meta-analysis. *Clinical Psychology Review, 39*, 1–15.

Biography.com (2015). *Howie Mandel.* Editors. https://www.biography.com/performer/howie-mandel

Borrell-Carrió, F., Suchman, A. L., & Epstein, R. M. (2004). The biopsychosocial model 25 years later: Principles, practice, and scientific inquiry. *Annuals of Family Medicine, 2*, 576–582.

Buhlmann, U., Glaesmer, H., Mewes, R., Fama, J. M., Wilhelm, S., Brähler, E., & Rief, W. (2010). Updates on the prevalence of body dysmorphic disorder: A population-based survey. *Psychiatry Research, 178*(1), 171–175.

Grant, J. E., Odlaug, B. L., Chamberlain, S. R., Keuthen, N. J., Lochner, C., & Stein, D. J. (2012). Skin picking disorder. *American Journal of Psychiatry, 169*, 1143–1149. https://doi.org/10.1176/appi.ajp.2012.12040508

Grant, J. E., & Chamberlain, S. R. (2016). Trichotillomania. *American Journal of Psychiatry, 173*, 868–874. https://doi.org/10.1176/appi.ajp.2016.15111432

Grant, J. G., Odlaug, B. L., & Chamberlain, S. R. (2016). *Why can't I stop?: Reclaiming your life from a behavioral addiction.* Johns Hopkins Press.

Haddad, J., Strauss, E. M., & Muir, D. (2009). Germs: "No deal" for host Howie Mandel. *ABC News.* https://abcnews.go.com/2020/howie-mandel-public-obsessive-compulisve-disorder-fear-germs/story?id=9153966

Hartmann, A. S., & Buhlmann, U. (2017). Body dysmorphic disorder. In S. Goldstein & M. DeVries (Eds.), *Handbook of DSM-5 disorders in children and adolescents* (pp. 233–248). Springer International Publishing.

Ivanov, V. Z., Mataix-Cols, D., Serlachius, E., Lichtenstein, P., Anckarsäter, H., Chang, Z., Gumpert, C. H., Lundström, S., Långström, N., & Rück, C. (2013). Prevalence, comorbidity and heritability of hoarding symptoms in adolescence: A population based twin study in 15-year olds. *PloS one, 8*(7), e69140.

March, J. S., & Benton, C. M. (2007). *Talking back to OCD.* The Guilford Press. https://doi.org/10.1371/journal.pone.0069140

National Institute of Mental Health (NIMH). (2020). *Obsessive-compulsive disorder.* https://www.nimh.nih.gov/health/topics/obsessive-compulsive-disorder-ocd/index.shtml

Nordsletten, A. E., Reichenberg, A., Hatch, S. L., de la Cruz, L. F., Pertusa, A., Hotopf, M., & Mataix-Cols, D. (2013). Epidemiology of hoarding disorder. *British Journal of Psychiatry, 203*, 445–452.

Odlaug, B. L., & Grant, J. E. (2008). Clinical characteristics and medical complications of pathologic skin picking. *General hospital psychiatry, 30*(1), 61–66. https://doi.org/10.1016/j.genhosppsych.2007.07.009

Pertusa, A., Frost, R. O., Fullana, M. A., Samuels, J., Steketee, G., Tolin, D., Saxena, S., Leckman, J. F., & Mataix-Cols, D. (2010). Refining the diagnostic boundaries of compulsive hoarding: A critical review. *Clinical Psychology Review, 30*(4), 371–386.

Ruscio, A. M., Stein, D. J., Chiu, W. T., & Kessler, R. C. (2010). The epidemiology of obsessive-compulsive disorder in the national comorbidity survey replication. *Molecular Psychiatry, 15*(1), 53.

Tierney, T. S., Abd-El-Barr, M. M., Stanford, A. D., Foote, K. D. & Okun, M. S. (2014). Deep brain stimulation and ablation for obsessive compulsive disorder: evolution of contemporary indications, targets and techniques, *International Journal of Neuroscience, 124*(6), 394–402, DOI: 10.3109/00207454.2013.852086

Veale, D., Miles, S., Smallcombe, N., Ghezai, H., Goldacre, B., & Hodsoll, J. (2014). Atypical antipsychotic augmentation in SSRI treatment refractory obsessive-compulsive disorder: A systematic review and meta-analysis. *BMC Psychiatry, 14*, 317.

World Health Organization (WHO). (2016). *International statistical classification of diseases and related health problems, 10th revision (ICD-10).*

Credits

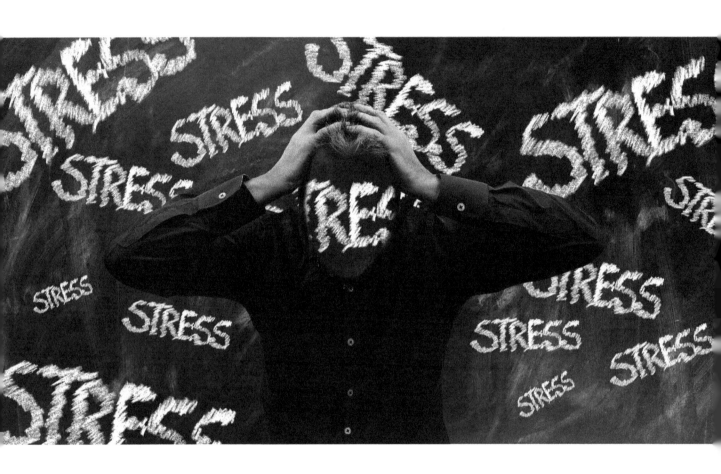

CHAPTER EIGHT

TRAUMA AND STRESSOR-RELATED DISORDERS

Brooke Wymer, Christopher J. Hipp, Liz Boyd, and David A. Scott

CASE STUDY 8.1 Lisbeth, 26, sits uneasily in the clinic waiting room. Her eyes are bloodshot from a lack of sleep, and her appearance is disheveled. As another client leaves the room, the door quietly clicks. Lisbeth jerks toward the noise with her full attention and braces until she ascertains that there is no threat. Once inside your office, she explains that 8 months ago she was walking home from the movies with a friend, Tatiana, when suddenly a man jumped out of an alley and began beating Tatiana. Lisbeth froze and watched as her friend was brutally beaten and then sexually assaulted in the alley. Only after the attacker ran away was Lisbeth able to call for help. Lisbeth has been reliving this event every night. She is ridden with guilt that it could have been her and that she should have gotten help for Tatiana sooner. Lisbeth has ceased going out at night because of her fear of another attack.

Overview

All of us will experience stress at some point in our lives, whether it manifests from an impending work deadline or exciting life event. From weddings and births to divorce and death and everything in between, stress happens. Stress is our body's protective response to stimuli, and it may cause physical, emotional, and mental reactions. This chapter provides an overview of trauma and stressor-related disorders identified in the *International Statistical Classification of Diseases* (ICD-10) and the *Diagnostic and Statistical Manual of Mental Disorders, 5th Edition* (DSM-5).

TABLE 8.1 *ICD-DSM* Comparison

ICD CODES	DSM-5 CODES
Disorders of social functioning with onset specific to childhood and adolescence (**F94**)	*Trauma and stressor-related disorders*
Reactive attachment disorder of childhood (F94.1) Symptoms are a result of severe social neglect or abuse and include irregularities and difficulty in the child's relating to caregivers and others, emotional reactivity	**Reactive attachment disorder (313.89)** Symptoms are a result of severe social neglect and could include the child not seeking and withdrawing from caregiver comfort when in distress

(continued)

Did You Know?

- In the United States, 7%–8% of the population will develop post-traumatic stress disorder in their lifetime (National Center for PTSD, 2019b).

- Women have a higher likelihood of developing post-traumatic stress disorder than men (NIMH, 2019).

- Following a traumatic experience, most individuals begin to experience post-traumatic stress disorder symptoms within 3 months. However, some develop symptoms later (NIMH, 2019).

- It has been found that post-traumatic stress disorder symptoms may intensify for aging veterans. A number of veterans report having symptoms 50 or more years after wartime (National Center for PTSD, 2020).

- Post-traumatic stress disorder and certain traumatic experiences have been linked to health conditions such as chronic pain and migraines (American Migraine Foundation, 2016). Of individuals who have chronic pain, around 15%–35% are also experiencing post-traumatic stress disorder (National Center for PTSD, 2019a).

- Having a strong support system and sound coping strategies to manage and resolve trauma symptoms as they arise are protective factors that may reduce the likelihood of a person developing post-traumatic stress disorder (NIMH, 2019).

TABLE 8.1 *Continued*

ICD CODES	*DSM-5* CODES
Disinhibited attachment disorder of childhood (F94.2) Symptoms could include deviations from normed social boundaries and indiscriminate social and physical contacts with unfamiliar adults, poor social skills with peers, and emotional/behavioral concerns	**Disinhibited social engagement disorder (313.89)** Symptoms are a result of severe deficits in care and could include deviations from normed social boundaries and indiscriminate social and physical contacts with unfamiliar adults
Reaction to severe stress, and adjustment disorders (**F43**)	
Post-traumatic stress disorder (F43.1) Symptoms could include intrusion, diminished emotional expression, withdrawal, avoidance, arousal, and impairment in cognitive and emotional functioning	**Post-traumatic stress disorder (309.81)** Symptoms could include intrusion, avoidance, arousal, and impairment in cognitive and emotional functioning
Acute stress reaction (F43.0) Symptoms could include hypervigilance, rumination, and fear	**Acute stress disorder (308.3)** Symptoms could include hypervigilance, rumination, and fear
Adjustment disorders (F43.2) **With depressed mood (F43.21)** Symptoms could include lethargy, apathy toward social activities, and negative thought patterns **With anxiety (F43.22)** Symptoms could include racing thoughts, nervousness, and physical reactions (e.g., increased heart rate) **With mixed anxiety and depressed mood (F43.23)** Symptoms could include any combination of symptoms from with depressed mood and with anxiety **With disturbance of conduct (F43.24)** Symptoms could include fighting, reenacting the traumatic event, and acting out (e.g., throwing things) **With mixed disturbance of emotions and conduct (F43.25)** Symptoms could include any combination of depressed mood, with anxiety, and with disturbance of conduct **Unspecified (F43.20)** Symptoms could include any other reaction not described by any other specifier	**Adjustment disorders (309.xx)** **With depressed mood (309.0)** Symptoms could include lethargy, apathy toward social activities, and negative thought patterns **With anxiety (309.24)** Symptoms could include racing thoughts, nervousness, and physical reactions (e.g., increased heart rate) **With mixed anxiety and depressed mood (309.28)** Symptoms could include any combination of symptoms from with depressed mood and with anxiety **With disturbance of conduct (309.3)** Symptoms could include fighting, reenacting the traumatic event, and acting out (e.g., throwing things) **With mixed disturbance of emotions and conduct (309.4)** Symptoms could include any combination of depressed mood, with anxiety, and with disturbance of conduct **Unspecified (309.9)** Symptoms could include any other reaction not described by any other specifier

Note: Adapted from ICD-10 (WHO, 2016); DSM-5 (American Psychiatric Association [APA], 2013)

Trauma and Stressor-Related Disorders

Trauma and stressor-related disorders have varying levels of symptom severity, diverse presentation, and a variety of effects on daily living and ability to cope. All the disorders in this chapter share one mutual criterion for diagnosis, which is that the person must have been exposed to a traumatic or stressful experience. For these disorders, the experienced trauma or stressor is considered to be the main cause of the person's symptomology.

Trauma and stressor-related disorders include the following:

- Reactive attachment disorder
- Disinhibited social engagement disorder
- Post-traumatic stress disorder
- Acute stress disorder
- Adjustment disorders

Reactive Attachment Disorder (F94.1) (313.89)

CASE STUDY 8.2 Amiir, 5, is brought to the clinic by his adoptive parents. His parents adopted him from a Somali orphanage 6 months prior. Somali is an extremely dangerous and war-torn country in east Africa. Amiir's birth father worked for Muslim warlords in his village and rarely interacted with Amiir. Amiir's mother, Sahro, was raped by Amiir's father and then forced to marry him against her will. She suffers from debilitating depression and pretended that Amiir did not exist. Most days, she would not feed Amiir, and he became malnourished. One day, Sahro left the hut and did not return, resulting in Amiir going to an orphanage. Amiir is withdrawn and appears listless most of the time. His adoptive mom cannot ever remember him smiling. His expression goes completely blank when either parent hugs him, and he does not hug them back. Last week, Amiir was pushed to the ground by one of his classmates. He refused to be comforted by teachers, peers, or his adoptive parents.

As is consistent across the *ICD-10* and *DSM-5*, reactive attachment disorder symptoms present and can be diagnosed between 9 months and 5 years old. The symptoms of reactive attachment disorder (RAD) are considered to be as a result of severe social neglect. However, these symptoms may occur when children have also experienced separation or abuse by parental caregivers early in their development. The most prominent *DSM-5* feature of reactive attachment disorder involves the child rarely seeking comfort from caregivers and withdrawing from caregivers' attempts to comfort them when distressed. As discussed in the *ICD-10*, reactive attachment disorder is also associated with irregularities and difficulties in the child's style of relating to others and can include emotional reactivity (e.g., increased irritability, aggression, despondence, being fearful and hyperalert to signs of danger), especially when their environment is altered. To be diagnosed using the *DSM-5*, the symptoms of reactive attachment disorder must be present for more than 12 months and can be specified as severe when the child is displaying all symptoms at substantial levels. Given that the cause of reactive attachment disorder is associated with severe neglect, developmental delays (e.g., language, cognition) and failure to thrive may also co-occur (World Health Organization [WHO], 2016).

The reactive attachment disorder diagnosis is controversial within the clinical field and has recently undergone changes to diagnostic criteria in the *DSM-5* and *ICD-10* (11), as previous versions have included both attachment and social behaviors that often led to misdiagnosis (Allen & Schuengel, 2020). Although reactive attachment disorder is actually exceptionally low in occurrence in children with adverse caregiving histories, the disorder is often overdiagnosed because of clinicians connecting it to significant child behavioral problems (Allen, 2018). Gleason and colleagues (2011) completed a study with 187 children under the age of 5 who spent an average of 86% of their lives living in Romanian orphanages and only 5% met the criteria for emotionally withdrawn/inhibited reactive attachment disorder at baseline. Studies also show that children diagnosed with reactive attachment disorder who are placed in sufficient and responsive caregiving environments show notable improvements over time (Zeanah & Gleason, 2015). In considering this disorder within the context of the case of Amiir, how will you relate to clients like Amiir who have experienced a great amount of suffering when you may not have experienced something similar? What are some things to consider in incorporating culture into your counseling with Amiir and his adoptive parents? Reactive attachment disorder is one of the only diagnoses given to young children. What other disorders might apply to children under 5 years of age?

Box 8.2　A Short History of Reactive Attachment Disorder and Disinhibited Social Engagement Disorder Diagnoses

- The reactive attachment disorder diagnosis in the *DSM-IV-TR* included two subtypes: inhibited and disinhibited subtype (Allen & Schuengel, 2020).
- The inhibited subtype in the *DSM-IV-TR* included symptoms similar to the current criteria for reactive attachment disorder, which involves a lack of seeking out or responding to caregivers' comfort (Gleason et al., 2011).
- The disinhibited subtype in the *DSM-IV-TR* included disorganized and inappropriate attachment to unknown adults (Gleason et al., 2011).
- The *ICD-10* separated these subtypes into two distinct disorders, which included reactive attachment disorder (with inhibited symptoms) and disinhibited attachment disorder of childhood (with disinhibited symptoms; Allen, 2018).
- The *DSM-5* followed suit and now separates the two subtypes into two distinct disorders: reactive attachment disorder and disinhibited social engagement disorder (Kliewer-Neumann et al., 2018).

Disinhibited Social Engagement Disorder (F94.2) (313.89)

Disinhibited social engagement disorder, also known in the *ICD-10* as disinhibited attachment disorder of childhood, presents before age 5. Across the *DSM-5* and *ICD-10*, disinhibited social engagement disorder is marked by deviations from normed social boundaries and includes indiscriminate social and physical contacts with unfamiliar adults (e.g., approaching strangers without apprehension, showing physical affection toward unknown individuals, readily leaving the presence of caregivers, and willingness to go away with unknown adults). According to the *ICD-10*, this disorder can also involve poor social skills with peers, as well as emotional and behavioral concerns. Similar to reactive attachment disorder, the *DSM-5* includes severe deficits in care (e.g., social neglect, frequent changes in parental caregivers, overcrowded institutional care) as being the cause of symptoms. Specifiers for disinhibited social engagement disorder in the *DSM-5* also involve the symptoms persisting for more than 12 months and can be considered severe if all symptoms are being exhibited at extreme levels. Consistent with reactive attachment disorder, cognitive and language delays, as well as physical signs of neglect may co-occur with disinhibited social engagement disorder. The prevalence of disinhibited social engagement disorder is also considered to be rare (Allen & Schuengel, 2020). In the aforementioned study by Gleason et al. (2011), only 32% of the children with inadequate early caregiving met the criteria for disinhibited social engagement disorder at baseline. Unlike reactive attachment disorder, disinhibited social engagement disorder symptoms are more likely to continue into childhood even when caregiving is enhanced (WHO, 2016). However, research around the prognosis of disinhibited social engagement disorder is inconclusive, with some children showing improvements with changes in adequate caregiving, while other children's symptoms persisted for longer periods of time (Zeanah et al., 2016).

CASE STUDY 8.3 Mia, 3, seems unable to differentiate between her foster parents and all other adults. Her foster father brings her to the clinic after an incident at the grocery store during the past week. While her mother was attending to the five other children with her on the shopping trip, Mia slipped away. They found her in the lap of a stranger at the front of the store. They were relieved that the stranger had told a manager about Mia and had the family paged over the intercom. If Mia had fallen into the wrong hands, things could have gone much worse. The current foster parents do not know much about Mia's upbringing. She was transferred to their family after child services had been called to Mia's previous foster home and the environment was found "unfit" for a child. It appeared the parents had not been there in several weeks, and there were animal feces everywhere.

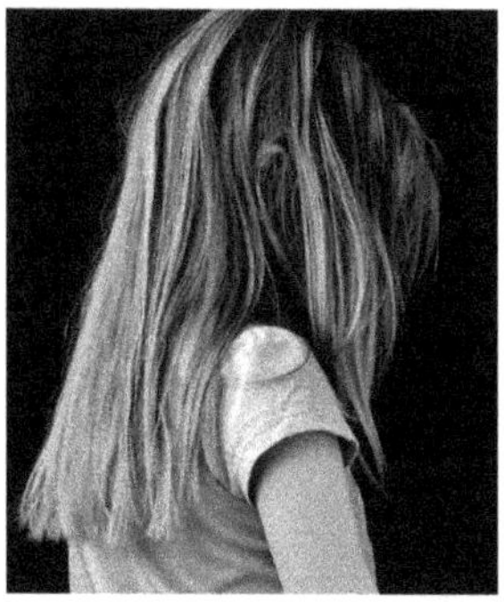

Given the case studies of Amiir and Mia, how is disinhibited social engagement disorder similar to reactive attachment disorder? If you had to make a diagnosis for these two children, what aspects of their cases would help you to identify the differences in the two disorders?

Image 8.2

Treatment Options

Zeanah et al. (2016) outlined treatment recommendations for reactive attachment disorder and disinhibited social engagement disorder with ratings based on empirical evidence of effectiveness. These recommendations included the need for extensive observational, diagnostic, and psychiatric assessment of attachment behaviors associated with reactive attachment disorder, disinhibited social engagement disorder, and other comorbid disorders for children who have a history of living in institutional settings, foster care, or adoptive placements (Zeanah et al., 2016). For reactive attachment disorder and disinhibited social engagement disorder, the intervention with the strongest empirical evidence is the child being in a safe placement with a committed, emotionally responsive caregiver. It is also recommended that therapeutic interventions should involve both the caregiver and child with a focus on building healthy attachments and positive parenting practices (Zeanah et al., 2016). Some treatments that show promise for intervention in cases of reactive attachment disorder and disinhibited social engagement disorder are child-parent psychotherapy (Ippen et al., 2014), circle of security (Humber, McMahon, & Sweller, 2016), and attachment and biobehavioral catch-up (Bick & Dozier, 2013). For children diagnosed with disinhibited social engagement disorder who also exhibit behavioral problems, the aforementioned attachment-focused interventions are indicated and may be enhanced by the addition of parent-child interaction therapy (Eyberg et al., 2008) or multisystemic therapy (Ogden & Hagen, 2006). There are no empirical studies to support the use of pharmacological interventions for children with reactive attachment disorder or disinhibited social engagement disorder (Zeanah et al., 2016). How would you apply these treatment recommendations to the cases of Amiir and Mia?

Post-Traumatic Stress Disorder (F43.1) (309.81)

Post-traumatic stress disorder occurs in individuals of any age who have experienced at least one extremely distressing event where they believed themselves or someone else was in a life-threatening, dangerous, or harmful situation (Substance Abuse and Mental Health Services Administration [SAMHSA], 2019). According to the National Center for PTSD, 60% of men and 50% of women will have at least one traumatic experience during their lifetimes. Women are at a greater risk for experiencing trauma in the form of sexual violence as an adult or child. Men are at a higher risk of experiencing trauma in the form of physical violence, a serious accident or disaster, combat during war, or witnessing someone dying or being seriously injured (U.S. Department of Veterans Affairs, 2019). Of the children who responded to the National Survey of Children's Exposure to Violence, approximately 61% reported experiencing or witnessing a traumatic event (Hamblen & Barnett, 2019). In a sample of children aged 12–17, they most frequently reported experiencing sexual abuse (8%), physical abuse (17%), and witnessing violence (39%; SAMHSA, 2015). While all individuals are likely to experience some psychological effects from trauma immediately following the experience, most will not develop post-traumatic stress disorder (National Institute of Mental Health [NIMH], 2019).

Both the *DSM-5* and the *ICD-10* require that a person has experienced a traumatic event to receive a diagnosis of post-traumatic stress disorder. The *DSM-5* also considers a person as meeting criterion for having experienced trauma when they witness a traumatic event, are made aware of the details of a loved one's traumatic experience or sudden death, or are exposed to the details of a person's trauma in their professional capacity (e.g., law enforcement, medical personnel, counselors, social workers). Symptoms included in the criteria for diagnosis across the *DSM-5* and the *ICD-10* include

Box 8.3 How Trauma Affects the Developing Brain

When trauma occurs in the early years, children's brain development can be affected (Klorer, 2011). Chronic trauma exposure causes constant activation of the stress hormone system ("fight or flight" response), which eventually leads to children experiencing persistent hyperarousal, increased sensitivity to stress, and changes in the brain's structure and functioning (Perry, 2009). Chronic trauma exposure can cause the brain to go into survival mode and decreases the brain's capacity to process new information for learning (Ford, 2009). Trauma affects children's brain function in the following areas:

- Effects on language and speech development (van der Kolk, 2003)
- Delays in cognitive and lower IQ (Hart & Rubia, 2012)
- Reduced size of the hippocampus and diminished memory retrieval (Bremner, 2001)
- Negative responses in the functioning of the amygdala and prefrontal cortex, which are responsible for emotional regulation and executive functioning (McLaughlin et al., 2014)
- Difficulty maintaining concentration and attention (DeBellis, Hooper, Spratt, & Woolley, 2009)

It is important to note that not all children who experience trauma will develop post-traumatic stress disorder or prolonged stress responses (National Child Traumatic Stress Network [NCTSN], 2016). For children with this disorder or long-term effects related to chronic stress, resilience is still possible. Children's resilience is enhanced when they have the following (NCSTN, 2016): (a) a close, healthy relationship with a primary caregiver; (b) other social, community, and familial supports; and (c) safe and supportive environments (e.g., school). Trauma-focused treatment interventions also significantly reduce long-term effects of trauma on children (Dorsey et al., 2017). How could you support the fostering of resilience in children who have experienced trauma in your work?

intrusive experiences related to the trauma (e.g., intrusive thoughts or memories, nightmares, feeling or acting as if one is reliving the traumatic event, emotional and physical reactivity to reminders). Avoidance symptoms are also common across both diagnostic tools and involve the individual avoiding thinking about the trauma and avoiding people, places, and things that remind them of the trauma. Moreover, both the *ICD-10* and *DSM-5* include criteria associated with significant impairment in cognitions and emotional functioning related to the trauma that may lead to depression, suicidal ideation, anxiety, and withdrawal from relationships and previously enjoyed activities. Finally, diagnostic criteria for post-traumatic stress disorder in both tools contain arousal symptoms, which may include hypervigilance, being alert to signs of danger, getting startled easily, irritability, difficulty concentrating, and risk-taking behaviors.

While post-traumatic stress disorder can be diagnosed in persons of any age, the *DSM-5* has criteria specific to children under the age of 6. Symptoms in children may differ in presentation and sometimes include regressive behaviors (e.g., enuresis, difficulty with verbal expression, clinging to a parent) and reenacting the traumatic experience in play (NIMH, 2019). In the *DSM-5*, symptoms must persist for longer than 1 month and cause substantial impairment in daily functioning not caused by substance use or other medical concerns. Specifiers in the *DSM-5* that can be included in the diagnosis of post-traumatic stress disorder include dissociative symptoms and a delay in symptom presentation at 6 months or later following the traumatic experience. The post-traumatic stress disorder diagnosis is given to approximately 10% of women and 4% of men at some point in their lifetimes (U.S. Department of Veterans Affairs, 2019). Around 15.9% of children and youth have a diagnosis of post-traumatic stress disorder (Alisic et al., 2014). For individuals who develop post-traumatic stress disorder, symptoms are prolonged and cause impairment for 10%–20% (Fletcher et al., 2010; Norris & Sloane, 2007). Therefore, effective treatments for post-traumatic stress disorder are essential. Reflecting back on Lisbeth, what symptoms is she exhibiting that indicate a potential post-traumatic stress disorder diagnosis? What additional information might be important to know before making a diagnosis? How would you go about gathering all of the information you need?

Box 8.4 Post-Traumatic Growth

Have you, or someone you know, faced a challenging life event and feel as though you, or they, came out stronger because of it? If so, you, or they, may have experienced post-traumatic growth. Tedeschi and Calhoun (2004) described post-traumatic growth as the "positive psychological changes experienced as a result of the struggle with highly challenging life circumstances" (p. 1). They also identified five areas, or domains, where growth typically occurs:

1   ***Personal Strength.*** Recognition of the strength and courage shown as moving through trauma
2   ***Relationships With Others.*** Typically close family and friends
3   ***New Possibilities.*** Finding new ways to fill roles and time
4   ***Appreciation of Life.*** Increased willingness to live spontaneously
5   ***Spiritual Changes.*** Seek meaning, reexamine how they are living

As a helping professional who is facilitating post-traumatic growth, it is critical to process the negative emotions while also focusing on growth. How do you think you could use post-traumatic growth in your work with clients who have experienced trauma?

Treatment Options

Outlined by Ostacher and Cifu (2019), evidence-based practice guidelines for the treatment of post-traumatic stress disorder include recommendations that interventions should include individual, trauma-focused psychotherapy that is manualized and incorporates exposure and cognitive restructuring techniques. These treatments are recommended over pharmacological intervention. In addition, there is little empirical evidence that pharmacotherapy is effective even when used in conjunction with trauma-focused psychotherapy for post-traumatic stress disorder (Ostacher & Cifu, 2019). In Cusack et al.'s (2016) meta-analysis and systematic review of adult post-traumatic stress disorder treatments, the following treatments were found to be sufficiently supported by empirical evidence: (a) exposure therapies (e.g., prolonged exposure therapy), (b) cognitive therapies (e.g., cognitive processing therapy), (c) cognitive behavioral therapies (CBT), (d) eye movement desensitization and reprocessing therapy (EMDR), and (e) narrative exposure therapy. For children diagnosed with post-traumatic stress disorder, clinical interventions that use individual and group CBT, as well as child-focused CBT with parental involvement (e.g., trauma-focused cognitive behavioral therapy [TF-CBT]) have the highest empirical evidence (Dorsey et al., 2017). In Dorsey and colleagues' review (2017), interventions with a developing empirical base for child post-traumatic stress disorder treatment included EMDR, integrated therapy for complex trauma responses, and child-centered play therapy. According to the California Evidence-Based Clearinghouse for Child Welfare (2020), EMDR, Prolonged Exposure Therapy for Adolescents, and TF-CBT have the highest evidence base for treatment of post-traumatic stress disorder in children and youth. If you were working with Lisbeth, which treatment modality do you think would be most effective?

CLINICIAN'S CORNER 8.1

Post-Traumatic Stress Disorder

Most of my clinical experiences have been working with children and families following trauma, specifically sexual abuse. One of the things that I believe makes this work so rewarding is witnessing the resilience of children despite having gone through such adverse experiences. Not only do children often greatly benefit from evidence-based, trauma-focused interventions, but they often thrive when they have *the support of a caregiver* during the treatment process. Sometimes this can be a challenge if the child is in foster care, living in a group home, or has a parent who is not far enough along in their own healing process to support them. Therefore, the clinician, in collaboration with child protection agencies, may have to be *creative in engaging supports* for the child in these circumstances, which could include involving peers, siblings, extended family members, case managers, foster parents, and mentors. The key here is to allow the child to have a *choice* in deciding who they trust and believe can support them during treatment.

Beyond support being a significant factor in the child's healing process, it is also important to assist the child in *making meaning of their experiences.* This often occurs during the termination phase of evidence-based treatment intervention. It can truly enhance the healing process when children are able to find purpose and meaning in moving forward after a traumatic event. This may look like the child wanting to help other children who have had a similar experience or wanting to do something to prevent another child from having this experience. Some examples of how I've seen children do this are creating their own public service announcements, writing and illustrating their own books, or developing a puppet show about how to be safe. It can be an empowering experience for the child to feel they are able to find meaning and purpose at the culmination of their treatment process. In addition, it is just as important for the clinician to find the same meaning and purpose in doing this type of work because it can be taxing. However, I believe there is no work more meaningful than this!

Brooke Wymer, PhD, MSW, LISW-CP/S

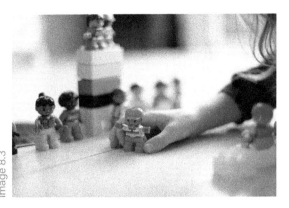

Image 8.3

Acute Stress Disorder (F43.0) (308.3)

Acute stress disorder (ASD) was added to the *DSM-IV* (APA, 1994) as there was no diagnosis that addressed the immediate psychological effects of experiencing traumatic events (Bryant, 2017). Post-traumatic stress disorder could not be diagnosed until 1 month after exposure to the traumatic event (APA, 1994). As such, acute stress disorder was originally introduced as a billable diagnosis for individuals to receive mental health treatment within the first month of experiencing a traumatic event and to hinder the potential development of post-traumatic stress disorder; however, more recent studies suggest a diagnosis of acute stress disorder does not automatically set a client up for a future diagnosis of post-traumatic stress disorder (Brown et al., 2016; Bryant, 2018; Meiser-Stedman et al., 2017).

A *DSM-5* (APA, 2013) diagnosis of acute stress disorder consists of (a) exposure to a traumatic event; (b) exhibiting nine out of 14 symptoms from any combination of negative mood, dissociative features, avoidance, or arousal; (c) symptom expression occurs within 3 days of the traumatic event and lasts between 3 days and 1 month; (d) traumatic stress; and (e) the symptoms cannot be better explained by another mental health or medical diagnosis. In the *ICD-10* (WHO, 2016), acute stress disorder is termed acute stress reaction, with similar symptomology to the *DSM-5*. Furthermore, *ICD-10* focuses acute stress reaction symptomology on the cognitive, emotional, and/or behavioral reactions to crises, traumas, and combat scenarios.

Acute stress disorder prevalence rates do not coincide with the experiencing of traumatic events. Individuals who experience the same traumatic event will not necessarily manifest trauma-based symptoms that require an acute stress disorder diagnosis or require treatment. Furthermore, Bryant (2017, 2018) reported that individuals who experience a traumatic event may not meet criteria for acute stress disorder but manifest symptomology that requires a post-traumatic stress disorder diagnosis in the future. Some individuals will experience short periods of stress and will recover without seeking professional assistance. Other individuals may require professional help and exhibit symptoms that require a diagnosis of acute stress disorder or another mental health diagnosis.

The prevalence of acute stress disorder diagnosis after experiencing a traumatic event is less than 20% (APA, 2013). Because people respond differently to traumatic events, prevalence rates vary depending on the traumatic event experienced by individuals. For example, prevalence rates of acute stress disorder range from 24% to 40.6% after experiencing violence (Ophuis et al., 2018), 38% following a bank robbery (Frans et al., 2018), 31% of children and adolescent burn victims (Saxe et al., 2005), and 62% of Hurricane Katrina survivors (Kavan et al., 2012).

Individuals diagnosed with acute stress disorder can exhibit a wide range of symptomology based on the client having to meet nine out of 14 descriptive symptoms. The effect of acute stress disorder on an individual's functioning depends on the specific symptoms reported. For example, a client with intrusive thoughts, negative mood, avoidance, and arousal symptoms can have impairment in their daily functioning. Intrusive thoughts can affect an individual's ability to process the traumatic event, which can snowball into focusing on the negative, which produces the inability to experience positive emotions or feelings. Adding avoidance and arousal symptoms to those intrusive thoughts and a negative mood would affect the client's behavioral responses, which would influence the client's experienced consequences. Without intervention, the individual's symptoms could evolve into chronic disorders (e.g., post-traumatic stress disorders or major depressive disorder). It is, therefore, recommended that early screening of individuals who experienced a traumatic event could reduce the risk of chronic symptomology (Meiser-Stedman et al., 2017).

Treatment Options

There are multiple treatment options for acute stress disorder. TF-CBT is highly recommended for an individual diagnosed with acute stress disorder (Bryant, 2017, 2018; Guay et al., 2018). In conjunction with TF-CBT, other forms of therapy include exposure therapies, cognitive restructuring from cognitive therapy, psychoeducation and normalization, and anxiety/stress management techniques (Bryant, 2018; Kavan et al., 2012). According to researchers, there are currently no recommended pharmacological interventions approved in the United States for acute stress disorder.

CASE STUDY 8.4 Clara, 24, works at a school full time and takes graduate classes part time for educational leadership. She hopes one day to be the vice president of a university. On her way to work 3 months ago, she experienced a traumatic event. A coworker was driving in front of her and was hit by a semitruck driver who ran a red light. The car rolled three times, and Clara saw her friend's body tossed around the car. Clara managed to call 911 and then rushed to her friend. The images of the accident haunt Clara. Her boyfriend tells her that she has seemed depressed since the accident. She has little interest in sex and no longer wants to go out to bars with her friends. Clara avoids the area where the accident took place, even though she has to drive several miles further to avoid it. She sleeps fitfully for 3 or 4 hours a night with nightmares before giving up and getting out of bed. Sometimes she feels like another person watching her life instead of an active participant. Upon her boyfriend's urging, she came to the clinic.

CASE STUDY 8.5 Harrison, 56, has been on the police force for more than 30 years. He has seen more than his fair share of trauma, working primarily with crimes involving children. In the last few years, his wife has noticed a change in his behavior. Harrison has been unable to get a good night's sleep, and when he does sleep, he is tortured by nightmares. He never seems to be happy, and things that once interested him do not seem to be important anymore. Harrison discloses that he keeps re-experiencing a memory of the coroner bringing a child's body out of a home. The parents chronically abused their children, but Department of Social Services never found enough proof to remove the children from the home. Harrison is "jumpy" and immediately alert in response to small noises. His wife encourages him to go to the clinic.

How is acute stress disorder different from post-traumatic stress disorder? Would you diagnose Clara with acute stress disorder or post-traumatic stress disorder? Would you diagnose Harrison with acute stress disorder or post-traumatic stress disorder? Why? Discuss some treatment options for Clara and Harrison. What are some ways to

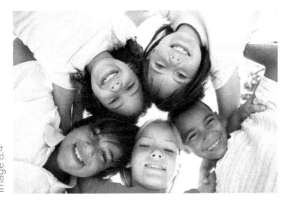

prevent burnout in professions like police work, counseling, and social work where individuals deal with vicarious trauma daily?

Adjustment Disorders (F43.2) (309.xx)

A diagnosis of adjustment disorder occurs when individuals experience a traumatic event and express a heightened response that exceeds the response that would typically occur (i.e., level of dysfunction, impairment, and behavioral change) within 3 months of the triggering event, and the symptoms do not meet any other disorder, particularly acute stress disorder or post-traumatic stress disorder (Strain, 2018; Yaseen, 2017). Also, once the stressor is removed, the client's symptoms subside within 6 months and cannot be culturally appropriate or normal expressions of bereavement (APA, 2013; Casey, 2009; O'Donnell et al., 2019). Specifiers include symptoms associated with depression, anxiety, behavioral changes, mixed depression and anxiety, mixed behavioral changes and mood changes, and an unspecified option (APA, 2013). The *ICD-10* specifies symptom expression within 1 month of the stressor. Furthermore, the *ICD-10* differentiates depressive symptomology to brief (<1 month) and prolonged (<2 years), while the *DSM-5* differentiates acute or chronic by symptoms occurring for less than or greater than 6 months, respectively (Bachem & Casey, 2018).

Adjustment disorders are some of the most commonly diagnosed mental health disorders (Ben-Ezra et al., 2018; Strain, 2018). The prevalence of adjustment disorder ranged between 0.5% and 2% of the population up to 50% in targeted population studies (O'Donnell et al., 2019; Strain, 2018). Females are diagnosed at higher rates than males (Casey, 2009). Have you ever experienced adjustment disorder or known someone who has? Explain what it looks like.

CASE STUDY 8.6 Emma, 19, does not remember being happy since moving away from home. After her senior year in college, she was excited to leave her hometown and go on to an exciting college environment. In high school, Emma did not have to try to make friends. It seemed like everyone knew each other, and she never struggled to make plans. She was well liked and excelled in school. College is a different story. The schoolwork is difficult, and making friends is even harder. After an initial attempt to meet people, Emma was left feeling even more alone. She went to a party but hardly talked to anyone, and the people she did talk to seemed more interested in partying than studies. Emma has always been introverted and studious and felt awkwardly out of place at the party. Since then, she has withdrawn into her studies and spends most of her time alone in her room. She goes home every weekend to see her parents and friends who are still around, but it doesn't feel like home anymore. She is considering dropping out and moving back home.

Adjustment disorder's effect on client functioning depends on the specifier. Individuals with the specifier *with depressed mood* may exhibit similar symptoms to a depressive episode, while individuals with the specifier *with anxiety* can exhibit similar symptoms to an anxiety disorder. Furthermore, disturbance of conduct can be seen through behavioral changes, such as acting out and fighting. As such, an individual diagnosed with an adjustment disorder can have decreased quality of life and a potential of legal issues if disturbance of conduct involves fighting and acting out that causes bodily or property harm. In the case of Emma, would you diagnose adjustment disorder? Which specifier matches her symptoms?

Another area that a diagnosis of adjustment disorder can affect is the heightened prevalence of suicidal ideation/behavior and self-harm behavior. Researchers reported individuals expressing adjustment disorder symptomology had earlier presentations of suicidal behavior, suicidal ideation with less symptom expression, and shortened elapsed time from ideation to attempts compared to individuals with major depressive disorder (Bachem & Casey, 2018; O'Donnell et al., 2019). Another study emphasized the importance of clinicians screening clients diagnosed with adjustment disorder, as 25% reported a history of suicide attempts and 60% reported a history of self-harm activities. In the case of Emma, consider what makes adjustment disorder different than just experiencing a change or a difficult life circumstance? What do you think happens if adjustment disorder is not dealt with?

Treatment Options

Several researchers suggested psychotherapy interventions focus on brief and symptom-focused therapies that build client awareness of how symptoms affect their lives and their role in building empowerment through resiliency techniques to reduce symptoms (e.g., Bachem & Casey, 2018; Eimontas et al., 2018). For example, CBT (found to be most efficacious; O'Donnell et al., 2018) focuses on the trigger to thoughts, emotions, and behaviors and how those behavioral responses create positive or negative consequences for the individual (Strain, 2018). If an individual can change their thoughts, emotions, and behavioral reactions to the trigger, then they can experience the consequences they wish.

Other forms of treatment recommended are client-centered psychotherapy, psychodynamic therapy, relaxation-based therapies, behavioral therapy, Gestalt psychotherapy, and meditation, while reality therapy and self-help treatments are building a research base (Bachem & Casey, 2018; O'Donnell et al., 2018). Future interventions may involve using software programs to provide support to the client through computer modules, along with psychological support from a clinician, if needed (Eimontas et al., 2018). Currently, there are no pharmacological interventions specifically for adjustment disorder (Greiner et al., 2020); however, Bachem and Casey (2018) suggested the potential use of medications that combat the target symptoms from the particular specifier. What do you think may be an effective treatment option for Emma?

Case Study Summary

One of this chapter's case studies reviewed the behaviors of Lisbeth. As you process the story and examine possible diagnostic criteria, take a few minutes to answer the following questions:

1. What would be the correct diagnosis for Lisbeth?

    _____

    _____

2. What are the specific symptoms or criteria that led you to this diagnosis?

_____

_____

3. What other possible disorders might you diagnose Lisbeth with and why?

_____

_____

4. Briefly discuss what types of treatment may be beneficial for Lisbeth. Could you see using a certain counseling theory and/or medication?

_____

_____

Guided Practice Exercises

Scenario 1

Solomon, 64, recently moved from Africa to the United States with his partner of 28 years. His partner discloses that Solomon is often awake at night and will occasionally rouse him, warning that a lethal African tribe is outside of the house. It turns out, when Solomon was a teenager, a neighboring tribe raided his village. Solomon was in the village with friends but returned home as his house was burning down with his family inside. He ran inside to try to save his parents, grandparents, and two siblings but to no avail. He was rescued and spent several weeks in the hospital with third-degree burns on his extremities. The helpless and hopeless feelings evoked from this experience have characterized his life for years. He blames himself for not being home to protect his family and for their deaths. He is ridden with guilt that he survived and nobody else did. He avoids all fires, including birthday candles and gas stoves, as they seem to trigger something negative in him. In addition, Solomon has flashbacks of the trauma from time to time. In response, he often drops to the ground and rocks in the fetal position.

What would be the correct disorder? What are the specific symptoms or criteria that led you to this diagnosis?

_____

_____

_____

What specific behaviors caused you to diagnose the disorder?

_____

_____

_____

What other possible disorders might you diagnose Solomon with and why?

_____

_____

_____

Scenario 2

Jacob, 26, has been living alone since Sherri, his wife of 4 years, moved out. They were high school sweethearts, and the early years of their relationship were filled with traveling and good times with friends and family. Since Jacob finished law school 2 years ago, their relationship has been on the rocks. Jacob is a successful and ambitious attorney, often working 12–14 hour days. He hopes to become a partner in his firm and has committed to working hard for as long as it takes. His dedication to his job appeared to be his priority, as he would often cancel plans with Sherri to finish projects at work. Sherri also wanted to have children, but Jacob did not feel that it was the right time. He would never suggest when the time would be right, leaving Sherri disheartened. When Sherri left, Jacob felt like his life was falling apart. His friends and family assured him that it was normal to feel this way in his situation. The problem is that it has been 5 months, and Jacob only seems to be getting worse. He has missed a lot of work deadlines recently, which is completely uncharacteristic of him. Beyond the concern in his workplace, several of his closest friends believe he is blowing them off. He is not up to doing anything, including golf, one of his favorite pastimes.

What would be the correct disorder? What are the specific symptoms or criteria that led you to this diagnosis?

_____

_____

_____

What specific behaviors caused you to diagnose the disorder?

_____

_____

_____

What other possible disorders might you diagnose Jacob with and why?

_____

_____

_____

Web-Based and Literature-Based Resources

Mental Health Provider Resources for Reactive Attachment Disorder and Disinhibited Social Engagement Disorder

https://childmind.org/guide/reactive-attachment-disorder/

http://circleofsecuritynetwork.org/

https://www.circleofsecurityinternational.com/

http://www.pcit.org/

https://www.childwelfare.gov/pubPDFs/f_interactbulletin.pdf

https://www.nctsn.org/interventions/child-parent-psychotherapy

https://childparentpsychotherapy.com/

https://youth.gov/content/multisystemic-therapy-mst

http://www.abcintervention.org/

Mental Health Provider Resources for Post-Traumatic Stress Disorder in Adults

https://www.integration.samhsa.gov/clinical-practice/trauma

https://www.acesconnection.com/

https://www.ptsd.va.gov/

https://www.integration.samhsa.gov/clinical-practice/SAMSA_TIP_Trauma.pdf

https://www.integration.samhsa.gov/clinical-practice/screening-tools#TRAUMA

https://www.nimh.nih.gov/health/topics/coping-with-traumatic-events/index.shtml

https://istss.org/home

https://www.nimh.nih.gov/health/publications/post-traumatic-stress-disorder-ptsd/index.shtml

Mental Health Provider Resources for Post-Traumatic Stress Disorder in Children

https://www.nctsn.org/

https://www.samhsa.gov/child-trauma/recognizing-and-treating-child-traumatic-stress

https://www.apsac.org/

https://www.nationalcac.org/

https://www.ncbi.nlm.nih.gov/books/NBK519712/table/ch3.t4/

https://www.cebc4cw.org/search/results/?keyword=PTSD

https://www.cdc.gov/childrensmentalhealth/ptsd.html

https://www.nctsn.org/resources/it-adhd-or-child-traumatic-stress-guide-clinicians

https://tfcbt.org/wp-content/uploads/2014/07/Your-Very-Own-TF-CBT-Workbook-Final.pdf

https://www.ptsd.va.gov/professional/treat/specific/ptsd_child_teens.asp

Mental Health Provider Resources for Stress

https://www.therapistaid.com/

Mental Health Provider Resources for Acute Stress Disorder

https://www.ptsd.va.gov/professional/treat/essentials/acute_stress_disorder.asp

https://childmind.org/guide/guide-acute-stress-disorder/

https://nami.org/Support-Education/Support-Groups

Mental Health Provider Resources for Adjustment Disorders

https://www.psychologytoday.com/us/conditions/adjustment-disorder

https://childmind.org/guide/guide-adjustment-disorder/treatment/

https://psychcentral.com/disorders/adjustment-disorder-symptoms/
adjustment-disorder-treatment/

Bibliotherapy Resources for Mental Health Providers

Armstrong, C. (2019). *Rethinking trauma treatment: Attachment, memory reconsolidation, and resilience.* W. W. Norton & Company.

Bryant, R. A. (2016). *Acute stress disorder: What it is and how to treat it.* Guilford Press.

Cohen, J. A., Mannarino, A. P., & Deblinger, E. (2006). *Treating trauma and traumatic grief in children and adolescents.* Guilford Press.

Deblinger, E., Cohen, J. A., & Mannarino, A. P. (2012). Introduction. In J. A. Cohen, A. P. Mannarino, & E. Deblinger (Eds.), *Trauma-focused CBT for children and adolescents: Treatment applications (pp 1-3.).* Guildford Press.

Friedman, M. J. (2015). *Posttraumatic and acute stress disorders* (6th ed.). Springer.

Van der Kolk, B. A. (2014). *The body keeps the score: Brain, mind, and body in the healing of trauma.* Viking.

References

Alisic, E., Zalta, A. K., Van Wesel, F., Larsen, S. E., Hafstad, G. S., Hassanpour, K., & Smid, G. E. (2014). Rates of post-traumatic stress disorder in trauma-exposed children and adolescents: Meta-analysis. *British Journal of Psychiatry, 204*, 335–340. https://doi.org/10.1192/bjp.bp.113.131227

Allen, B. (2018). Misperceptions of reactive attachment disorder persist: Poor methods and unsupported conclusions. *Research in Developmental Disabilities, 77*, 24–29. https://doi.org/10.1016/j.ridd.2018.03.012

Allen, B. & Schuengel, C. (2020). Attachment disorders diagnosed by community practitioners: A replication and extension. *Child and Adolescent Mental Health, 25*(1), 4–10. https://doi.org/10.1111/camh.12338

American Migraine Foundation. (2016). Abuse, maltreatment, and PTSD and their relationship to migraine. https://americanmigrainefoundation.org/resource-library/abuse-maltreatment-and-ptsd-and-their-relationship-to-migraine/

American Psychiatric Association. (1994). *Diagnostic and statistical manual of mental disorders* (4th ed.).

American Psychiatric Association (APA). (2013). *Diagnostic and statistical manual of mental disorders* (5th ed.).

Bachem, R., & Casey, P. (2018). Adjustment disorder: A diagnosis whose time has come. *Journal of Affective Disorders, 227*, 243–253.

Ben-Ezra, M., Mahat-Shamir, M., Lorenz, L., Lavenda, O., & Maercker, A. (2018). Screening of adjustment disorder: Scale based on the ICD-11 and the adjustment disorder new module. *Journal of Psychiatric Research, 103*, 91–96.

Bick, J., & Dozier, M. (2013). The effectiveness of an attachment-based intervention in promoting foster mother's sensitivity toward foster infants. *Infant Mental Health Journal, 34*(2), 93–103.

Bremner, J. D. (2001). A biological model for delayed recall of childhood abuse. *Journal of Aggression, Maltreatment and Trauma, 4*(2), 165–183. https://doi.org/10.1300/J146v04n02_08

Brown, R. C., Nugent, N. R., Hawn, S. E., Koenen, K. C., Miller, A., Amstadter, A. B., & Saxe, G. (2016). Predicting the transition from acute stress disorder to posttraumatic stress disorder in children with severe injuries. *Journal of Pediatric Health Care, 30*(6), 558–568.

Bryant, R. A. (2017). Acute stress disorder. *Current Opinion in Psychology, 14*, 127–131.

Bryant, R. A. (2018). The current evidence for acute stress disorder. *Current Psychiatry Reports, 20*(12), 111.

California Evidence-Based Clearinghouse for Child Welfare. (2019). *Program registry: Programs.* https://www.cebc4cw.org/search/results/?keyword=&scientific_rating%5B%5D=1&program_topics%5B%5D=45&program_topics%5B%5D=46&q_search=Search&realm=advanced

Casey, P. (2009). Adjustment disorder: Epidemiology, diagnosis and treatment. *CNS Drugs, 23*(11), 927–938.

Cusack, K., Jonas, D. E., Forneris, C. A., Wines, C., Sonis, J., Middleton, J. C., Feltner, C., Brownley, K. A., Olmsted, K. R., Greenblatt, A., Weil, A., & Gaynes, B. N. (2016). Psychological treatments for adults with posttraumatic stress disorder: A systematic review and meta-analysis. *Clinical Psychology Review, 43*, 128–141. https://doi.org/10.1016/j.cpr2015.10.003

DeBellis, M. D., Hooper, S. R., Spratt, E. G., & Woolley, D. P. (2009). Neuropsychological findings in childhood neglect and their relationships to pediatric PTSD. *Journal of the International Neuropsychological Society, 15*, 868–878.

Dorsey, S., McLaughlin, K. A., Kerns, S., Harrison, J. P., Lambert, H. K., Briggs, E. C., Revillion Cox, J., & Amaya-Jackson, L. (2017). Evidence Base Update for Psychosocial Treatments for Children and Adolescents Exposed to Traumatic Events. *Journal of clinical child and adolescent psychology : the official journal for the Society of Clinical Child and Adolescent Psychology, American Psychological Association, Division 53, 46*(3), 303–330. https://doi.org/10.1080/15374416.2016.1220309

Eimontas, J., Gegieckaite, G., Dovydaitiene, M., Mazulyte, E., Rimsaite, Z., Skruibis, P., Zelviene, P., & Kazlauskas, E. (2018). The role of therapist support on effectiveness of an internet-based modular self-help intervention or adjustment disorder: A randomized controlled trial. *Anxiety Stress Coping, 31*(2), 146–158. https://doi.org/10.1080/10615806.2017.138506

Eyberg, S., Nelson, M., & Boggs, S. (2008). Evidence-based psychosocial treatments for children and adolescents with disruptive behavior. *Journal of Clinical Child & Adolescent Psychiatry, 37*, 215–237.

Fletcher, S., Creamer, M., & Forbes, D. (2010). Preventing post-traumatic stress disorder: Are drugs the answer? [Review]. *Australian and New Zealand Journal of Psychiatry, 44*(12), 1064–1071.

Ford, J. D. (2009). Neurobiological and developmental research: clinical implications. In C. A. Courtois & J. D. Ford (Eds.), *Treating complex traumatic stress disorders: An evidence-based guide* (pp. 31–58). Guilford Press.

Frans, Ö., Åhs, J., Bihre, E., & Åhs, F. (2018). Distance to threat and risk of acute and posttraumatic stress disorder following bank robbery: A longitudinal study. *Psychiatry Research, 267*, 461–466.

Gleason, M. M., Fox, N. A., Drury, S., Smyke, A., Egger, H. L., Nelson III, C. A., Gregas, M. C., & Zeanah, C. H. (2011). Validity of evidence-derived criteria for reactive attachment disorder: Indiscriminately social/disinhibited and emotionally withdrawn/inhibited types. *Journal of the American Academy of Child & Adolescent Psychiatry, 50*(3), 216-231.

Greiner, T., Haack, B., Toto, S., Bleich, S., Grohmann, R., Faltraco, F., Heinze, M., & Schneider, M. (2020). Pharmacotherapy of psychiatric inpatients with adjustment disorder: Current status and changes between 2000 and 2016. *European Archives of Psychiatry and Clinical Neuroscience, 270*(1), 107–117.

Guay, S., Sader, J., Boyer, R., & Marchand, A. (2018). Treatment of acute stress disorder for victims of violent crime. *Journal of Affective Disorders, 241*, 15–21.

Hamblen, J., & Barnett, E. (2019). *PTSD in children and adolescents.* National Center for PTSD. https://www.ptsd.va.gov/professional/treat/specific/ptsd_child_teens.asp

Hart, H., & Rubia, K. (2012). Neuroimaging of child abuse: a critical review. *Frontiers in Human Neuroscience, 6*, 52.

Humber, A., McMahon, C., & Sweller, N. (2016). Improved parental emotional functioning after circle of security 20-week parent-child relationship intervention. *Journal of Child and Family Studies, 25*, 2526–2540.

Ippen, C. G., Norona, C., & Lieberman, A. (2014). Clinical considerations for conducting child-parent psychotherapy with young children with developmental disabilities who have experienced trauma. *PCSP: Pragmatic Care Studies in Psychotherapy, 10*(3), 196–211.

Kavan, M. G., Elsasser, G. N., & Barone, E. J. (2012). The physician's role in managing acute stress disorder. *American Family Physician, 86*(7), 643–649.

Kliewer-Neumann, J. D., Zimmerman, J., Bovenschen, I., Gabler, S., Lang, K., Spangler, G., & Nowacki, K. (2018). Assessment of attachment disorder symptoms in foster children: Comparing diagnostic assessment tools. *Child and Adolescent Psychiatry and Mental Health, 12*(43), 109. https://doi.org/10.1186/s13034-018-0250-3

Klorer, P. G. (2011). Expressive therapy with severely maltreated children: Neuroscience contributions. *Art Therapy, 22*(4), 213–220. https://doi.org/10.1080/07421656.2005.10129523

McLaughlin, K. A., Sheridan, M. A., & Lambert, H. K. (2014). Childhood adversity and neural development: Deprivation and threat as distinct dimensions of early experience. *Neuroscience and Biobehavioural Review, 47*, 578–591. https://doi.org/10.1016/j.neubiorev.2014.10.012

Meiser-Stedman, R., McKinnon, A., Dixon, C., Boyle, A., Smith, D., & Dalgleish, T. (2017). Acute stress disorder and the transition to posttraumatic stress disorder in children and adolescents: Prevalence, course, prognosis, diagnostic stability, and risk markers. *Depression and Anxiety, 34*(4), 348–355.

National Center for PTSD. (2019a). *Chronic pain and PTSD: A guide for patients.* https://www.ptsd.va.gov/understand/related/chronic_pain.asp

National Center for PTSD. (2019b). *How common is PTSD in adults?* https://www.ptsd.va.gov/understand/common/common_adults.asp

National Center for PTSD. (2020). *Aging veterans and posttraumatic stress symptoms.* https://www.ptsd.va.gov/understand/what/aging_veterans.asp

National Child Traumatic Stress Network (NCTSN). (2016). *Resilience and child traumatic stress.* https://www.nctsn.org/resources/resilience-and-child-traumatic-stress

National Institute of Mental Health (NIMH). (2019). *Post-traumatic stress disorder.* https://www.nimh.nih.gov/health/topics/post-traumatic-stress-disorder-ptsd/index.shtml

Norris, F., & Sloane, L. B. (2007). The epidemiology of trauma and PTSD. In M. J. Friedman, T. M. Keane, & P. A. Resick (Eds.), *Handbook of PTSD: Science and practice* (pp. 78–80). Guilford Press.

O'Donnell, M. L., Agathos, J. A., Metcalf, O., Gibson, K., & Lau, W. (2019). Adjustment disorder: Current developments and future directions. *International Journal of Environmental Research and Public Health*, *16*(14).

O'Donnell, M. L., Metcalf, O., Watson, L., Phelps, A., & Varker, T. (2018). A systematic review of psychological and pharmacological treatments for adjustment disorder in adults. *Journal of Traumatic Stress*, *31*(3), 321–331.

Ogden, T., & Hagen, K. A. (2006). Multisystemic therapy of serious behavior problems in youth: Sustainability of therapy effectiveness two years after intake. *Journal of Child & Adolescent Mental Health*, 11, 142–149.

Ophuis, R. H., Olij, B. F., Polinder, S., & Haagsma, J. A. (2018). Prevalence of post-traumatic stress disorder, acute stress disorder, and depression following violence related injury treated at the emergency department: A systematic review. *BMC Psychiatry*, *18*(1), 311–320.

Ostacher, M. J., & Cifu, A. S. (2019). Management of posttraumatic stress disorder. *JAMA Clinical Guidelines Synopsis*, *321*(2), 200–201. https://doi.org/10.1001/jama.2018.19290

Perry, B. D. (2009). Examining child maltreatment through a neurodevelopmental lens: Clinical applications of the neurosequential model of therapeutics. *Journal of Loss and Trauma*, 14, 240–255.

Saxe, G., Stoddard, F., Chewla, N., Lopez, C. G., Hall, E., Sheridan, R., King, D., & King, L. (2005). Risk factors for acute stress disorder in children with burns. *Journal of Trauma & Dissociation*, *6*(2), 37–49.

Strain, J. J. (2018). Adjustment disorders. *Psychiatric Times*, *35*(2), 25–27.

Substance Abuse and Mental Health Services Administration (SAMHSA). (2015). *Recognizing and treating child traumatic stress.* http://www.samhsa.gov/child-trauma/recognizing-and-treating-child-traumatic-stress

Substance Abuse and Mental Health Services Administration (SAMHSA). (2019). *Trauma and Violence.* https://www.samhsa.gov/trauma-violence

Tedeschi, R. G., & Calhoun, L. G. (2004). Target Article: "Posttraumatic Growth: Conceptual Foundations and Empirical Evidence". *Psychological Inquiry*, *15*(1), 1–18. https://doi.org/10.1207/s15327965pli1501_01

U. S. Department of Veterans Affairs, National Center for PTSD. (2019). *How common is PTSD in adults?* Retrieved from https://www.ptsd.va.gov/understand/common/common_adults.asp

van der Kolk, B. A. (2003). The neurobiology of childhood trauma and abuse. *Child and Adolescent Psychiatric Clinics of North America*, *12*(2), 293–317. https://doi.org/10.1016/S1056

World Health Organization (WHO). (2016). *International statistical classification of diseases and related health problems, 10th revision (ICD-10).*

Yaseen, Y. A. (2017). Adjustment disorder: Prevalence, sociodemographic risk factors, and its subtypes in outpatient psychiatric clinic. *Asian Journal of Psychiatry*, 28, 82–85.

Zeanah, C. H., & Gleason, M. M. (2015). Annual research review: Attachment disorders in early childhood—clinical presentation, causes, correlates, and treatment. *Journal of Child Psychology and Psychiatry*, *56*(3), 207-222. https://doi.org/10.1111/jcpp.12347

Zeanah, C. H., Chesher, T., Boris, N. W., & the American Academy of Child and Adolescent Psychiatry Committee on Quality Issues. (2016). Practice parameter for the assessment and treatment of children and adolescents with reactive attachment disorder and disinhibited social engagement disorder. *Journal of the American Academy of Child & Adolescent Psychiatry*, *55*(11), 990–1003.

Credits

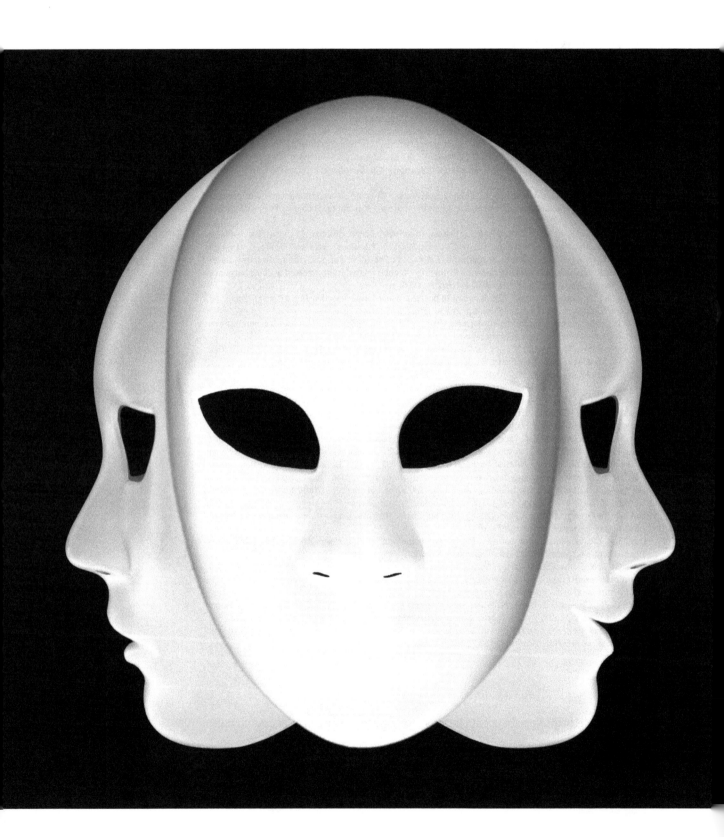

CHAPTER NINE

SOMATIC SYMPTOM AND DISSOCIATIVE DISORDERS

Theresa C. Allen and David A. Scott

CASE STUDY 9.1 Sidney, 24, limps slowly into the clinic. The receptionist is surprised at Sidney's young age because it appears difficult for Sidney to even walk. As the counselor conducts the intake interview, he is unable to move past the health section. Sidney talks at length about her many health problems. She suffers from severe stomach cramping, indigestion, lower back pain, chronic migraines, sudden fits of dizziness, nausea, double vision, hip pain, diarrhea, and, recently, her left calf has been so sore that she cannot walk without a limp. When asked about doctor assessments, Sidney confides that she sees her primary care physician about twice a week and about seven other specialists monthly. Her boyfriend complains about the astronomical medical bills and Sidney's inability to work, but Sidney argues that it is worth it to try to control the pain. The doctor has never found anything directly wrong but has "been on the right track a few times" according to Sidney. Her health problems began around the time she was 19 years old when she was a freshman at a large public university. When questioned further about school, Sidney admits that she never felt she fit in at college. After becoming a date rape victim at a party freshmen year, Sidney withdrew from others and kept to herself.

Did You Know?

- Between 26% and 75% of people have experienced a depersonalization/derealization moment in their lives (Hunter et al., 2004).
- Conversion disorder is mostly diagnosed in females.
- Dissociative identity disorder was once called multiple personality disorder.

Overview

Look at you … you are just faking it! Oh … you "pulled your hamstring" just before your big sporting event. You are such a hypochondriac!

I'm sure we have all either said these things to someone or heard someone say them to another person. A lot of the time, we may be just joking around, but other times we may think to ourselves, *this person is ALWAYS getting sick at specific times. What is going on with this person!* Somatic symptom disorders are an attempt to try to understand and explain why some people have physical symptoms but do not have an official medical diagnosis. Most of the time, people with somatic disorders go to a medical doctor and do not seek mental health treatment; they believe that their issues must be of a physical nature.

This chapter will explore various somatic disorders and dissociative disorders, including dissociative identity disorder. Dissociative disorders are a fascinating group of disorders that have been made famous in movies and the news. Unfortunately, the majority of these movies portray people with dissociative disorders as out of control and even monsters. This misconception only adds to the difficulty in treating and providing support for people dealing with dissociative identity disorder.

Somatic Symptom Disorder (F45.1) (300.82)

People with somatic symptom disorder experience abnormal bodily sensations or feel physical discomfort, yet their symptoms are inconsistent with any clear medical explanation (Cozzi & Barbi, 2019). These people often seek medical attention first but may subsequently be referred to mental health professionals. As a result, people diagnosed with somatic symptom disorder may feel dismissed, misunderstood, or not believed.

The *International Statistical Classification of Diseases* (*ICD-10;* WHO, 2016) describes symptoms of somatization disorder as the presentation of recurrent and frequent physical symptoms that last 2 years or more. These clients will have a lengthy history of seeking medical care, which usually results in negative physical findings. These clients can become frustrated and even depressed when they are unable to find a cause for their aliments. Clients can also be resistant to seeking assistance from a mental health provider because they believe their concerns are medically based. There are so many stories of clients going to a medical doctor after medical doctor but refusing to visit a mental health professional.

According to the *Diagnostic and Statistical Manual of Mental Disorders, 5th Edition* (*DSM-5;* American Psychiatric Association [APA], 2013), an individual must meet three basic criteria to be diagnosed with somatic symptom disorder. They are as follows:

- One or more distressing physical symptoms that may impair daily functioning
- Excessive amounts of time are spent appraising or worrying about the physical symptoms
- Symptoms must be present for 6 months or longer

Somatic symptom disorder in the *DSM-5* (APA, 2013) replaced the category of somatoform disorders found in previous editions (Limburg et al., 2017). A major change in the diagnosis included the fact that individuals with both structural and functional symptoms can receive the diagnosis of somatic symptom disorder (Limburg et al., 2017). This means that a person with somatic symptom disorder has authentic somatic symptoms that may or may not relate to a medically explainable condition as long as Criterion B of psychological impairment is present. Research has shown that about 75% of patients who would have previously met the criteria for hypochondriasis are now believed to be diagnosed with somatic symptom disorder (Hedman et al., 2016).

The most frequent types of these subjective somatic complaints are headaches, abdominal pain, or fatigue (Cozzi & Barbi, 2019). In severe cases, a person becomes consumed with appraising their health to the extent that it becomes a part of their identity and negatively affects daily functioning, such as work or interpersonal relationships.

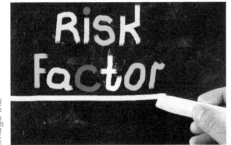

Image 9.2

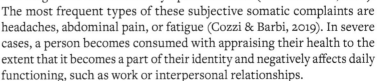

Think about what you know concerning Sydney. Would you diagnosis her with somatic symptom disorder?

Risk Factors

There are gender and age groups that are at higher risk for somatic symptom disorder (Limburg et al., 2017). Females are more likely than males to develop somatic symptom disorder. Older adults are more likely than younger people to develop the disorder, although children can receive the diagnosis. In addition, those in lower socioeconomic populations are more susceptible to a somatic symptom disorder diagnosis (APA, 2013; Limburg et al., 2017). Other risk factors include the following:

1. History of depression or anxiety
2. Having an above-average family history of a specific disease
3. Past trauma
4. Problems maintaining healthy relationships (Mayo Clinic, 2018)

Conversion Disorder (F44.4) (300.11)

Conversion disorder, also known as functional neurological symptom disorder, is a condition whereby a person experiences impairment in sensory functioning or motor functioning yet without a viable neurological explanation (Voon et al., 2016). Nevertheless, these individuals experience severe disability. Loss of sensory functioning might include visual, hearing, or olfactory disturbances; mutism or slurred speech; or abnormal sensations of the skin, such as tingling or numbness. Impairment in motor functioning could result in uncontrolled movement, tremors, gait issues, difficulty swallowing, or paralysis in the body. According to the *ICD-10* (WHO, 2016), conversion disorder is diagnosed in the following instances:

- Abnormal or involuntary movement in motor functioning or sensory functioning
- Neurological symptoms do not match a known medical condition
- Involuntary neurological symptoms cannot be explained by another medical condition
- Symptoms result in significant distress and impairment in daily functioning

In addition, a clinician must confirm evidence of preserved physiological function, even with the presence of such abnormal neurological symptoms prior to assigning a diagnosis of conversion disorder (O'Neal & Baslet, 2018; Voon et al., 2016).

Risk Factors

There are several predisposing factors associated with conversion disorder, including genetics, early childhood experiences, and temperament (Voon et al., 2016). According to O'Neal and Baslet (2018), between 78% and 93% diagnoses of conversion disorder are women. The majority of these patients have a history or comorbid diagnosis with depression, anxiety, or trauma (O'Neal & Baslet, 2018). In addition, a history of child abuse, neglect, or maladaptive personality traits are all risk factors for developing this functional neurological disorder (APA, 2013).

Illness Anxiety Disorder (F45.21) (300.7)

Illness anxiety disorder and somatic symptom disorder both involve an excessive preoccupation with physical health, yet there are specific differences in the two disorders. Primarily, somatic symptom disorder focuses on the experience of physical pain with one or more somatic symptoms, while illness anxiety disorder is more mentally fear based with the preoccupation of having or developing a serious illness (Arnáez et al., 2020; Axelsson et al., 2016; Scarella et al., 2019).

People with illness anxiety disorder will either engage in health-related check-ing behaviors, such as requesting medical tests or making doctor appointments, or avoidance behaviors, such as not going to the doctor to avoid bad news to reduce their anxiety about having an illness (Arnáez et al., 2020). Therefore, the core identifier of illness anxiety disorder is this pattern of worry and reassurance-seeking behaviors instead of the pursuit of relief from painful somatic symptoms as in somatic symptom disorder (Scarella et al., 2019). These people are often accused of being hypochondriacs by others.

Would you diagnosis Sydney with illness anxiety disorder?

According to the *DSM-5* (APA, 2013), the criteria for an illness anxiety disorder diagnosis are as follows:

- Excessive thinking about having or catching a disease or illness
- Physical symptoms are absent or minimal
- Intense anxiety about one's personal health and well-being
- Excessive checking (going to the doctor) or avoiding (staying away from the doctor) behaviors to help ease anxiety about having an illness
- This type of thinking has been present for at least 6 months, but the specific disease or illness can change over time
- The irrational preoccupation with one's health is not better explained by another disorder

Risk Factors

People with a history of child abuse or exposure to a health-related trauma are at higher risk for developing illness anxiety disorder (APA, 2013). Research has shown that people with this disorder often experience intrusive memories of an earlier life event that represented a potential health threat (Arnáez et al., 2020), thus seeding the origin and the development of the disorder.

Dissociative Disorders

Dissociative disorders are a group of disorders that are characterized by a break with reality, sometimes as a response to a traumatic event. Hunter et al. (2004) reported that between 26% and 75% of people have experienced a depersonalization/derealiza-tion moment in their lives. Symptoms of dissociation are included in numerous other disorders, including borderline personality disorder and post-traumatic stress disorder (Ellickson-Larew et al., 2020). The National Alliance on Mental Health (2020) describes some of the symptoms of dissociative disorders as emotional numbness, feelings of having an out-of-body experience, and memory loss related to people, places, and times. Patients describe these symptoms as if they are watching themselves from another location. An example of this phenomenon is when people describe their memories of surviving a traumatic event. Clients with dissociative disorders frequently visit emer-gency care settings, but many times they receive other diagnoses because of the nature of their presenting complaints (Loewenstein, 2018). This lack of a clear diagnosis can be severely demoralizing and can lead to chronic mental illness (Loewenstein et al., 2017).

TRUE LIFE 9.1

Some know him as one of the most talented and powerful running backs in college football history. This is evidenced by his 3-year collegiate campaign where he amassed a total of 5,259 rushing yards in 994 carries with 49 touchdowns (Griffith, 2020). During his breakout freshman season, he led the University of Georgia to its second national championship title, and 2 years later, he received the most esteemed award in college football as the 1982 Heisman Trophy winner. However, much of Herschel Walker's life was not as decorated as his collegiate and professional careers.

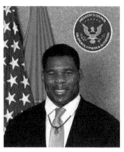
Image 9.3

As a young child, Walker struggled in school with his weight, as well as a speech impediment. He shared, "I didn't love myself. I didn't love who I was," and so he decided to make a change in seventh grade. "You create your Incredible Hulk inside you. In the sense that you create somebody that's going to take control, somebody that's never going to give up," Herschel said (CBN, 2013). During this time, Walker created a daily routine that consisted of him reading aloud and doing 1,500 push-ups and 2,500 sit-ups. This is where some suspect Walker's first encounter with an alter may have occurred, but it would be after his retirement from professional football in 1997 that he would receive a dissociative identity disorder diagnosis.

Walker became unable to separate his football self from his home self. He said, "When you start wearing a hat—that you wear this red hat for football, you wear the white hat for home, you wear the blue hat for work. But all of a sudden when you leave home, you put on the red hat; you put it on at home. The hat's all screwed up. So now, that aggressive nature that you had in football is now at home because you put on the wrong hat" (CBN, 2013). Walker went on to take his anger out on himself and his wife at the time. Walker held a gun to his wife Cindy's head a handful of times and threatened her life with knives and razors on numerous occasions. All of which he does not remember. He shared times where his alters had him play Russian roulette with his own life. Walker does not remember many of his aggressive acts, which is not uncommon for a person with dissociative identity disorder because of blackouts. Dr. Sanjay Gupta suspected that the emergence of Walker's alters stemmed from his retirement from football (Falco, n.d.). The alters no longer had one common goal that they were working toward, so they unraveled, so to speak.

Unfortunately, the numerous accolades and achievements Walker earned were not enough to keep his wife, Cindy DeAngelis Grossman, around. Walker's marriage of 19 years ultimately came to an end when his ex-wife came to the conclusion that she was unable to live with her husband because of his mental health diagnosis. Walker has continued to interact with the sports community and keeps the public informed of how he lives with his mental illness. He released a book titled *Breaking Free*, which documents his life with dissociative identity order. Through his book, he wanted to educate people on what dissociative identity disorder really is and break down the stigma behind it. Walker told CNN, *"I'm okay. I love me—Herschel Walker. You know, 10 years ago I probably couldn't say that. But today, I can say that. I'm not going to say I'm great or I'm good, but I'm okay."*

The *ICD-10* lists several disorders within the category of dissociative (conversion) disorders. Table 9.1 lists some of the disorders and symptoms.

TABLE 9.1 Dissociative [Conversion] Disorders

Dissociative amnesia	Memory loss, mostly around important events. Not connected with organic disorders
Dissociative fugue	Symptoms of dissociative amnesia with unplanned/ unknowingly travel
Dissociative stupor	Marked inability to move or react to external stimuli (noise, touch, or light)
Trance and possession disorders	Loss of a sense of identity. Disorder is outside a religious or culturally accepted situation
Dissociative motor disorders	Inability to move a limb
Dissociative convulsions	Similar to epileptic seizures. Can include behaviors like a trance
Dissociative anesthesia and sensory loss	Inability to feel pain or temperature
Mixed dissociative (conversion) disorders	Can be a combination of disorders within this category
Other dissociative (conversion) disorders	This section includes multiple personality disorder and Ganser syndrome (deliberately acting as if a person has a mental or physical condition)

Note: Adapted from ICD-10 (WHO, 2016).

Dissociative Identity Disorder (F44.81) (300.14)

Dissociative identity disorder (DID), previously referred to as multiple personality disorder, is a complex condition whereby an individual experiences a minimum of two distinct and abiding personality states. While the symptoms of dissociative identity disorder are well defined, the etiology of the disorder is still a topic of research and great deliberation (Reinders et al., 2016). There is still a general thought that dissociative identity disorder is just "made up" and not really a diagnosable condition.

Dissociation is a break in the normal integration of the mind and body, including consciousness, memory, behavior, emotion, and even identity (APA, 2013). There are competing theories for the answer to why this happens to a person. Two such theories are the fantasy model and the trauma model (Reinders et al., 2016). The fantasy or sociocognitive model of dissociative identity disorder postulates that it is instigated in individuals who are highly susceptible to suggestibility or fantasy (Giesbrecht et al., 2007; Reinders et al., 2016). Fantasy proneness and suggestibility in a person can be correlated with many factors, such as cognitive impairment, sleep deprivation, cultural or religious beliefs, and even media exposure (Reinders et al., 2016). Contrarily, the trauma model is correlated with negative environmental factors, neglect or abuse in childhood, or attachment disorder and a child's failure to develop emotion regulation (Reinders et al., 2016).

Would you diagnose Sydney with dissociative identity disorder?

The *DSM-5* (APA, 2013) criteria for a dissociative identity disorder diagnosis are as follows:

- A disruption in the normal integration of mind and body that results in two or more distinct personality states that are a fully integrated entity possessing unique memories, personalities, and behaviors
- Gaps in recall that are beyond normal forgetting
- Symptoms cause severe distress and impairment in normal areas of functioning (work, school, relationships)
- The disruption in the normal integration of mind and body is not a result of child's play (such as imaginary friends)

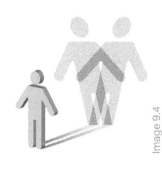

Image 9.4

RISK FACTORS

As discussed earlier, negative early childhood experiences may be a high-risk factor for the development of a dissociative identity disorder. Spiegel et al. (2011) reported that children with higher rates of abuse and neglect more associated with dissociative identity disorder. This may be due to the fact that personality is still developing in childhood (Rutkowski et al., 2016). Therefore, a child may be able to step outside more easily of themselves and view personal trauma as though it is happening to someone else. Subsequently, the development of the skill to dissociate can become a habitual coping skill throughout one's life in moments of great distress (Mayo Clinic, 2020).

Other risk factors include having a diagnosis of post-traumatic stress disorder, borderline personality disorder, depression, anxiety, or substance use disorders (APA, 2013).

Dissociative Amnesia (F44.0) (300.12)

Dissociative amnesia involves marked memory gaps, with clients not able to remember personal information. The memory loss must not be due to an existing organic medical condition and not a part of general forgetfulness. The *ICD-10* reports that many times, this condition is focused on factors such as accidents or other traumatic events. A similar condition is known as *dissociative fugue*. Both the *ICD-10* and *DSM-5* discuss a category of dissociative amnesia named dissociative fugue. This condition is where the person actually travels away from home but does not remember how or why they are traveling or who they are at the time. Even though they appear normal to others, the person will be unable to identify themselves or provide any information about themselves. From time to time, the news will report a person who was declared missing only to show up days later miles from home with no idea how they got there. While dissociative fugue is very rare, dissociative amnesia is one of the more common dissociative disorders. Dissociative amnesia differs from organic memory loss in that dissociative amnesia is usually after a traumatic event, and the client retains the ability to learn new information and function in a normal capacity (Leong et al., 2006).

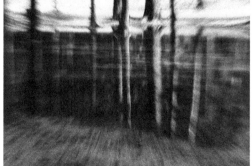

Image 9.5

Depersonalization Disorder (F48.1) (300.6)

The *DSM-5* lists depersonalization disorder within the dissociative disorders chapter. The *ICD-10* places depersonalization disorder within the "Other Neurotic Disorders" section. The *ICD-10* explains that a person with depersonalization disorder exhibits symptoms of loss of emotions and a sense of detachment from their bodies and the real world. Even with these thoughts, the person remains aware of reality and acknowledges the abnormality of their condition. Patients often state that they felt like they were watching themselves inside a movie or like a robot and worry that the condition will become permanent. While most researchers believe that depersonalization disorder is related to a person's autonomic nervous system, the exact cause is unknown. Factors that could affect a person include genetic or environmental issues and increased stress or traumatic events.

Treatment Options

Diagnosing somatic and dissociative disorders may be the most challenging part of treatment. On the surface, the general public may question whether the person truly has a mental health issue or is just faking it. Even in the field of mental health, there may be some trepidation and concern that the client may be malingering for some type of personal gain. Researchers suggest that a continuum of care (including primary care and mental health therapists) is currently viewed as the treatment of choice. Without including the person's primary care professional, the client may continually think their problem is medically based and not a mental health issue. Clients who present with somatic or dissociative disorders are considered by some to be difficult to treat. Initially, one of the first steps is to actually rule out any physical conditions that may be the cause. Henningsen (2018) suggested that one focus of treatment is to try to stay away from saying that the issue is either physical or mental. Another factor to consider is a person's culture. It will be important for the diagnosing clinician to make sure they take into account any cultural or religious traditions that may be similar to a mental health condition.

Treatment mainly consists of traditional mental health therapy and can include cognitive behavioral therapy, mindfulness, and eye movement desensitization and reprocessing (NAMI, 2020). Medications such as antidepressants, pregabalin, and gabapentin offer only low to moderate results as treatment options. Surprisingly, tricyclic antidepressants have shown a moderate effective rate (Henningsen, 2018).

Case Study Summary

One of this chapter's case studies reviewed the behaviors of Sidney. As you process the story and examine possible diagnostic criteria, take a few minutes to answer the following questions:

1. What would be the correct diagnosis for Sidney?

    _____

    _____

2. What are the specific symptoms or criteria that led you to this diagnosis?

    _____

    _____

3. What other possible disorders might you diagnose Sidney with and why?

    _____

    _____

4. Briefly discuss what types of treatment may be beneficial for Sidney. Could you
    see using a certain counseling theory and/or medication?

    _____

    _____

Guided Practice Exercises

Scenario 1

Seji, 62, is a Chinese man who moved with his parents to the United States when he was
16 years old. He worked as the manager of a successful family restaurant in a large city
for many years. Around age 50, Seji started experiencing extensive health problems.
It first began with episodes of insomnia, dizziness, and headaches. When he went to
the doctor, no medical explanation for his problems was found. He was put on sleep
aids, and his condition improved for a time. Now the insomnia has returned, along
with symptoms of constipation, bowel pain, and erectile dysfunction. The doctor has
referred him to a therapist. Upon questioning by the therapist, Seji remains stoic and
denies any symptoms of anxiety or depression.

What would be the correct disorder? What are the specific symptoms or criteria that
led you to this diagnosis?

_____

_____

_____

_____

What specific behaviors caused you to diagnose the disorder?

_____

_____

_____

What other possible disorders might you diagnose Seji with and why?

_____

_____

_____

_____

Scenario 2

Mina, 25, is a Japanese American woman who abruptly lost her sight 6 months ago. With the help of her sister, Mina went to the local medical clinic for help. After an examination, the doctor could not find any medical reason for her blindness. She had had no eye or brain trauma, and everything appeared to be working correctly. The doctor told her, "This condition is only in your head." But to Mina, the condition is not only in her head. She has had to quit her job as an accountant, as well as cease her night courses at a community college for a business degree. She now needs assistance in even simple life tasks. Mina decides to get psychological help. Soon after presenting at the counseling center, the therapist finds out that Mina was the victim of a brutal rape about 7 months ago. The rapist was never found and thus charges were never pressed.

What would be the correct disorder? What are the specific symptoms or criteria that led you to this diagnosis?

_____
_____
_____
_____

What specific behaviors caused you to diagnose the disorder?

_____
_____
_____
_____

What other possible disorders might you diagnose Mina with and why?

_____
_____
_____
_____

Scenario 3

Stephen, 29, sits in a wheelchair in your office. His girlfriend, Carrie, sits next to him and assists him in any way he asks. Stephen has been court ordered to go to counseling because of multiple drug charges, several domestic violence offenses, and sudden leg paralysis. He first begins to tell you that his probation officer treats him brutally, even beating him at times. Suddenly, Carrie nudges Stephen and tells him to tell the truth. She knows his probation officer does no such thing. He gives her an extremely angry look before continuing with accurate information. Stephen discloses that about 3 months ago he lost the ability to use his legs suddenly. When he went to the doctor, he was told that there was no neurological cause or explanation for the paralysis. When questioned about other events that happened 3 months ago, Stephen says he does not remember any. Carrie interjects and says that they were involved in a domestic dispute, and she ended up moving out but decided to move back in after seeing Stephen's condition. Throughout the interview, Stephen expresses little remorse for any of the charges brought against him. He even admits that most of them are true but with more pride than regret.

Do you believe that Stephen genuinely has conversion disorder or is he malingering?

_____

_____

_____

_____

What would be the correct disorder? What are the specific symptoms or criteria that led you to this diagnosis?

_____

_____

_____

_____

What specific behaviors caused you to diagnose the disorder?

_____

_____

_____

_____

What other possible disorders might you diagnose Stephen with and why?

_____

_____

_____

_____

Scenario 4

Salim, 25, has given up on going to the doctor. He knows that it will be a waste of time and money, as the doctor always tells him, "You are perfectly healthy. I can't find anything physically wrong with you." Salim has been convinced at times that he has had chlamydia, tuberculosis, influenza, and, recently, Ebola. These concerns started around the time he was 18 years old. Salim watched his mother die from brain cancer and has trouble coping even years after her death. He usually hears about ailments on the nightly news, internet, or from his coworkers at a local factory. It seems that there is always a connection for Salim. For example, one of his friends was describing COVID-19, and Salim remembered coughing earlier in the day. He then became pre-occupied with the thought that he must have COVID-19. He spent hours that night researching COVID-19 and was unable to sleep. Salim went for a run the next day and as he rounded the corner home, he felt short of breath and was sweating. He knew that this meant he had COVID-19. He must again fight the misery of feeling that death was certain and refrain from going to the doctor.

What would be the correct disorder? What are the specific symptoms or criteria that led you to this diagnosis?

_____

_____

_____

_____

What specific behaviors caused you to diagnose the disorder?

_____

_____

_____

_____

What other possible disorders might you diagnose Salim with and why?

_____

_____

_____

_____

Web-Based and Literature-Based Resources

National Alliance on Mental Illness: https://www.nami.org/About-Mental-Illness/
Mental-Health-Conditions/Dissociative-Disorders

International Society for the Study of Trauma and Dissociation: https://www.isst-d.
org

References

American Psychiatric Association (APA). (2013). _Diagnostic and statistical manual of mental disorders_ (5th ed.).

Arnáez, S., García-Soriano, G., López-Santiago, J., & Belloch, A. (2020). Illness-related intrusive thoughts and illness anxiety disorder. _Psychology and Psychotherapy: Theory, Research and Practice._ https://doi.org/10.1111/papt.12267

Axelsson, E., Andersson, E., Ljótsson, B., Wallhed Finn, D., & Hedman, E. (2016). The health preoccupation diagnostic interview: Inter-rater reliability of a structured interview for diagnostic assessment of _DSM-5_ somatic symptom disorder and illness anxiety disorder. _Cognitive Behaviour Therapy, 45_(4), 259–269. https://doi.org/10.1080/16506073.2016.1161663

CBN. (2013, September 17). _Herschel Walker's battle with D.I.D._ https://www1.cbn.com/700club/herschel-walkers-battle-did

Cozzi, G., & Barbi, E. (2019). Facing somatic symptom disorder in the emergency department. _Journal of Paediatrics and Child Health, 55_(1), 7–9. https://doi.org/10.1111/jpc.14246

Ellickson-Larew, S., Stasik-O'Brien, S. M., Stanton, K., & Watson, D. (2020). Dissociation as a multidimensional transdiagnostic symptom. _Psychology of Consciousness: Theory, Research, and Practice, 7_(2), 126–150. https://doi.org.libproxy.clemson.edu/10.1037/cns0000218.supp

Falco, M. (n.d.). _Herschel Walker reveals many sides of himself._ https://www.cnn.com/2008/HEALTH/conditions/04/15/herschel.walker.did/index.html

Giesbrecht, T. , Merckelbach, H. , Kater, M., & Sluis, A. F. (2007). Why dissociation and schizotypy overlap. _Journal of Nervous and Mental Disease, 195_(10), 812-818. https://doi.org/ 10.1097/NMD.0b013e3181568137.

Griffith, M. (2020, January 14). _Georgia legend Herschel Walker No. 2 on ESPN's Top 150 all-time college player list._ https://www.dawgnation.com/football/georgia-uga-herschel-walker-espn-all-time

Hedman, E., Erland, A., Andersson, E., Mats, L., & Brjánn, L. (2016). Exposure-based cognitive–behavioural therapy via the internet and as bibliotherapy for somatic symptom disorder and illness anxiety disorder: Randomised controlled trial. _British Journal of Psychiatry, 209_(5), 407–413. http://dx.doi.org.ezproxy.liberty.edu/10.1192/bjp.bp.116.181396

Henningsen, P. (2018). Management of somatic symptom disorder. _Dialogues in Clinical Neuroscience, 20_(1), 23–31.

Hunter, E. C., Sierra, M., & David, A. S. (2004). The epidemiology of depersonalisation and derealisation. A systematic review. _Social Psychiatry and Psychiatric Epidemiology, 39_(1), 9–18. https://doi.org/10.1007/s00127-004-0701-4

Leong, S., Waits, W., & Diebold, C. (2006). Dissociative amnesia and DSM-IV-TR cluster c personality traits. *Psychiatry, 3*(1), 51–55.

Limburg, K., Sattel, H., Dinkel, A., Radziej, K., Becker-Bense, S., & Lahmann, C. (2017). Course and predictors of *DSM-5* somatic symptom disorder in patients with vertigo and dizziness symptoms-A longitudinal study. *Comprehensive Psychiatry, 77*, 1–11. doi:http://dx.doi.org.ezproxy.liberty.edu/10.1016/j.comppsych.2017.05.003

Loewenstein, R. J. (2018). Dissociation debates: Everything you know is wrong. *Dialogues in Clinical Neuroscience, 20*, 229–242.

Loewenstein, R. J., Frewen, P. A., & Lewis-Fernández, R. (2017). Dissociative disorders. In B. J. Sadock, V. A. Sadock, & P. Ruiz (Eds.), *Kaplan & Sadock's comprehensive textbook of psychiatry* (10th ed., Vol. 1, pp. 1866–1952). Wolters Kluwer/Lippincott Williams & Wilkens.

Mayo Clinic. (2018). *Somatic symptom disorder.* https://www.mayoclinic.org/diseases-conditions/somatic-symptom-disorder/symptoms-causes/syc-20377776

Mayo Clinic. (2020). *Dissociative disorders.* https://www.mayoclinic.org/diseases-conditions/dissociative-disorders/symptoms-causes/syc-20355215

National Alliance on Mental Illness (NAMI). (2020). *Dissociative disorders.* https://www.nami.org/About-Mental-Illness/Mental-Health-Conditions/Dissociative-Disorders

O'Neal, M. A., & Baslet, G. (2018). Treatment for patients with a functional neurological disorder (conversion disorder): An integrated approach. *American Journal of Psychiatry.* https://doi.org/10.1176/appi.ajp.2017.17040450

Reinders, A., Willemsen, A., Vissia, E., Vos, H., den Boer, J., & Nijenhuis, E. (2016). The psychobiology of authentic and simulated dissociative personality states: The full monty. *Journal of Nervous and Mental Disease, 204*(6), 445–457. https://doi.org/10.1097/NMD.0000000000000522

Rutkowski, K., DembiAska, E., & Walczewska, J. (2016). Effect of trauma onset on personality traits of politically persecuted victims. *BMC Psychiatry, 16*(149). https://link-gale-com.ezproxy.liberty.edu/apps/doc/A452641704/AONE?u=vic_liberty&sid=AONE&xid=7202e730.

Scarella, T., Boland, R., & Barsky, A. (2019). Illness anxiety disorder. *Psychosomatic Medicine, 81*(5), 398–407. https://doi.org/10.1097/PSY.0000000000000691

Spiegel, D., Loewenstein, R. J., Lewis-Fernández, R., Sar, V., Simeon, D., Vermetten, E., Cardeña, E., & Dell, P. F. (2011). Dissociative disorders in *DSM–5. Depression and Anxiety, 28*, 824–852. https://doi.org/10.1002/da.20874

Voon, V., Cavanna, A., E., Coburn, K., Sampson, S., Reeve, A., & LaFrance, W. C. (2016). Functional neuroanatomy and neurophysiology of functional neurological disorders (conversion disorder). *Journal of Neuropsychiatry.* https://doi-org.ezproxy.liberty.edu/10.1176/appi.neuropsych.14090217

World Health Organization (WHO). (2016). *International statistical classification of diseases and related health problems, 10th revision (ICD-10).*

Credits

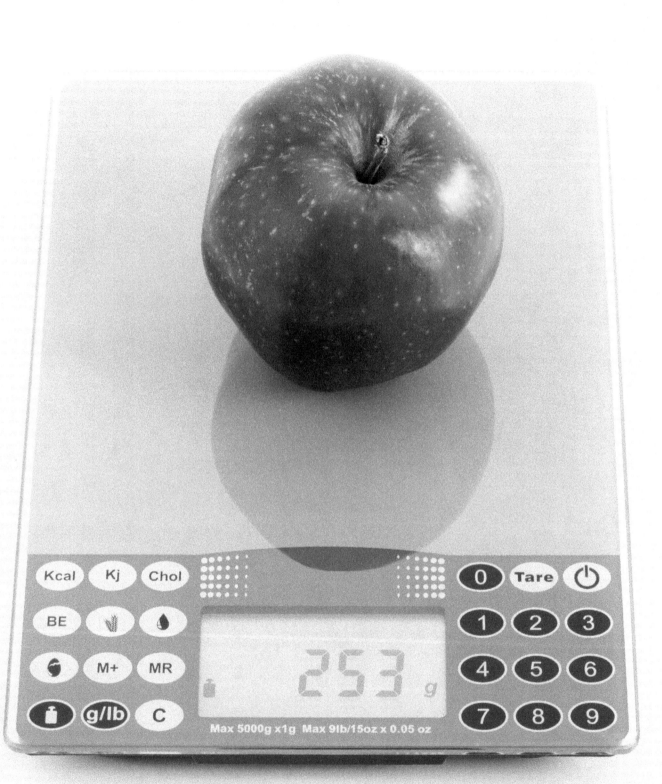

CHAPTER TEN

FEEDING AND EATING DISORDERS

Melanie Burgess, Liz Boyd, and David A. Scott

CASE STUDY 10.1 Ruby, 18, has wanted to be a gymnast for as long as she can remember. Her earliest childhood memories are of time spent in the gym practicing balance, form, and agility. When she was seven, Ruby was mocked and criticized by her coach for being a "chubby" child. Although the coach stated the criticisms in a joking form, they continue to haunt her today. In high school, the media reinforced Ruby's obsession with the importance of being skinny. Her sophomore year of high school, her eating habits changed drastically. She felt powerful when she was able to skip a meal and squeeze three workouts into one day. She felt her confidence rise as she was able to fit into size 0 leotards. By her senior year of high school, her body mass index dipped below underweight and has continued to fall. While family and friends have suggested concern related to her size, Ruby has always been adamant that she is "fine." Now in her freshman year of college, her coach has told her she has to get help at the university counseling center. If she does not comply, the coach has told her she will not be on the team. Ruby thinks her coach is crazy and completely overreacting. Ruby firmly believes that she is overweight. Her worst fear is becoming fat, and she doesn't understand why nobody else can see this.

Overview

Although we all rely on food to sustain ourselves, for more than 30 million people in the United States, the relationship they have with food goes beyond sustenance in the form of a feeding or eating disorder (ANAD, n.d.). Since food can represent power and control, individuals with feeding or eating disorders feel like they are able to exert control over their body's size, shape, or image through food intake, or lack thereof. Just think: how frequently do we reflect on food and eating habits in our own lives? Whether it's a meal out with friends, heading to the grocery store, seeing advertisements for weight loss programs, or viewing dieting "before and after" pictures on social media, we experience food-related content in many mediums in our lives. Therefore, eating and feeding disorders can feel all-encompassing as they affect many facets of life.

Box 10.1 Cultural Considerations

Feeding and eating disorders know no cultural boundaries. They can be life-threatening disorders that affect individuals regardless of age, gender, race, and ethnicity. Here are just a few cultural factors to consider:

- It is estimated that one in three individuals with an eating disorder is male.
- It is estimated that males represent 25% of individuals with anorexia nervosa.
- The number of incidences of anorexia nervosa has increased in females aged 15–24 over the past 50 years while remaining steady in other age groups and with men.
- Thirteen percent of women over the age of 50 engage in behaviors related to eating disorders.
- Nearly 20% of individuals with avoidant/restrictive food intake disorder have an autism spectrum diagnosis.
- Although rates of eating disorders are fairly similar, people of color are significantly less likely to receive help for an eating disorder.
- Individuals who identify as transgender experience eating disorders at significantly higher rates than individuals who identify as cisgender.
- Sixteen percent of transgender college students report having an eating disorder (ANAD, n.d.; NEDA, 2018).

Did any of these facts surprise you? If so, what was surprising, and if not, why do you think the facts aligned with your expectations? While we can see that eating disorders do not discriminate, access to treatment can be an issue for marginalized populations. As a counselor, how could you address marginalized populations affected by eating disorders?

This chapter will explore the most common feeding and eating disorders, including anorexia nervosa, bulimia nervosa, binge eating disorder, avoidant/restrictive food intake disorder, pica, and rumination disorder. While all of these disorders are mentioned in detail in the *Diagnostic and Statistical Manual of Mental Disorders, 5th Edition (DSM-5)*, only anorexia nervosa, bulimia nervosa, and pica are specifically included in the *mental and behavioral disorders* chapter of the *International Statistical Classification of Diseases (ICD-10*; see Table 10.1). The remaining disorders can be diagnosed in the *ICD-10* using specifiers such as "atypical" or "unspecified disorder." A recent movement has advocated to include additional feeding and eating disorders in the *ICD-11*, with an expected release date of early 2022. It is also important to note that each of these disorders, with the exception of pica, are mutually exclusive. This means that a client can only be diagnosed with one eating disorder at a time. The disorders we will discuss in this chapter all have different clinical courses, outcomes, and treatment needs, making the differentiation critical to the treatment process.

TABLE 10.1 *ICD-DSM* Comparison

***ICD* CODES** Eating disorders (F50)	***DSM-5* CODES** Feeding and eating disorders
Anorexia nervosa (F50) Symptoms could include dread of gaining weight, intentional weight loss through restricted diet, excessive exercise, and various forms of purging.	**Anorexia nervosa** (307.1) Symptoms could include restriction of food intake leading to low body weight/malnutrition, dread of gaining weight, and negative body image. *Specify if restricting type or binge eating/purging type.*
Bulimia nervosa (F50.2) Symptoms could include episodes of overeating followed by purging, significant weight change, overconcern with body image.	**Bulimia nervosa** (307.51) Symptoms could include recurrent episodes of overeating followed by purging and negative body image.
Not included in *ICD-10*	**Binge eating disorder** (307.51) Symptoms could include recurrent episodes of binge eating, lack of control of eating, eating fast, eating until overfull, embarrassment about, and distress related to food intake. This disorder does not include any compensatory behaviors.
Not included in *ICD-10*	**Avoidant/restrictive food intake disorder** (307.59) Symptoms can include lack of interest in eating or avoidance toward food based on sensory characteristics that are not attributed to a lack of available food and concern about negative consequences of eating.
Pica (F98.3) **children,** (F50.8) **adults** Symptoms could include persistent eating of non-nutritive substances.	**Pica** (307.52) Symptoms could include ingestion of non-food, non-nutritive substances.
Rumination (F98.2) **in infancy and childhood** Symptoms could include food refusal and food regurgitation.	**Rumination Disorder** (307.53) Symptoms could include repeated regurgitation of food that is not attributed to other gastrointestinal or medical conditions.
Atypical anorexia nervosa (F50.1) Symptoms could include some, but not all, of the features of anorexia nervosa. **Atypical bulimia nervosa** (F50.3) Symptoms could include some, but not all, of the features of bulimia nervosa.	**Other Specified Feeding or Eating Disorder** (307.59) Any eating or feeding disorder that does not meet the full criteria for disorders listed above.
Other eating disorders (F50.8) (See Pica in adults above) Psychogenic loss of appetite **Eating disorder, unspecified** (50.9)	

Note: Adapted from ICD-10 (WHO, 2016); DSM-5 (APA, 2013)

Anorexia Nervosa (F50) Restricting Type (F50.01); Binge Eating/Purging Type (F50.02) (307.1)

When people think of eating disorders, anorexia nervosa is often one of the first to come to mind. An image of an extremely skinny, high school–age female may even come to mind. This is somewhat appropriate in that the prevalence of anorexia among adolescent females is 0.4% and only 0.1% among adolescent males (NEDA, 2018). Although anorexia is less common among males, they have a higher risk of severe health consequences, including death, compared to females (Mond et al., 2014). Why do you think this is?

CLINICIAN'S CORNER

When working with teenagers in school settings, it was shockingly common to encounter folks who had unhealthy relationships with food. Whether it involved "cutting weight" for a sports team, restricting food intake during lunch, or taking diet pills to shed a few pounds, teenagers may associate a lot of shame with their diet and are likely to either justify and minimize their unhealthy eating habits or hide their harmful relationship with food altogether. It can be a challenge for a teenager to open up to an adult about this topic; therefore, if a teenager trusts us enough to disclose their eating disorder, it is exceedingly important to respond in a nonjudgmental manner.

Unfortunately, many teens are exposed to a multitude of negative food-related messages from social media, tv/movies, magazines, and celebrities. Teens are under an enormous amount of peer pressure to "fit in," which might involve looking a certain way. Teens can therefore be highly critical of their own bodies. Teens can even experience these negative messages about food in their own household. Some teens mention how their own negative internal dialogue related to food mirrors their parent/guardians' relationship with food. These messages can influence their body image in such strong ways. When treating eating disorders in teenagers, it can be beneficial to include their family members in the treatment process, allowing everyone to get onboard with a clear and consistent message of support. It is also important for practitioners, family members, and individuals with eating disorders to recognize the dangers of anorexia nervosa and jump to action to prevent serious medical risks associated with the disorder.

Liz Boyd, PhD

Anorexia nervosa is characterized by constant weight loss and low body weight. According to the *DSM-5* and the *ICD-10*, common symptoms that an individual with anorexia may exhibit include low calorie intake, distorted body image, fear of gaining weight, and/or taking actions to ensure no weight gain. For diagnostic coding, the *DSM-5* distinguishes between two subtypes: restricting and binge eating/purging. The restricting type achieves a low body weight and/or loses weight through excessive exercise, fasting, or diet. In contrast, the binge eating/purging type engages in elimination behaviors, such as vomiting or the use of laxatives or diuretics after eating (APA, 2013;

WHO, 2016). In addition, counselors should specify the severity from mild to extreme, which is based primarily on the client's body mass index. It is important to note that body mass index is not the best indicator of overall health and should never be used as the sole determinant in diagnosing anorexia.

Let's think back to Ruby in Case Study 10.1. After rereading her scenario, which type of anorexia nervosa would you diagnose Ruby with? What led you to your decision?

Box 10.2 Did You Know?

American singer Taylor Swift opened up about her struggles with an eating disorder in the 2020 documentary *Miss Americana.* Swift thinks back to her photo on the cover of a popular magazine with the headline "Pregnant and 18?" and notes that her stomach wasn't completely flat. From there, she remembers being commended for being able to fit into sample size clothing without alterations to increase the size. How do you think these comments from media may have affected Swift? Similarly, actress Jameela Jamil started *I Weigh*, an online movement that embraces radical body positivity and self-worth to combat the harmful effects of social media. She has openly shared her struggle with anorexia during her teenage years. Through her activism, Facebook and Instagram have adjusted their policies regarding diet and detox products being shown to minors. What form of advocacy can counselors take to try to curb these types of influences from news, marketing, and social media outlets?

You may notice that the binge eating subtype of anorexia sounds rather similar to bulimia nervosa. While there are several similarities, there are also two stark differences. First, anorexia is characterized by a significantly low body weight, whereas bulimia does not have any guidelines related to body weight. Second, a person with anorexia has an intense fear of gaining weight. The individual may be obsessed with not becoming fat, regardless of their already low body weight. As we mentioned early in the chapter, these disorders are mutually exclusive, so it is critical to pay attention to details like these to differentiate between the disorders.

The medical health risks related to anorexia nervosa can be severe. The lack of nutrients and low body weight associated with anorexia nervosa can lead to amenorrhea, low bone density, and cardiovascular and gastrointestinal complications (Mehler et al., 2015). In fact, anorexia nervosa has the highest mortality rate among all mental health disorders. Because of the dangerous nature of anorexia nervosa, inpatient or outpatient treatment may be necessary for safety reasons. Research suggests that family-based treatments and cognitive behavioral therapy (CBT) are most effective for individuals with an early onset of anorexia, such as during childhood and adolescence (Hurst et al., 2012; Mittnacht & Bulik, 2015). Clinical teams composed of mental health practitioners, medical providers, and registered dietitians can develop treatment plans that may involve the use of medical care (e.g., hydration and nutritional rehabilitation)

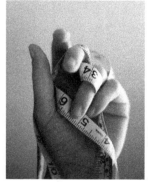

Image 10.2

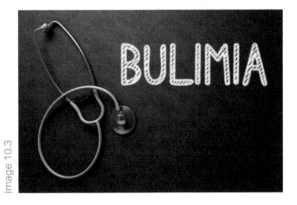

Image 10.3

and pharmacotherapy (e.g., antidepressants or anxiolytics) to combat malnourishment and manage symptoms (Brockmeter et al., 2017; Mittnacht & Bulik, 2015).

Knowing what you know now, why do you think Ruby's coach was so adamant about her scheduling a counseling session at the university counseling center? What other steps do you think Ruby will need to take to support her treatment and well-being?

Bulimia Nervosa (F50.2) (307.51)

Bulimia nervosa is primarily characterized by both the *ICD-10* and *DSM-5* as binge eating and inappropriate compensatory behaviors. Binge eating is defined as eating more food in a short amount of time than most people would, along with a sense of not being in control of one's eating. Inappropriate compensatory behaviors are used to prevent weight gain and include vomiting, laxatives, fasting, or excessive exercise. For a diagnosis, these behaviors have been occurring on average at least once a week for a minimum of 3 months. Bulimia is also characterized by a negative self-evaluation that is highly influenced by body shape and weight (APA, 2013; WHO, 2016).

As mentioned in the earlier section about anorexia nervosa, you will notice two characteristics of anorexia not included in the criteria for bulimia: low body weight and fear of gaining weight. It is often challenging to notice when a friend or family member suffers from bulimia because there is not typically a rapid change in weight, if any at all. It is common for individuals with bulimia to engage in binging and purging while alone, adding to the challenge of identifying the behaviors. Finally, a person with bulimia may be overly concerned about their body weight, shape, or image, but it does not reach the point of intense fear of gaining weight.

Physical symptoms such as acid reflux and electrolyte abnormalities are frequently seen in individuals with bulimia nervosa (Mehler et al., 2015). Depending on the severity, individuals with bulimia nervosa may need to seek inpatient or outpatient treatment for comprehensive medical and mental health care. Alternatively, short-term treatment, such as CBT and other forms of counseling/psychotherapy, can be effective in reducing binging and purging, as well as improving self-reports of bulimia and body dissatisfaction; however, research indicates that long-term treatments to prevent relapse are widely inconclusive (Erford et al., 2013; Slade et al., 2018). Guided self-help can produce positive short-term results and is particularly appealing because of convenience and low cost, making it more accessible to clients. Lastly, pharmacotherapy, including the use of antidepressants can be used in combination with psychotherapy to further manage symptoms (Walsh et al., 2016).

CASE STUDY 10.2 Elle, 42, tries to eat her way out of her unhappiness in life. She has been married for 14 years, but it has always been a rocky relationship. Elle considered leaving after her husband admitted to an affair a year ago but stayed for the sake of their children (ages 5 and 8). There hasn't been intimacy in the marriage for over a year, and honestly, Elle doesn't even care. She is grossly overweight and knows she needs to start taking better care of herself. Elle is a stay-at-home mom. Now that the youngest is in school during the day, Elle has little to stay busy with. During the day, Elle finds her escape in consuming large amounts of food. There have been days where she went through an entire pan of brownies, a package of Oreos, and a gallon of milk, in addition to the meals she shares with her family. Elle knows her eating habits are hurting her health, but food is her sole source of contentedness. Once she starts eating, she finds it difficult to stop. Elle knows that she needs to stop eating and make changes to improve her health, but she doesn't know how to stop eating or where to go for help.

Binge Eating Disorder (F50.8) (307.51)

A national survey found that binge eating disorder is the most common eating disorder in the United States, affecting 3.5% of women, 2% of men, and 1.6% of adolescents (Swanson et al., 2011). Interestingly, the *DSM-5* is the first version of the *DSM* to include binge eating disorder as a recognized and diagnosable disorder. Prior to this, it was included in the *DSM-IV* as a provisional diagnosis. The *ICD-10* does not have a specific diagnosis for binge eating disorder. According to the *DSM-5*, diagnostic markers for binge eating disorder include recurrent episodes of binge eating where a person feels out of control with their eating and is eating more than most people would in a certain amount of time.

These binge eating episodes have to include at least three of the following: (1) eating faster than usual, (2) feeling uncomfortably full, (3) eating a lot of food when not hungry, (4) eating alone to avoid embarrassment, and (5) feeling disgusted with self after the binge. To determine a binge eating disorder diagnosis, these symptoms must occur at least once a week for 3 months, and the individual must exhibit distress in regard to their eating habits (APA, 2013). Binge eating disorder does not include any compensatory behaviors, and a person with the disorder is often somewhere between

Box 10.3 Obesity

According to the 2017–2018 National Health and Nutrition Examination Survey conducted by the Center for Disease Control and Prevention, the prevalence of obesity in adults in the United States was 42.4% (Hales et al., 2020). A body mass index of 30 or higher indicates obesity. The 2017–2018 survey did not find a significant difference between obesity rates in males and females. Obesity is noted as a medical diagnosis in the *ICD-10*, but it is not considered a disorder in the *DSM-5*. That said, there appears to be a link between obesity and mental health diagnoses. Rajan and Menon (2017) found that there is a relationship between depression and eating disorders, with either one potentially leading to the other. Similarly, Tagay and colleagues (2014) found that out of 2,400 individuals hospitalized for an eating disorder, 94% had a co-occurring disorder. The most common co-occurring disorder was depression, followed closely by anxiety disorders.

As counselors, we emphasize the importance of holistic wellness. How can we incorporate more holistic wellness into our sessions to help combat obesity? What can we do to advocate for our clients who are struggling with weight, whether over or under?

average and obese in regard to weight. Box 10.3 provides information on obesity. Let's reflect on Elle from the beginning of this section. What symptoms does she exhibit that seem to align with binge eating disorder? Are there any other disorders you would consider in this case?

Treatment for binge eating disorder can include psychotherapy and pharmacotherapy, aimed at reducing the frequency of binge eating episodes, promote healthy weight and metabolism, maintain stable mood, and develop healthier cognitions related to eating habits (Brownley et al., 2016). Psychological and behavioral interventions can include CBT and dialectical behavior therapy with an emphasis on self-monitoring and mindfulness. In addition to counseling, pharmacotherapy is seen as a useful treatment, including the use of psychotropic medications, such as antidepressants (Brownley et al., 2016; Walsh et al., 2016).

What would your treatment plan for Elle include?

Avoidant/Restrictive Food Intake Disorder (F50.8) (307.59)

Avoidant/restrictive food intake disorder (ARFID) is another new diagnosis in the *DSM-5*. The diagnosis replaces "feeding disorder of infancy or early childhood" from the *DSM-IV*, which was only used for children under the age of 6 and lacked a clear definition. Avoidant/restrictive food intake disorder does not have any age restrictions and is characterized by a failure to meet nutritional and energy needs. This could be signified by significant weight loss or nutritional deficiency, a dependence on enteral feedings, or interference with psychosocial functioning. For the diagnosis, these symptoms should not be related to a lack of available food or a cultural practice (APA, 2013). The primary distinction between avoidant/restrictive food intake disorder and anorexia or bulimia is that the former does not include a negative body image. In fact, it is common that individuals with avoidant/restrictive food intake disorder want to eat and are frustrated that they cannot get themselves to do so. There is not currently a related disorder in the *ICD-10*.

Pediatricians are often the first to diagnose avoidant/restrictive food intake disorder, as it is most common in older children and younger adolescents. This diagnosis goes beyond the 8-year-old "picky eater" who leaves the green vegetables on their plate every night. Avoidant/restrictive food intake disorder reflects severe nutritional deficiencies and/or a persistent inability to meet energy needs (Zimmerman & Fisher, 2017). The disorder is a hot topic in eating disorder research, as clinicians and researchers are constantly trying better to understand the etiology to best inform treatment modalities. The etiology of this disorder is broad, and a few suggested reasons for the behaviors can be found in Box 10.4.

Treatment methods for avoidant/restrictive food intake disorder include pharmacotherapy, psychological treatment, and multimodal methods to meet a wide range of needs. Anxiolytics and antidepressants may be beneficial to relieve stress, support appetite, and promote weight gain; however, more medical trials are needed to further examine the effectiveness of these treatment methods (Bourne et al., 2020; Walsh et al., 2016). CBT can help address thought patterns and anxiety relating to food consumption, weight, and shape. In addition, family-based therapy can be used to empower parents/

guardians and caregivers of individuals with avoidant/restrictive food intake disorder. Family-based therapy can help reduce feelings of guilt and improve the recovery environment in the home. Lastly, multimodal approaches may be needed for more severe cases of avoidant/restrictive food intake disorder, where multidisciplinary teams of practitioners can provide a wide range of interventions to comprehensively address many needs (Bourne et al., 2020).

Pica (F98.3) in Children and (F50.8) in Adults (307.52)

Pica, or the eating of non-nutritive, nonfood substances for at least 1 month, is considered to be one of the most common, yet most underreported, mental health disorders. Frequently, a person with pica will present with a health-related concern caused by ingesting a nonfood. Most reports of pica indicate a childhood onset, although developmental levels should be considered. For example, a toddler who is chalking their driveway for the first time and decides to stick the chalk in their mouth should not be sending up red flags. However, if an elementary-age child was eating chalk from their classroom daily, this would be a concern. Pica is also seen in adults, primarily in those who have intellectual disabilities or other mental health disorders.

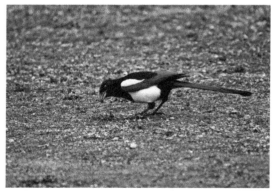

Image 10.4

The word pica is derived from the Latin word magpie, which is a crow that is known for eating just about anything.

The substances that individuals with pica eat vary from non-nutritive, yet mostly benign substances, such as paper, to potentially life-threatening poisons, such as household cleaners or laundry detergents. Often, it is discovered that individuals with pica have underlying nutritional deficiencies (e.g., low zinc or iron) or malnutrition, and although the bodies crave nutrients to fill these voids, rarely do non-nutritive or nonfood substances alleviate these deficiencies.

Historically, there have been a wide range of treatments for pica that are presently considered socially unacceptable, including punitive measures or aversive techniques, such as spraying lemon juice or water in a child's face when they exhibit pica-related behaviors (Matson et al., 2013). Treatments have also included physical restraint or time-outs; however, there is currently little evidence supporting these treatments. Most frequently, positive reinforcement and biological interventions have been used successfully to manage pica-related behaviors (Matson et al., 2013). Starting with the least intrusive method, positive reinforcement can be used to both acknowledge when appropriate behaviors occur and interrupt pica-related behaviors and substitute a nonfood item with appropriate edibles, such as a bite-size candy. In addition, biological interventions, such as providing nutritional supplements to counteract deficiencies, have been shown to modestly improve pica behaviors. Pharmacotherapy, while potentially promising, has limited research to warrant its use (Matson et al., 2013). Individuals with pica may also require treatment from medical doctors, such as being monitored for other health conditions, such as malnutrition, bowel obstruction, infection, poisoning, or other complications because of ingesting harmful items.

Rumination Disorder (F98.21) (307.53)

Often the earliest feeding and eating disorder to manifest, rumination disorder is characterized by the unintentional regurgitation of food shortly after eating. A person may then rechew and swallow the food or spit it out. Typically seen in infants or children, this disorder is incredibly rare in adults. While there is no evidence of underlying triggers, it is hypothesized that rumination disorder may be brought on by illness, injury, or emotional distress (Walsh et al., 2016). Presently, very little is known about this disorder. As mentioned previously, the *DSM-5* notes that many eating disorder diagnoses are mutually exclusive. While many other eating disorders involve elements of rumination (e.g., anorexia nervosa and bulimia nervosa), an additional diagnosis of rumination disorder is prohibited. Therefore, this stand-alone disorder is increasingly rare, as there is a paucity of information available about its actual prevalence.

Another reason why rumination disorder is uncommon is due to difficulty differentiating rumination disorder from other gastrointestinal concerns and medical disorders. While people with rumination disorder often experience esophageal reflux, it important to note that reflux, gastrointestinal diagnoses, and medical conditions do not sufficiently explain the symptoms of this disorder, and therefore, rumination disorder cannot be successfully treated with interventions for these concerns (Walsh et al., 2016). People may also feel nauseous or experience belching, bloating, heartburn, abdominal pain, or pressure prior to, during, and after rumination. In more severe cases, people can experience malnutrition, weight loss, electrolyte imbalances, halitosis, or dental erosion (Walsh et al., 2016).

Similar to other eating disorders, CBT is an important tool in the treatment of rumination disorder. Because of the rare nature of this diagnosis, limited treatment information is readily available; however, other strategies, such as mindfulness, diaphragmatic breathing, biofeedback, and operant conditioning, can be useful when managing symptoms (Vanzhula & Levinson, 2020; Walsh et al., 2016). Pharmacotherapy interventions, such as antidepressants and antianxiety medications, have shown limited positive effects (Walsh et al., 2016).

Case Study Summary

One of this chapter's case studies reviewed the behaviors of Ruby. As you process the story and examine possible diagnostic criteria, take a few minutes to answer the following questions:

1. What would be the correct diagnosis for Ruby?

    _____

    _____

2. What are the specific symptoms or criteria that led you to this diagnosis?

    _____

    _____

3. What other possible disorders might you diagnose Ruby with and why?

    _____

    _____

4. Briefly discuss what types of treatment may be beneficial for Ruby. Could you see using a certain counseling theory and/or medication?

    _____

    _____

Guided Practice Exercises

Scenario 1

EJ, a 19-year-old male, is a sophomore in college and was referred to you by the health center on campus. When EJ was in high school, he was deeply invested in the wrestling team. His coach was optimistic that he could receive a college scholarship because of his level of talent. He was proud of this and wanted to do everything in his power to secure a scholarship. EJ had a serious exercise regimen and monitored his weight obsessively. Just before competitions, EJ would engage in purging to lose a few pounds, which would hopefully place him in a lower weight class during weigh-ins, making it easier for him to win matches. He knew this wasn't a good habit, but several teammates were also purging, and he was not doing this very frequently. Plus, when he looked in the mirror, he saw the epitome of health, so he didn't second guess this decision.

During his senior year of high school, EJ discovered that he did not receive a scholarship. When EJ went off to college as a regular student and not a college athlete, he was disappointed in himself. He continued to eat typically; however, he no longer maintained his exercise regimen. Since he was living a more sedentary lifestyle now, he began to gain a noticeable amount of weight. Disgusted by how he looked, he turned back to purging. At first, he would only purge after eating a high-calorie meal. Over time, he began to schedule a routine of purging multiple times each day, obsessively weighing himself, and looking in the mirror to see how his clothes fit on his changing body. Both his high school and college friends commented on how good he looked, but he did not tell them how he was losing the weight.

Almost a year into developing this habit, he noticed his teeth changing color and twinges of stomach pain. When he could no longer take the pain in his stomach, he went to the health center on campus. The physician asked many questions about his eating habits upon hearing about the symptoms. EJ denied inquiries until the doctor directly asked if he had been throwing up his food. After a conversation about health risks and the scheduling of follow-up appointments, he referred EJ to you as well.

What would be the correct disorder? What are the specific symptoms or criteria that led you to this diagnosis?

_____

_____

_____

_____

What specific behaviors caused you to diagnose the disorder?

_____

_____

_____

_____

What other possible disorders might you diagnose EJ with and why?

_____

_____

_____

_____

Scenario 2

Bianca is a 5-year-old girl who just recently started kindergarten. Her parents shared that Bianca was always a quirky, curious child. When they would play together, she would always want to investigate different objects and textures. For instance, she would enjoy putting glue, dirt, or paper in her mouth. Her parents once found a recipe to make slime at home together but quickly caught Bianca trying to eat it. They all laughed and thought nothing more about it. When Bianca began having some stomach issues, her parents became concerned. She would experience bouts of constipation and diarrhea and frequently experienced stomach pain. Her parents assumed she had food allergies like her mom and began elimination diets to identify which foods were giving her trouble.

When Bianca was enrolled in kindergarten, her new teacher quickly noticed that Bianca had a habit of eating crayons and glue. She mentioned this to her parents, who dismissed the idea that she was eating those objects. Instead, they shared that she has always been orally fixated, but they were convinced that she didn't eat the objects she put in her mouth. Later that day, Bianca experienced intense stomach pain. She had blood in her stool and was constipated. Her parents took her to the doctor immediately and were hoping to ask more about food allergies since this had been a long-term problem that recently became more severe. Bianca's bloodwork showed that she was anemic (i.e., iron deficiency) and had a blockage in her intestines. When the doctor spoke with Bianca, she seemed ashamed but admitted that she regularly ate crayons and glue but recently ate several marbles.

What would be the correct disorder? What are the specific symptoms or criteria that led you to this diagnosis?

_____

_____

_____

_____

What specific behaviors caused you to diagnose the disorder?

_____

_____

_____

_____

What other possible disorders might you diagnose Bianca with and why?

_____

_____

_____

_____

Web-Based and Literature-Based Resources

Academy for Eating Disorders: https://www.aedweb.org/resources/about-eating-disorders

Eating Disorders Coalition: http://www.eatingdisorderscoalition.org/

National Association of Anorexia Nervosa and Associated Disorders: https://anad.org/

National Eating Disorders Association: http://www.nationaleatingdisorders.org

National Institute of Mental Health: https://www.nimh.nih.gov/health/topics/eating-disorders/index.shtml

Project Heal: https://www.theprojectheal.org/

The Center for Eating Disorders at Sheppard Pratt: http://www.eatingdisorder.org/

The International Association of Eating Disorders Professionals Foundation: http://www.iaedp.com/

Trans Folx Fighting Eating Disorders: https://www.transfolxfightingeds.com/

References

American Psychiatric Association (APA). (2013). *Diagnostic and statistical manual of mental disorders* (5th ed.).

Bourne, L., Bryant-Waugh, R., Cook, J., & Mandy, W. (2020). Avoidant/restrictive food intake disorder: A systematic scoping review of the current literature. *Psychiatry Research, 288,* 112961. https://doi.org/10.1016/j.psychres.2020.112961

Brockmeyer, T., Friederick, H. C., & Schmidt, U. (2018). Advances in the treatment of anorexia nervosa: A review of established and emerging interventions. *Psychological Medicine, 48*(8), 1228-1256. http://dx.doi.org/10.1017/S0033291717002604

Brownley, K. A., Berkman, N. D., Peat, C. M., Lohr, K. N., Cullen, K. E., Bann, C. M., & Bulik, C. M. (2016). Binge-Eating Disorder in Adults: A Systematic Review and Meta-analysis. *Annals of Internal Medicine, 165*(6), 409–420. https://doi.org/10.7326/M15-2455

Erford, B. T., Richards, T., Peacock, E., Voith, K., McGair, H., Muller, B., Duncan, K., & Chang, C. (2013). Counseling and guided self-help outcomes for clients with bulimia nervosa: A meta-analysis of clinical trials from 1980 to 2010. *Journal of Counseling & Development, 91,*152–172.

Hales, C. M., Carroll, M. D., Fryar, C. D., & Ogden, C. L. (2020). *Prevalence of obesity and severe obesity among adults: United States, 2017–2018.* NCHS Data Brief: National Center for Health Statistics. https://www.cdc.gov/nchs/data/databriefs/db360-h.pdf

Hurst, K., Read, S., & Wallis, A. (2012). Anorexia nervosa in adolescence and Maudsley family-based treatment. *Journal of Counseling & Development, 90*(3), 339-345.http://dx.doi.org/10.1002/j.1556-6676.2012.00042.x

Matson, J. L., Hattier, M. A., Belva, B., & Matson, M. L. (2013). Pica in persons with developmental disabilities: Approaches to treatment. *Research in Developmental Disabilities, 34,* 2564–2571.

Mehler, P. S., Krantz, M. J., & Sachs, K. V. (2015). Treatment of medical complications of anorexia nervosa and bulimia nervosa. *Journal of Eating Disorders, 3,* 15. https://doi.org/10.1186/s40337-015-0041-7

Mittnacht, A. M., & Bulik, C. M. (2015). Best nutrition counseling practices for the treatment of anorexia nervosa: A delphi study. *International Journal of Eating Disorders, 48,* 111–122.

Mond, J. M., Mitchison, D., & Hay, P. (2014). Prevalence and implications of eating disordered behavior in men. In L. Cohn & R. Lemberg (Eds.), *Current findings on males with eating disorders* (pp. 195–215). Routledge.

National Association of Anorexia Nervosa and Associated Disorders (ANAD). (n.d.). *Eating disorder statistics.* https://anad.org/education-and-awareness/about-eating-disorders/eating-disorders-statistics/

National Eating Disorders Association (NEDA). (2018). *Statistics & research on eating disorders.* https://www.nationaleatingdisorders.org/statistics-research-eating-disorders

Rajan, T. M., & Menon, V. (2017). Psychiatric disorders and obesity: A review of association studies. *Journal of Postgraduate Medicine, 63*(3), 182–190. https://doi.org/10.4103/jpgm.JPGM_712_16

Slade, E., Keeney, E., Mavranezouli, I., Dias, S., Fou, L., Stockton, S., Saxon, L., Waller, G., Turner, H., Serpell, L., Fairburn, C. G., & Kendall, T. (2018). Treatments for bulimia nervosa: A network meta-analysis. *Psychological Medicine. 48*(16), 2629–2636. https://doi.org/10.1017/S0033291718001071

Swanson, S. A., Crow, S. J., Le Grange, D., Swendsen, J., & Merikangas, K.R. (2011). Prevalence and correlates of eating disorders in adolescent: Results from the national comorbidity survey replication adolescent supplement. *Archives of General Psychiatry, 68*(7), 714–723.

Tagay, S., Schlottbohm, E., Reyes-Rodriguez, M. L., Repic, N., & Senf, W. (2014). Eating disorders, trauma, PTSD, and psychosocial resources. *Eating Disorders, 22*(1), 33–49.

Vanzhula, I. A., & Levinson, C. A. (2020). Mindfulness in the treatment of eating disorders: Theoretical rationale and hypothesized mechanisms of action. *Mindfulness, 11,* 1090–1104.

Walsh, T. B., Attia, E., Glasofer, D. R., & Sysko, R. (2016). *Handbook of assessment and treatment of eating disorders.* American Psychiatric Association.

World Health Organization (WHO). (2016). *International statistical classification of diseases and related health problems, 10th revision (ICD-10).*

Zimmerman, J., & Fisher, M. (2017). Avoidant/restrictive food intake disorder (ARFID). *Current Problems in Adolescent Health Care, 47*(4), 95–103.

Credits

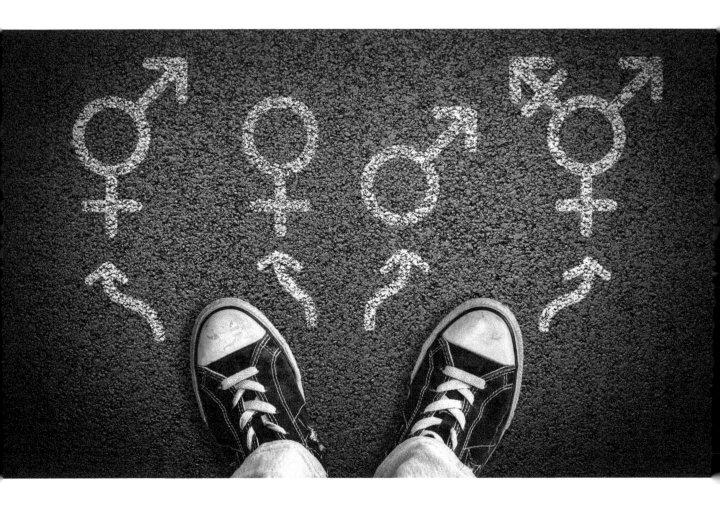

CHAPTER ELEVEN

SEXUAL DISORDERS AND GENDER DYSPHORIA

Sonja Lund, T'Airra Belcher, and David A. Scott

CASE STUDY 11.1 John is a 25-year-old male who was court ordered to come to counseling after being arrested for the fourth time for sexual harassment. When John was in college, he would attend parties with his buddies and hit the bars afterward. While he was at the bars, he mentioned that he would fight the urge to grab women's breasts as they walked by. One night while dancing with a woman, he could no longer fight his urge, so he fondled her. The women's friends witnessed the unconsented fondling and immediately had the man removed from the bar. The police were called, and John was arrested for harassment.

Since that first time, John's urges have been harder and harder to fight. He regularly finds himself walking past women in the grocery store and brushing his hand up against their body parts. He would always apologize if confronted, saying that the act was accidental. Also, when John is in bed at night, he fanaticizes about rubbing up on women he cannot identify in public places, such as the park or at a sporting event. He always gets away before police arrive in his fantasies.

John says to you, "I can no longer fight the urges, and it's becoming a big problem." John's girlfriend has begun to notice the incidents and threatened to leave him after the last arrest. He loves her and does not want to lose her.

Overview

What is normal sexual behavior? How do we know when our sexual behaviors become abnormal? Do we let society define sexual behavior or is it up to us to define? Procreation is genetically programmed in our brains. Passing on our genetic code is one of the basic premises for our existence. When does sex become abnormal? What does the *Diagnostic and Statistical Manual of Mental Disorders, 5th Edition (DSM-5)* and *International Statistical Classification of Diseases (ICD-10)* say about what constitutes sexual disorders? This chapter will explore sexual disorders and the evolution of what were once considered sexual disorders. Sexual issues are located in several different chapters (*DSM-5*) and categories (*ICD-10*) but will be discussed in this one overarching chapter.

This chapter comprises three classes of disorders: (1) sexual dysfunction, (2) gender dysphoria, and (3) paraphilic disorders. Overlooking these issues is common and may be an unintentional or intentional act when working with clients. Clinicians may lack competence in the subject area or may find it to be an unfavorable and uncomfortable topic of discussion. When diagnosing and treating these disorders, awareness and

Did You Know?

- Erectile dysfunction is one of the leading sexual disorders in the United States. With global sales of erectile disorder medications at $4.82 billion in 2017 and expected to reach $7.10 billion in 2024 (Zion Market Research, 2019).

- Forty-three percent of women and 31% of men report experiencing sexual dysfunction (Cleveland Clinic, 2015).

- Roughly 67% of transgender individuals experience some type of workplace harassment directly related to being a transgender individual (James et al., 2016).

assessment of our own knowledge, comfort, bias, morals, and beliefs are essential to provide quality care. Reading this chapter and applying your critical thinking skills is an example of one way you begin to explore these factors.

Treatment of sexual issues requires an accepting and nonjudgmental approach, as these are highly personal, socialized, and, often, stigmatized topics of discussion. An individual's sexual health and expression is an important part of holistic care. Frequently, issues of a sexual nature will not only affect the person experiencing them but others, such as romantic partners, as well. Making a person's sexual history a part of the standard screening/interviewing process aids in collecting background information and demonstrates a clinician's willingness to discuss sexual issues.

Sexual Dysfunctions

Sexual dysfunctions include a wide range of issues and are some of the more prevalent disorders within the population. Sexual dysfunctions can be grouped into four categories:

1. Sexual Desire/Interest

   ICD-10 terms: Lack or loss of sexual desire, sexual aversion and lack of sexual enjoyment, excessive sexual drive (nymphomania, satyriasis)

   DSM-5 terms: Male hypoactive sexual desire disorder

2. Arousal

   ICD-10 terms: Failure of genital response (female sexual arousal disorder, male erectile disorder, psychogenic impotence)

   DSM-5 terms: Female sexual interest/arousal disorder, erectile disorder

3. Orgasm

   ICD-10 terms: Orgasmic dysfunction (inhibited orgasm, psychogenic anorgasmy), premature ejaculation

   DSM-5 terms: Female orgasmic disorder, premature ejaculation, delayed ejaculation

4. Sexual Pain

   ICD-10 terms: Nonorganic vaginismus, nonorganic dyspareunia

   DSM-5 terms: Genito-pelvic pain/penetration disorder

Also included in sexual dysfunctions are substance/medication-induced sexual dysfunction, other specified sexual dysfunction and unspecified sexual dysfunction (*DSM-5*) and other sexual dysfunction, not caused by an organic disorder or disease and unspecified sexual dysfunction, not caused by organic disorder or disease.

As we begin this chapter, can you think of a possible diagnosis for John?

Sexual desire/interest disorders describe a group of disorders that encompass a person's sexual interest or lack thereof and how it is affecting them. Typically, a psychological issue, such as depression or anxiety, contributes to these disorders. Relationship problems, including poor communication with one's partner, can also contribute to these disorders. Other possible factors include drinking excessive amounts of alcohol and taking antidepressants and other recreational drugs in excess.

Arousal disorders involve a lack of response to sexual stimulation. Sexual stimulation varies from person to person but typically could include kissing, touching the genitals, or watching erotic videos. Many of the same causes of arousal disorders are similar to sexual desire/interest disorders.

Sexual dysfunctions are commonly associated with older age. Indeed, youth is fleeting, and our bodies naturally deteriorate and encounter more issues as we age. However, we also want to acknowledge that younger populations experience sexual dysfunctions so as not to overlook reported symptoms and complaints simply because of age. One study of 2,309 French individuals between the ages of 15 and 24 found that 31% of females and 9% of males reported experiencing at least one sexual dysfunction that significantly hindered their sexuality (Moreau et al., 2016). These experiences resulted in reported sexual dissatisfaction in both genders.

In addition to specified presenting symptoms, most sexual dysfunctions can be further categorized. A dysfunction may be lifelong or acquired, generalized or situational, and range in severity from mild to moderate to severe. A lifelong dysfunction occurs during one's first sexual experience and continues with subsequent sexual experiences. Conversely, if onset follows a period of relatively normal sexual functioning, then it is acquired. A generalized dysfunction consistently persists regardless of varying stimulation, situations, or partners. When it only occurs with specific types of stimulation, situations, or partners, then it is situational. To meet diagnostic criteria, all sexual dysfunctions must be present for approximately 6 months and cause significant distress for the individual.

This section on sexual dysfunctions provides an overview of each dysfunction, along with diagnostic standards and currently researched treatment options. Compared to other psychological disorders, research on sexual dysfunctions is sparse. Your own research skills will be important in continually examining emerging and evidence-based research and treatment options. It is important to note that most of the existing research on sexual dysfunctions has focused on heterosexual males and females, resulting in an imbalance of knowledge of prevalence rates, impacts, and treatment options for individuals of other sexual orientations.

Male Hypoactive Sexual Desire Disorder (F52.0) (302.71)

The Western perspective of male sexual desire tends to view it in an almost compulsory nature. How many times have you heard the phrase, "Men only want one thing"? Despite this common line of thinking, male sexuality is multifaceted, and sexual socialization, cultural factors, and relationship factors must be taken into consideration when exploring desire issues (McCarthy & McDonald, 2009). Sexual desire concerns in males may often be overlooked and instead medical and mental health professionals may focus more on performance issues, such as premature ejaculation or erectile dysfunction. Male hypoactive sexual desire disorder is new to the *DSM-5* as previous editions listed hypoactive sexual desire disorder as a gender nonspecific disorder. The *ICD-10* includes this disorder under F52.0 (lack or loss of sexual desire) in which sexual desire is the primary issue and is not secondary to other sexual difficulties, such as erectile failure. Estimated prevalence rates are relatively low, with one study reporting that 4.8% of men occasionally lacked sexual desire and 3.3% frequently lacked sexual desire (Laumann et al., 2009). Male hypoactive sexual desire disorder is more likely to be acquired rather than lifelong. Desire is subjective and may include elements such as sexual or erotic thoughts, fantasies, and overall desire for sexual activity (McCarthy

& Ginsberg, 2007). From a psychological standpoint, the core issue of primary male hypoactive sexual desire disorder usually revolves around a secret or shameful pattern of desire or arousal. At the individual level, this might include a preference for masturbatory sex, unprocessed sexual trauma, or conflicts regarding sexual orientation.

When diagnosing male hypoactive sexual desire disorder, the clinician will define what is considered to be "deficient." Thus gathering accurate information during the clinical interview is essential in making an accurate diagnosis and establishing treatment. Box 11.2 provides screening factors for male hypoactive sexual desire disorder.

Would John be diagnosed with hypoactive sexual desire disorder?

Box 11.2 Screening Factors: Male Hypoactive Sexual Desire Disorder

- Childhood and adolescent sexual history, as many early sexual experiences affect future sexual preferences and interactions
- Quantitative data, such as the number of monthly orgasms
- Qualitative data, such as how the client typically reaches orgasm
- History of sexual abuse
- Concerns or incongruity in sexual orientation

Note: Suggested by McCarthy & McDonald (2009).

In the therapeutic treatment setting, it is important to consider the difficulty males may have discussing issues related to sexual desire. When assessing and treating male hypoactive sexual desire disorder, the clinician must first work to destigmatize the problem before attempting to explore any material that is secretive or sensitive. Once rapport and feelings of safety are increased, sexual vulnerabilities and strengths can be explored. Cognitive behavioral therapy, acceptance therapy, and behavioral activation strategies are all possible treatment considerations (Meana & Steiner, 2014). It is not unusual for sexual desire to fade in long-term relationships, so unsurprisingly, male hypoactive sexual desire disorder is a common complaint in couples' therapy. During

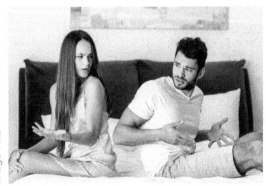

the course of couples' treatment, alternative ways of satisfying desire may be revealed, including masturbation, extramarital affairs, paraphilias, and pornography. Relationship skill building, conflict resolution, and communication training are important for those in intimate relationships. While there is no magic pill to suddenly make sexual experiences more desirable, pharmacological treatment may be a consideration in certain instances of this disorder. For example, individuals with low testosterone may experience desire issues, and thus testosterone replacement therapy may be helpful (Allan et al., 2008). Certain medical conditions, such as hyperthyroidism and psychological disorders like depression, can contribute to desire issues. Lifestyle changes to diet and exercise may be beneficial for some. Box 11.3 asks you to consider several relevant factors associated with sexual desire.

Image 11.2

Box 11.3 Consider

- How does gender socialization affect males' comfort in discussing sexual desire issues?
- Is a sexual desire/interest dysfunction diagnosis applicable for someone who identifies as asexual?

Female Sexual Interest/Arousal Disorder (F52.2)(302.72)

Female desire complications can be attributed to psychological, biological/medical, and social/relational causes (McCarthy et al., 2017). Female sexual interest/arousal disorder is the most common sexual dysfunction in females, affecting approximately 10% of American women aged 18–44 (Parish et al., 2019). Primary care physicians and mental health specialists may diagnose female sexual interest/arousal disorder, but it is important to remember that female clients may also discuss these issues with their obstetricians/gynecologists. When a woman lacks sexual desire, thoughts, or fantasies, it does not necessarily mean she has this disorder (Basson, 2014). Because of the complexity presentation in females, desire and arousal are not usually separate factors. Sexual motivation and interest are often larger than desire alone. Activating that desire or urge may only happen once sexual activity has started. The *ICD-10* includes this disorder under F52.2 (failure of genital response). Physical indications of female sexual interest/arousal disorder (Box 11.4) include vaginal dryness or failure of lubrication.

Box 11.4 Did You Know?

Female sexual interest/arousal disorder is a new addition to the *DSM-5* and was formerly categorized as hypoactive sexual desire disorder. This separate diagnosis recognizes that female sexual desire is different from the male model of hypoactive sexual desire disorder. Compared to their male counterparts, female sexual desire is seen as more variable and complex.

Psychological factors that may be of focus in therapy include anticipatory anxiety, viewing intercourse as a pass-fail test where you only pass if you reach orgasm, feelings of embarrassment and frustration, and patterns of avoidance (McCarthy et al., 2017). Narrative therapy may be particularly helpful, as it allows the client to restore their current narrative. Pharmacological options, such as filbanserin (Addyi) may help boost female libido; however, as a solo intervention, it does not address the psychological factors associated with sexual desire. Often, when a client uses a medical intervention and does not see dramatic differences or results, they infer that they have "failed." This may then lead to additional negative thoughts, such as, "I'm broken," or "Nothing is going to help me." Thus concurrent therapy is recommended, along with any medical treatment to challenge such thoughts. As with male hypoactive sexual desire disorder, female desire issues often have a larger effect on those who are in partnered relationships.

Erectile Disorder (F52.2)(302.72)

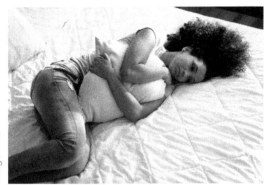

Image 11.3

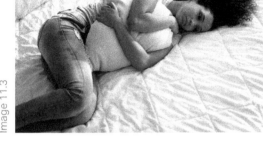

Image 11.4

The *ICD-10* includes erectile disorder under F5.2 (failure of genital response), which is marked by difficulty in developing or maintaining an erection to perform sexually satisfying intercourse. Erectile disorder (ED) is estimated to occur in 16%–22% of men with susceptibility to the disorder increasing with age (Muhall et al., 2018). An erection occurs when blood flows into the penis, thus anything that affects that blood flow can result in erectile disorder (Najari & Kashanian, 2016). The two most common medical conditions related to erectile disorder are hardening of the arteries (erosclerosis) and diabetes. Physiological or psychological factors may underlie erectile disorder, but often, it is a combination of both.

Treatment for erectile disorder will vary based on individual factors. Usually, the course of treatment is implementing lifestyle changes, such as smoking cessation, reducing alcohol intake, dietary changes, and weight loss (Muhall et al., 2018; Najari & Kashanian, 2016). While these changes may be helpful, only focusing on lifestyle changes will typically not cure erectile disorder, and client compliance with these changes is typically low. While male hypoactive sexual desire disorder and erectile disorder are separate conditions, they can overlap for some men (Millner & Ullery, 2002). Medications for erectile disorder, like sildenafil, increase blood flow to the penis (Najari & Kashanian, 2016). Other forms of medical treatment include injection therapy, vacuum erectile devices, and penile implants. It is important to note that because erectile disorder is so common, solutions to resolve this issue are highly marketable and not all products available online or in stores are proven to be effective or safe.

Before engaging in therapeutic care, it is important that a full medical examination is conducted (Millner & Ullery, 2002). Collaborative care between physicians and mental health providers can have positive effects on client outcomes. As part of holistic care, the psychological and psychosocial factors of erectile disorder should be addressed. These may include performance anxiety, depression, stress, satisfaction and communication with one's partner, and levels of self-confidence. Cognitive behavioral techniques can be helpful when dealing with negative thought patterns tied to performance anxiety or stress. In couples, teaching effective communication skills can address issues of emotional withdrawal and performance anxiety.

Female Orgasmic Disorder (F52.3)(302.73)

The *ICD-10* includes this disorder under F52.3 (orgasmic dysfunction) in which orgasm is absent or delayed after normal sexual excitement. The *DSM-5* diagnostic criteria for female orgasmic disorder further states that there may be a reduced intensity or infrequency of orgasm (Salmani et al., 2015). The diagnosis of female orgasmic disorder can be quite complex. What constitutes "a normal sexual excitement phase" may be difficult to define (Laan & Rellini, 2011). Further, anatomically, women can experience orgasm through penile-vaginal intercourse and clitoral stimulation or a combination of both. There is some skepticism in diagnosing an orgasmic disorder in females, as the majority of women (40%–60%) do not reach orgasm during normal sexual activity, and approximately 10% never reach orgasm at all (Zietsch et al., 2011). The estimated prevalence rate of female orgasmic disorder is between 20%–40% (Salmani et al., 2015). Not surprisingly, orgasmic difficulties can coexist with issues in sexual desire. Box 11.5 explores multicultural considerations around female orgasmic disorder.

Box 11.5 Multicultural Considerations

Diagnosis of female orgasmic disorder is complicated by the sociocultural context in which women exist, and treatment will vary based on this. The second "wave" of feminism brought issues of sexual liberation to the forefront, including the right of women to experience and enjoy an orgasm (Laan & Rellini, 2011). To get an idea of our current sociocultural context, at least in Western society, think of television shows or songs that glorify female orgasm, along with a partner's performance resulting in that orgasm. Conversely, some cultures dominated by heterosexual relationships may emphasize the sexual needs of a man and the biological purpose of reproduction over a woman's personal sexual satisfaction (Salmani et al., 2015). Discussing sex or sexual concerns may be seen as taboo for women of certain cultures or religions. When deciding the proper course of treatment, it is imperative to discuss and consider these factors with the client.

The medicalization of the absence of orgasm is often linked to sociocultural experiences, and it may be necessary to normalize this experience and provide psychoeducation to the client (Lavie-Ajayi, 2005). Pharmacological options are available to treat female orgasmic disorder, including testosterone, estrogen, and sildenafil (Salmani et al., 2015). Other treatments and psychological interventions include cognitive behavioral therapy, directed masturbation, Kegel exercises, bibliotherapy, and trauma therapy. Therapy for couples in which female orgasmic disorder is a central issue often focused on communication strategies. It may also be helpful to examine a partner's reaction to a woman's absence of orgasm and what role that plays in the woman labeling herself as dysfunctional (Lavie-Ajayi, 2005).

Delayed Ejaculation (F52.3)(302.74)

Delayed ejaculation is one of the least reported sexual complaints by males with an estimated prevalence rate of 1%–4% of sexually active men (Di Sante et al., 2016). As a diagnosable sexual dysfunction, delayed ejaculation lacks a clear diagnostic definition. For example, a delayed ejaculation diagnosis based on the *DSM-5* criteria requires that there either be a delay in or infrequency/absence of ejaculation at least 75%–100% of the time (Abdel-Hamid & Ali, 2018). Alternatively, the Third International Consultation on Sexual Medicine uses intravaginal ejaculation latency time to define delayed ejaculation. This is a measure of how long it takes a male to ejaculate during vaginal sex. In this case, delayed ejaculation is measured by one's intravaginal ejaculation latency time threshold exceeding 20–25 minutes (approximately two standard deviations above the mean) of sexual activity. The *ICD-10* includes this disorder under F52.3 (orgasmic dysfunction) in which orgasm is absent or markedly delayed. While ejaculation is often associated with orgasm, it is important to note that the two do not always coincide. Thus this disorder can occur in both the presence and absence of orgasm.

Depending on the individual, etiological factors of delayed ejaculation may be psychosexual/psychosocial and or organic/biological in nature. Collecting a comprehensive history of the individual and experienced symptoms is essential for diagnosis.

TABLE 11.1 Factors Contributing to Delayed Ejaculation

Psychogenic factors	• Insufficient mental and physical sexual stimulation • Unusual masturbation patterns and fantasies • A preference for solo masturbation over partnered sex • Mental conflicts, such as certain fears, feelings of hostility toward a partner, issues surrounding vulnerability, and guilt as a result of strong religious beliefs
Organic/biological factors	• Aging • Genetic factors • Neurobiological factors • Pharmacological side effects (multiple drugs, including alcohol, may result in delayed ejaculation, individuals taking selective serotonin reuptake inhibitors have a sevenfold increased risk for delayed ejaculation) • Medical procedures/treatment (individuals with pelvic or prostate cancer who are receiving radiation therapy may experience delayed ejaculation with the likelihood increasing with the length of treatment) • Other medical conditions (individuals with multiple sclerosis and diabetes mellitus are likely to experience delayed ejaculation)

Note: Proposed factors compiled by Abdel-Hamid & Ali (2018)

Treatment for delayed ejaculation may include psychological interventions, such as cognitive behavioral therapy, psychoeducation; masturbatory retraining; adjustment of sexual fantasies; sexual anxiety reduction by means of techniques, including mindfulness and progressive relaxation; and couples sex therapy (Abdel-Hamid & Ali, 2018). While an approved drug specifically for delayed ejaculation does not exist, there are multiple pharmacological options for managing delayed ejaculation. Some options include testosterone, bupropion, oxytocin, cabergoline, and cyproheptadine. The type of drug selected should be based on the individual's history, clinical evidence, and patient preference.

Premature Ejaculation (F52.4) (302.75)

According to the *ICD-10*, premature ejaculation is defined by the inability to control ejaculation sufficiently for both partners to enjoy sexual interaction. Premature ejaculation is the most common sexual dysfunction in men, affecting around 20% to 30% of the population (Brewer & Tidy, 2017; Corona et al., 2015). Lifelong premature ejaculation is marked by ejaculation that occurs prior to or approximately within 1 minute of vaginal penetration from the first sexual experience one has. Acquired premature ejaculation is defined by a clinically significant and bothersome reduction in latency time, approximately 3 minutes or less. The inability to delay ejaculation can be frustrating, and some individuals may choose to avoid sexual intimacy altogether. As such, premature ejaculation may result in dissatisfaction in relationships and avoidance of relationships for those who are not partnered (Brewer & Tidy, 2017).

Psychological factors, such as anxiety, and biological factors, such as genetics and hormonal abnormalities, can underlie premature ejaculation. Approximately one third of individuals with premature ejaculation also reported erectile disorder (Corona et al., 2015). The majority of men with lifelong premature ejaculation, however, do not have associated erectile disorder. Underlying factors that link premature ejaculation and erectile disorder are still unknown. Depressive and anxiety symptoms are significantly linked to the risk of individuals who have premature ejaculation also having erectile disorder. Men often find themselves in a cycle where they try to control ejaculation, which then reduces levels of excitation, leading to erectile disorder. Conversely, attempting to form an erection increases excitement, which can then lead to premature ejaculation.

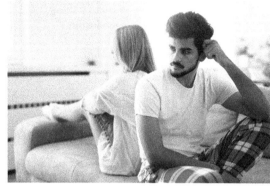

Image 11.5

Individuals with premature ejaculation often don't seek treatment and instead are frequently coaxed into treatment by their partners, often when they wish to conceive (Brewer & Tidy, 2017). Addressing the existing self-esteem of the individual experiencing premature ejaculation is an important part of therapy, along with any criticisms from the individual's partner that may contribute to lower confidence. Cultural views of masculinity can affect male self-esteem. Pornography often impacts an individual's view of what a typical sexual experience looks like and commonly paints an unrealistic picture. This may cause men to feel inadequate in their performance. Cognitive behavioral approaches can assist in addressing performance or general anxiety and distorted and unrealistic sexual expectations. Psychoeducation can also aid in normalizing sexual experiences and managing expectations. Religion is an important factor to consider in treatment, as it can affect the treatment approach. For example, some individuals may be reluctant to engage in masturbation as a form of treatment.

Genito-Pelvic Pain/Penetration Disorder (F52.6) (302.76)

Another new addition to the *DSM-5* is genito-pelvic pain/penetration disorder, which combines the previously separated disorders of dyspareunia and vaginismus (Conforti, 2017). The *ICD-10* includes this disorder under F52.6 (nonorganic dyspareunia), which occurs in both women and men. Pain during intercourse is often attributed to local pathology, and when applicable, it should be properly categorized under the pathological condition. While genito-pelvic pain/penetration disorder can be categorized as either lifelong or acquired and varies in severity, it is not categorized as generalized or situational.

The cause of genito-pelvic pain/penetration disorder is multifactorial and can be attributed to biological, psychological, and relational factors or any combination of such factors (Conforti, 2017). Many medical conditions can cause pain during intercourse, and it is important to rule them out before diagnosing a client with this disorder. Some medical conditions include infections, such as sexually transmitted infections; skin allergies, such as an allergy to semen; neoplastic and neurologic conditions; trauma, such as female genital mutilation; and hormonal issues, such as menopause, endometriosis, and pain resulting from operations and chemotherapy or radiation. Chemical irritation from soaps or douches can also contribute to pain.

TABLE 11.2 Diagnostic Requirements of Genito-Pelvic Pain/Penetration Disorder

Persistent or recurrent:	• Difficulty in vaginal penetration with intercourse • Vulvovaginal or pelvic pain present during vaginal intercourse or attempts at penetration • Fear or anxiety surrounding vulvovaginal or pelvic pain present prior to, during, or after vaginal penetration • Tensing or tightening of pelvic floor muscles when attempting vaginal penetration

Note: Adapted from ICD-10 (World Health Organization [WHO], 2016); DSM-5 (APA, 2013)

Naturally, when something causes us pain, we have a tendency to avoid the activity in the future. Pain and anticipation of pain affect mental and physical sexual arousal and decrease vaginal lubrication and pelvic muscle relaxation (Conforti, 2017). Anxiety and depression can negatively contribute to pain and further exacerbate symptoms. In addition, childhood trauma may contribute to genito-pelvic pain/penetration disorder symptoms. One study found that rates of childhood sexual abuse, emotional abuse, and emotional neglect were higher for women with a genito-pelvic pain/penetration disorder diagnosis compared to a control group (Özen et al., 2019). Psychoeducation is an important part of therapeutic treatment, along with cognitive behavioral therapy. Examining and replacing maladaptive or unhelpful cognitions contributing to pain or feelings of fear and anxiety are often effective (Conforti, 2017). Pelvic floor therapy aids in pain reduction by increasing awareness of pelvic muscles and providing relaxation techniques. In terms of medical treatments, more research is needed; however, options do exist. Local anesthetics and anti-inflammatory agents have been found to be minimally helpful in the treatment of pain. Botox may be a helpful treatment for those struggling with pelvic floor hyperactivity, as it causes local muscle paralysis lasting for approximately 3–6 months. Topical estradiol and testosterone gels have shown some promise in reducing pain, but more research is needed. The most effective treatment, vulvar vestibulectomy, is also the most invasive. This surgical procedure completely removes the vestibular mucosa. However, 88% of patients reported partial relief of sexual pain, and 78.5% reported significant relief of pain.

Gender Dysphoria

Gender Dysphoria (F64.2)(302.6)

One of the most publicly debated disorders within sexual disorders is that of gender dysphoria. Gender dysphoria, a new chapter, has journeyed through several name changes in both the *DSM* and *ICD* over the past 30 years. More importantly than a name change is the perception and updated knowledge concerning gender dysphoria among the general population and researchers. Unlike other chapters, gender dysphoria is the only disorder included. Yes, that's it! Although it may seem small, this one disorder, like many others, varies in classification based on age of onset.

In 2019, the WHO officially reclassified the name of *gender identity disorder* to *gender incongruence*. The WHO went a step further when it decided to move this diagnosis from the mental disorders chapter to the sexual health chapter. This change is pivotal, as the degree of severity is significant between gender identity and gender incongruence. Gender identity was viewed simply as the lack of congruence between assigned gender and the gender one may actually identify. Gender dysphoria is the marked and distressing lack of congruence between a person's assigned gender and the gender with which they identify (Ashley, 2019; Kuyper & Wijsen, 2014).

Gender dysphoria is diagnosed as F64.1 in the *ICD-10*. The diagnosis includes classifications for children, adolescents, and adults. The onset of gender dysphoria is between 2 and 4 years old. Family members report even earlier signs than the 2 to 4 age range through early behaviors of dressing as the opposite gender. Gender dysphoria consists of specific criteria occurring for a minimum of 6 months.

TABLE 11.3 Gender Dysphoria in Adolescents and Adults

Gender dysphoria in adolescents and adults
Marked incongruence between your experienced and expressed gender and your primary or secondary sex characteristics
Strong desire to be rid of your primary or secondary sex characteristics
Strong desire to be of the other gender
Strong desire to be treated as the other gender
Strong conviction that you have the typical feelings and reactions of the other gender

Note: DSM-5 (APA, 2013)

TABLE 11.4 Gender Dysphoria in Children

Gender dysphoria in children
Strong desire to be of the other gender or an insistence that they are the other gender
Strong preference for wearing clothes typical of the opposite gender
Strong preference for cross-gender roles in make-believe play or fantasy play
Strong preference for the toys, games, or activities stereotypically used or engaged in by the other gender
Strong preference for playmates of the other gender
Strong rejection of toys, games, and activities typical of their assigned gender
Strong dislike of their sexual anatomy
Strong desire for the physical sex characteristics that match their experienced gender

Note: DSM-5 (APA, 2013)

Often, when the topic of gender dysphoria comes up, there is confusion; however, some may think of transgender issues. The term transgender is not the official language supported by the World Health Organization, and this is a portion of the long-standing history around the medical and mental health professions over the past 3 decades. The inconsistency in language creates confusion and continues to feed into the mistrust and shame. For better understanding, please see the following common terms and definitions that may be, but are not always, affiliated with gender dysphoria:

- Transgender: an umbrella term for all individuals who, to varying degrees, do not align with their assigned gender.
- Cisgender: a term indicating that an individual aligns with their assigned gender.

- Gender binary: commonly shortened to binary, this term represents individuals who identify their gender as clearly male or female.
- Nongender binary: commonly shortened to nonbinary, this term represents individuals who identify their gender as beyond the social constructs of males and females.
- Sex: a term referencing your chromosomal makeup, which produces features that socially have been deemed male or female.
- Gender: the expression of one's identity and historically has been confined within the socially constructed dichotomy of male and female traits.
- Gender-affirming procedures: medical procedures that affirm an individual's physical body to their identified gender.

This long-awaited shift has the ability to provide hope and begin to improve the trust of lesbian, gay, bisexual, transgender, queer/questioning, intersex, ally, asexual, and pansexual (LGBTQ*) individuals and specifically transgender-identifying individuals and mental health professionals. Longhofer (2013) highlighted the lack of alliance and negative connotation that have existed between LGBTQ*-identifying clients, potential clients, and mental health providers. Shame has been affiliated with providers and the LGBTQ* community (Longhofer, 2013). The move by the World Health Organization from mental illness to sexual health has the ability to generate space for all of the voices that have felt silenced or had shame associated with who they are (Longhofer, 2013). The shame is possibly a connection to the low amounts of data that researchers have obtained (Kuyper & Wijsen, 2014; Longhofer, 2013). As cultural understanding and proper education on gender dysphoria continue to improve, the rates of individuals seeking services globally continues to rise (Thrower et al., 2019). Hopefully, there will continue to be an incline in individuals seeking care and eventually without fear and shame.

TRUE LIFE 11.1

Caitlyn Jenner

Caitlyn Jenner is an Olympic Gold medalist track star who was born on October 28, 1949, in Mount Kisco, New York. Ranging from the early '70s to the early 2000s, Jenner made appearances in several television series, and on October 14, 2007, she debuted the series *Keeping Up With the Kardashians. I Am Cait* was a docuseries that documented her life as a transgender woman; however, the series was canceled after 1 year (Biography, 2018). She is also known as a sports commentator, the author of *Decathlon Challenge: Bruce Jenner's Story* and *Finding the Champion Within*, and a

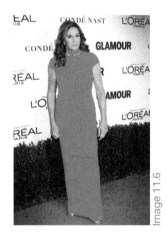

Image 11.6

motivational speaker. Jenner's voice gained more recognition when in 2015 she revealed to the public that she identified as a female and would no longer be referred to as Bruce Jenner.

For 65 years, Caitlyn was recognized by the world as Bruce Jenner, one of the greatest decathletes of his time, but in 2015, Bruce Jenner reintroduced himself to the world as Caitlyn Jenner, thus changing the manner in how we would refer to her in the current day. Caitlyn claims to have struggled her entire life with gender identity issues. Caitlyn has been vocal on the difficulties of being transgender but does not relish in the limelight. "I do it very quietly because I have been so criticized by the liberal side of the media. I can get more things done if I don't stick my nose into everything publicly" (Setoodeh, 2018). What made publicizing her transition even more controversial was being a Republican in Hollywood. However, Caitlyn aims to do more for the trans community, and one example includes employing an all-transgender cast on her show (Setoodeh, 2018), as well as knowing her fair share of statistics concerning the community. Caitlyn shared that "48 per cent of trans people in the UK have attempted suicide, and 85 per cent have thought about it," and "55 percent of trans people in the UK have been diagnosed with depression and 27 per cent of trans people aged 15–25 have attempted suicide. 72 per cent have self-harmed at least once" (Newman, 2018).

Caitlyn has also shared her struggles with an eating disorder, suicidal ideation, and depression. In her autobiography, *Secrets of My Life*, she reveals a time when she thought of ending it all. The purpose behind her sharing this intimate moment was to raise awareness for suicide among the transgender population. One of the reasons behind the suicidal ideation stemmed from years of harassment from the paparazzi questioning her gender identity and photoshopping pictures of her face onto the body of women. One evening months before Bruce was to announce his transition, he received a phone call threatening to post a picture of him in the tabloids revealing his transition. Bruce responded to the threat, "Harvey, don't even talk about this. It's none of your business and please, when you do stuff like that it affects people's lives." Bruce thought about getting his gun from the other room and ending his "pain" (Newman, 2018). After a night's rest, Bruce reflected on his thought of suicidality and came to the following conclusion: "Wasn't that like the stupidest thing you could possible do?" Bruce understood and accepted that there would be low points and that instance happened to be one of them.

June 1, 2015, marks the day that Caitlyn Jenner was introduced to the world via tweet: "I'm so happy after such a long struggle to be living my true self. Welcome to the world Caitlyn. Can't wait for you to get to know her/me." Caitlyn has received much backlash since coming out as transgender, but she has rolled with the punches. Upon accepting the Arthur Ashe Award for Courage, Caitlyn released the following media statement: "This transition has been harder on me than anything I could imagine, and that's the case for so many others, besides me. For that reason alone, trans people deserve something vital, they deserve your respect." Caitlyn has made progress in her goal to serve as an advocate for the transgender community. We leave you with Caitlyn's message to all: "I know I'm clear with my responsibility going forward, to tell my story the right way—for me, to keep learning, to do whatever I can to reshape the landscape of how trans issues are viewed, how trans people are treated. And then more broadly to promote a very simple idea: accepting people for who they are. Accepting people's differences" (Biography, 2018).

Treatment Options

Gender dysphoria can be treated from a systems approach, including mental health counselors, mental health specialists, physicians, and community agencies. Each individual with gender dysphoria may want to proceed differently with varying forms of treatment. It should be noted that every individual may not want to use hormone replacement or any gender-affirming procedures. There are also age considerations that should be explored prior to the start of any type of treatment.

Gender dysphoria in children can be treated by varying degrees of engagement and acceptance of dysphoria. Some providers will attempt to revert the child back to the assigned gender, while others will use community-based interventions to safely provide support while the child affirms their gender. Specifically, psychodynamic behavior modification and family therapy/groups can be used. In addition to the support provided to the child and family combined, there are also support groups and therapy groups for the parents/guardians to process their experience as well.

There are multiple comorbid diagnoses with gender dysphoria. The emerging literature shows that gender dysphoria has comorbidity with a variety of other disorders. When treating gender dysphoria, it would behoove providers to consider both when identifying the best course of treatment. Neurodevelopmental disorders, such as autism spectrum disorder and attention deficit hyperactivity disorder; dissociative disorders; anxiety disorders; and depressive disorders are a few of the comorbid disorders connected to gender dysphoria (Thrower et al., 2019). However, the research is limited, and at this time, comorbid disorders are only to be considered, not held as direct correlations. Similar to any other individuals, those with gender dysphoria benefit from early acknowledgment, being accepted and loved, and individualized treatment.

CASE STUDY 11.2 Leslie is a 9-year-old assigned female at birth who resides in the southern portion of the United States. Leslie presents at your office in loose-fitting jeans, a slightly oversized T-shirt, and hair pulled back under a hat. Leslie sits in the chair across from their father and mother and seems to match the body language of the father despite not being quite as big. Leslie sits back in the chair with legs wide and hands laying on top of their knees. Leslie presents calmly and seemingly content with the appearance and first impressions. Leslie's parents provide historical context and indicate that Leslie has the same gift request each Christmas: help them become a boy. Initially, Leslie's parents believed Leslie was going through some sort of phase, but after Leslie's feelings persisted for several years, they decided to seek a therapist's help. Leslie informs you that their favorite activities include helping out with cutting grass and lawn care, assisting with fixing cars, climbing trees, playing football, and wrestling. They show no interest in the barbies, kitchen sets, or stuffed animals in your office. Leslie has one older brother, Tony, who is 11. They often sneak into their brother's room and borrow his clothes. Leslie's parents are confused about whether they should punish this sort of behavior. Leslie's friends are all boys, and whenever they play games involving imagination, Leslie wants to be a male. Leslie's parents do not know how to react to Leslie's actions.

What is your clinical opinion about Leslie's presentation?

What concerns arise within you based on this case?

Would you work with this child and their family?

CASE STUDY 11. 3 Lance is a 35-year-old, able-bodied adult. Lance frantically enters your office dressed in a tank top, low-rise jeans, flip-flops, and crossbody bag. This is your 27th session with Lance, and this has been deemed a typical presentation. Lance asks if you remember the big savings account. Lance has been saving money for months, which will all be used to afford a sex reaffirming procedure. They believe that after the procedure, they will finally be comfortable in their own body and have freedom. Lance perceives this surgery as the first step to officially obtaining a name change and experiencing their true gender. Ever since Lance was ten, Lance has known that a cosmic mistake occurred at birth. They state, "I was supposed to be born a female." Lance expressed this desire to their parents during their 18th birthday celebration. Their parents had already suspected this because of Lance's tendency to cross-dress and spend time primarily with females. They were disowned by their parents and kicked out of the house. This forced Lance into homelessness for 2 years until steady employment was secured. Despite all of the pain of rejection, Lance feels that they are finally in a good place in life. Lance has steady work as a hairdresser and is happily dating Kevin. From the age of 10, Lance has been romantically interested in boys, but it usually ended in confusion or heartbreak. Kevin understands Lance's struggles and strives to support Lance completely.

What is your clinical opinion about Lance's presentation?

_____

What concerns arise within you based on this case?

_____

Would you work with this individual?

_____

Did you notice any differences in your thoughts and considerations about Leslie and Lance?

_____

Paraphilic Disorders

Paraphilic disorders are a class of disorders that traditionally are viewed within society as culturally unacceptable sexual behaviors. Frequently, behaviors housed within this class of disorders are viewed as sexually deviant to the degree of potential incarceration (Caldeano, 2016; Garcia et al., 2013). The limited data on these disorders seem to be skewed toward males being the primary individuals meeting full criteria. Considering the prevalence of males, readers are cautioned to consider how social constructs shape expectations of sexuality based on gender. Some research using nonclinical samples online shows that men are much more likely to be accepting of uncommon and paraphilic sexual interests than women (Downing, 2015; Ventriglio et al., 2019). This leads researchers to believe that sex drive is a sole contributor to this variation.

Countless clinicians and future providers shy away from treating paraphilic disorders out of ignorance of the disorders. However, a key helping skill is using empathy, and this is necessary when working with clients diagnosed with paraphilic disorders. It should be remembered that all individuals deserve compassion, and it is best to take the time to acknowledge our biases prior to engaging in any form of treatment. Currently, there are eight disorders within this class that are commonly identified. Each of these disorders describes a variety of sexual behaviors deemed socially unacceptable; however, they all have a minimum time requirement of 6 months prior to an official diagnosis.

The paraphilic disorders include the following:

1. Voyeuristic disorder
2. Exhibitionistic disorder
3. Frotteurism disorder
4. Sexual masochism disorder
5. Sexual sadism disorder
6. Pedophilic disorder
7. Fetishistic disorder
8. Transvestic disorder

A main point of contention around paraphilic disorders is the idea that nonreproductive sexual acts are all paraphilic; however, participating in same-sex relationships and consensual sexual behaviors is not a mental health disorder. Even though homosexuality is no longer classified as a mental disorder, heteronormativity still dictates what is deemed normal as it pertains to sexual preferences (Downing, 2015). With such a restrictive view of sexuality, those who report deviant sexual behavior will downplay the amount of admitted occurrences. The second concern that has emerged is the use of the word *nonconsenting* in this class of disorders. Paraphilic disorders include engaging with a person who is nonconsenting. The use of the word *nonconsenting* can include acts such as rape and molestation.

Often, incarceration is the first form of treatment for individuals diagnosed with paraphilic disorders (Alper, 2019; Caldeano, 2016; Garcia et al., 2013). However, research indicates that recidivism rates are high for individuals who have been incarcerated for any crime and higher for those with paraphilic disorders (Alper, 2019). Recidivism is the process of obtaining an additional arrest or violation after prior legal infraction within a 3-year period of release (National Institute of Justice, 2019). Other forms of treatment include the use of pharmacology, empathy, cognitive behavioral therapy, attachment therapy, and empirically tested treatment for sexually acting out (Garcia et al., 2013). Throughout the long history of this class of disorders, it appears there is a continued need for exploration, consideration, and implication behind what is grouped together as it influences culture and society. Now let's take a deeper dive into each paraphilic disorder.

CLINICIAN'S CORNER 11.1

Throughout my clinical experience I have noticed that clients tend to focus on the physical symptoms associated with sexual concerns and often overlook psychological aspects. While medication can be a "quick fix" for some, many have more complex underlying behaviors, emotions, and thoughts connected to their sex life. For those in relationships, I often find break downs in communication (i.e., of needs, desires, and preferences). Another common issue I notice is the connection of self-worth to sexual performance. As humans, in general, we tend to place a lot of pressure on ourselves. Pressure related to sexual performance can be exacerbated by social constructs like gender and portrayals of people in a variety of mediums (i.e., television, music, pornography, and social media). One's sex life can be a sensitive topic of conversation, especially when there are significant concerns. I find that an established, trusting, and nonjudgmental relationship with your client often provides the best environment for them to open up and discuss their concerns. It is also important for your client to experience this moment of vulnerability in a safe environment, such as therapy, in order to increase confidence in their ability to do the same outside of the session. As a final note, some beginning or even established therapists may not be entirely comfortable with or have faith in their ability to help those with sexual concerns. I believe that therapists are more equipped to help these clients than they often think they are. In therapy we commonly work on improving communication skills, increasing self-worth, and identifying and challenging negative thought patterns with our clients. Transferring your existing knowledge of theories, skills, and techniques is a great place to start when working with clients presenting concerns related to sex.

Sonja Lund, PhD

Voyeuristic Disorder (F65.3)(302.82)

A person with voyeuristic disorder is most commonly thought of as a peeping tom. This image is depicted as a person in a high-rise apartment sitting with the lights out and looking out the window with binoculars at their neighbors. This view is a bit dated, as the realm of what is socially acceptable continues to be stretched by the ever-faster exchange of information through the use of technology. The voyeuristic disorder is the process of an individual who gains sexual satisfaction from watching individuals disrobe or engage in sexual acts. Someone engages in this act through various means. They may go the route of peeking through a window or hanging out in the dressing room at a local department store, but as the world is quarantined, these urges are still being fulfilled. Currently, individuals with paraphilic disorders still need to engage in these various behaviors. Despite being seemingly trapped in the house, individuals are seeking ways to fulfill their sexual urges. Research shows that there are some correlations between voyeuristic disorder and exhibitionistic disorder, and some have indicated that they are both variations of the same disorder (Downing, 2015).

Exhibitionistic Disorder (F65.30)(302.4)

Continuing the exploration of paraphilic disorders includes expanding on the conversation around what's deemed acceptable and unacceptable as a society. The exhibitionist disorder includes behaviors associated with exposing genitals to unsuspecting individuals and masturbating to the idea or memories of the victim's expressions (McNally & Fremouw, 2014; Potik & Rozenberg, 2020). These events may happen in countless public places, such as train stations, parking lots/decks, malls, or amusement parks (Clark et al., 2016). Now, these events are typically depicted in sitcoms and horror movies as a man standing in a raincoat and top hat in the rain waiting for the unsuspecting victim to emerge from around the low-lit corner, but in reality, this behavior is far more common than these extremes. Any person can meet the criteria of this disorder, as it could be intentional positioning of a penis/phallic object in lighter colored cotton pants or low-cut pants that reveal the upper thigh. Often, individuals who engage in these behaviors appear average, and research shows that to a degree, an exhibitionist and voyeur may intentionally try to appear more average to not be noticed (Hopkins et al., 2016). The type of pleasure that one could seek and gain while in a crowd are limitless when you have no idea what degree of exposure or visibility is needed to achieve satisfaction.

There are countless factors that have been correlated to exhibitionist disorder, and other paraphilic disorders, such as poor child-parent attachment, distorted derivatives of courtship, injuries to fragile masculine identity, family upbringing, cultural factors, and biological factors (Hopkins et al., 2016; Potik & Rozenberg, 2020). These events involve early developmental moments where shame, fear, and confusion are connected with sexual urges and fantasies. During these moments, exhibitionists, primarily males, needed to be validated and experience empathy to form healthy connections; instead, they were taught to feel negative about themselves or their urges.

Exhibitionistic and voyeuristic disorders, which have been found to have similarities in the past, are both linked to courtship. Physical touch is a form of courtship and attraction. Hopkins et al. (2016) highlight how voyeurism and exhibitionism are the first and second forms of courtship. This perspective highlights the depth of the possibilities of human expression. These are various levels of behaviors that are deemed socially acceptable.

Frotteurism Disorder (F65.81)(302.89)

From walking down a crowded hallway, to being in a shopping center, to making your way through a busy terminal, there is a general understanding that sometimes people bump into others. But what if it wasn't an accident? This is not to make you alarmed but to draw attention to how specific each of the paraphilic disorders is to certain behaviors. Every time this happens, you are not the victim of frotteurism disorder, yet the act can be as normal as passing each other in a busy grocery store. Frotteurism disorder is the act of making contact with any portion of someone's body, specifically the genitals, who is not aware or consenting (Clark et al., 2016). In attempts to study frotteurism and other paraphilic disorders, the shift must go to those who have experienced/witnessed the act. As mentioned, many individuals with these disorders have discrepancies in the numbers they report and may often simply report lower occurrences to seem more socially acceptable. Research links frotteurism to exhibitionism through the expression of courtship gestures (Clark et al., 2016; Potik & Rozenberg, 2020). It is believed that for some individuals with frotteurism disorder, they are acting out what they would hope the individual would do to them willingly. In addition, frotteurism has correlated to the following early life experiences: poor child-parent attachment, distorted derivatives of courtship, injuries to fragile masculine identity, family upbringing, cultural factors, and biological factors (Clark et al., 2016; Hopkins et al., 2016; Potik & Rozenberg, 2020).

Sexual Masochism Disorder and Sexual Sadism Disorder

It may appear that we are going deeper and maybe even darker into the span of human sexuality. Viewing all of these behaviors on a spectrum is beneficial. It is important as a counselor to be empathic with individuals diagnosed with paraphilic disorders. As we continue to stretch our understanding and consideration of this spectrum, we enter the next level: sexual masochism disorder. Sexual masochism and sexual sadism disorders have been depicted in countless films and novels throughout history with secret rooms, leather, whips, chains, and countless other items. These disorders include six key traits: (1) bondage, (2) discipline, (3) domination, (4) submission, (5) sadism, and (6) masochism; this is more commonly known by the acronym BDSM. These behaviors are a spectrum, and individuals can enjoy them individually or shift between the two extremes. As society continues to expand its perspective on sexual fluidity, behaviors housed in these disorders are shifting. Society and thus the profession is moving away from pathologizing sexual masochism disorder and sexual sadism disorder behaviors (Dahan, 2019). Despite the growth, the disorders still stand as criminal offenses when connected to more aggressive and abusive levels of control manipulation (Nitschke et al., 2009).

SEXUAL MASOCHISM DISORDER (F65.51)(302.83)

Sexual masochism disorder (Box 11.6) is the enjoyment and pleasure experienced through being the recipient of pain, bondage, suffering, or humiliating actions from a partner. Sexual masochism disorder involves the relinquishing of control, which allows for a physically and emotionally detached experience (Dahan, 2019; Kurt & Ronel, 2017). These feelings of detachment are similar to the experiences of individuals who self-mutilate. One of the most dangerous associated conditions that may possibly occur with masochism is asphyxiophilia (Coluccia et al., 2016). This is achieved by various strategies aimed at depleting an individual's level of oxygen to enhance sexual arousal. Methods may include self-strangulation, hanging, and suffocation with an object, such as a plastic bag. In the United States, approximately 250–1,000 annual deaths occur as a result of autoerotic asphyxia. These rates may actually be underestimated because many are accidentally categorized as suicide cases. This is especially true for certain cultures, as family members who discover the victims often try to disguise the autoerotic behaviors.

> ## Box 11.6 Masochism and Addiction
>
> Research by Kurt and Ronel (2017) found behaviors and experiences similar to individuals with addictions in those who practice masochism. This study found that the first masochistic experience is often highlighted with individuals attempting to reach those intense sensations again. Because of this, they engage in more frequent and extreme masochistic experiences, usually failing to reexperience the sensations of their first encounter. After the masochistic experience has ceased, the intense positive feelings usually fade quickly, which reinforces the individual to seek those sensations out again despite major consequences.

SEXUAL SADISM DISORDER (F65.52)(302.84)

Sexual sadism disorder is the enjoyment of inflicting pain, bondage, and suffering, which leads to pleasure. Sexual sadism disorder involves the enforcement of control over another person, thus making them nonconsenting (Dahan, 2019; Nitschke et al., 2009). Difficulty in diagnosis occurs because there is no universal description of required behavior or cutoffs for severity cutoffs (Longpré et al., 2018). Because of this prevalence, rates vary by study, categorizing anywhere from 5% to 50% of sexual offenders as sadists. One dimension that is fairly consistent among different studies is that sexual sadism in sex offenders often predicts sexual recidivism. Music (2016) wrote about violent and sadistic behavior in children and adolescents, finding that those who were perpetrators of sexually sadistic behavior often lacked an environment where they could experience empathy and care. Typically, these children came from high-conflict backgrounds, environments of neglect, and had been victims of sexual abuse themselves. Manifestations of sexually sadistic behaviors may start as a way to avoid and regulate core complex anxieties, trauma, and feelings of inadequacy in children. Often, the pleasure provided by these defenses becomes addictive, especially during adolescence when dopamine circuits are rapidly developing.

While less common, sexually sadistic behavior can also be present in women. As perpetrators, women may engage in coercive behaviors, such as lying or attacking a man's sexuality after refusing a sexual advance, or aggressive behaviors, such as the use of physical force and intoxicants. Research examining maladaptive personality traits and adversarial sexual attitudes in both a university and national sample found that 10% of women surveyed reported perpetrating sexual violence (Russell et al., 2017). It is notable that the rates in the national sample were significantly higher than rates in the university sample. This study also found personality traits of hostility, eccentricity, and grandiosity are most commonly associated with sexually violent acts in women. The researchers suggested that women with these personality traits may obtain pleasure from controlling men and frequently view sex as a competition rather than a display of affection.

Pedophilic Disorder (F65.4)(302.2)

The pedophilic disorder is the act of engaging in sexual acts with prepubescent minors (Jordan et al., 2020; Tenbergen et al., 2015). Sexual child abuse can affect the rest of a person's life. It is a singular traumatic event that has the capacity to impact an individual's social development, hinder their ability to navigate life stages, and, generally, affect their overall intrapersonal communication skills. Pedophilia is commonly interchanged with child sexual offenders; however, only 50% of child sex abuse is done by an individual who meets the full criteria (Jordan et al., 2020; Tenbergen et al., 2015). When individuals do not meet the full diagnostic criteria, this may simply mean that they are not in any distress at that current time. It should be mentioned that individuals who meet criteria may also never act on the sexual urges and simply can satisfy the pedophilic disorder with fantasies alone (Jordan et al., 2020; Tenbergen et al., 2015). In addition to the field of counseling, neurology, psychology, psychiatry, and other professions are researching pedophilia (Jordan et al., 2020; Tenbergen et al., 2015). Biomarkers, biofeedback, and imaging are currently being used to gain a better understanding of the nuances surrounding pedophilic disorder (Tenbergen et al., 2015).

In the same manner that society wants to know the prevalence of other paraphilic disorders, individuals want the same for pedophilic disorder; unfortunately, the numbers are skewed. The individuals who are willing to report their acts or fantasies often report lower and inaccurate accounts. Reports show that gender is not an indicator of being susceptible; although male-identifying bodies have historically been viewed as pedophiles, female-identifying people have reported close to 25% of the cases of pedophilic behavior (Tenbergen et al., 2015). Studying and treating individuals includes discussions around masturbation. In treatment, clients use the following forms of trauma-focused care:

- Family therapy
- Individual therapy
- Group therapy

During therapy sexual urges, desires, and fantasies are discussed to assist the client to identify what is healthy and unhealthy sexual behavior.

Fetishistic Disorder (F65.0)(302.81)

The word "fetish" describes an inanimate object that can arouse sexual desire (Ventriglio et al., 2019). The sexual act is related to sexual attraction, fantasy, and behavior. A fetish may also apply to parts of the body, situations, or activities. Fetishes vary widely, and those surrounding objects may be linked to the object itself, shapes, consistencies, or surfaces. There may also be an attraction around sensory input, including touch, feel, or vision. Often, fetishes are very specific in nature. There is one case of a man from the United Kingdom who was arrested for having sex with 450 tractors. During the investigation, 5,000 tractor images were discovered on his laptop. He was particularly attracted to green John Deere and Massey Ferguson tractors. The theories behind the development of a fetish include a psychoanalytic perspective that encompasses "perversions" and regression and behavioral perspectives, such as classic conditioning, social learning, operant conditioning, and social cognition. A few biological theories also exist. One proposed theory is that the region in the brain that processes sensory input from the feet is next to the region that processes genital stimulation, and the two become accidentally linked.

The two main reasons people enter treatment for a fetish are because it is affecting their current relationship, or they have gotten into some legal trouble in which treatment was ordered. When assessing for a fetish, comorbid psychiatric conditions should be excluded (Box 11.7).

Box 11.7 Areas of Exploration for Fetishistic Disorder

Ventriglio et al. (2019) recommend gathering more detailed information on the following:

- The developmental path and context of the fantasies (including the age they started and masturbatory practices)
- Exploring various fetishistic tendencies in detail
- Pornography use
- Any history of violent sexual assaults
- General and sexual delinquency

Transvestic Disorder (F65.1)(302.3)

Similar to other disorders pertaining to sex and/or gender, transvestic disorder is not new to the mental health community. Transvestic disorder, also known as transvestic fetishism, has been discussed among helping professionals for decades. During this long history, individuals who have met the criteria have been viewed as having personality disorders, as well as simply being identified as sexually deviant. Transvestic disorder is the process of gaining sexual arousal from dressing as the nonassigned gender for a minimum duration of 6 months. Similarly to other paraphilic disorders, transvestic disorder has been assumed to primarily affect males; however, this is not true. Transvestic disorder is simply the arousal associated with dressing in different attire that is not socially deemed to match one's assigned presentation. Studies show that this happens more frequently than many assume.

Conclusion

This chapter highlighted the importance of sex, sexuality, and gender and their connection to our mental and physical health. Often, we have our own opinions, comfort levels, and preferences when it comes to these topics, so it is important to examine those in relation to the treatment we provide to reduce instances of countertransference. As clinicians, gaining competence in this area is essential, as it is part of holistic treatment. Disorders such as sexual dysfunctions and gender dysphoria will likely require collaborative care with physicians, psychiatrists, and other specialists, while paraphilic disorders may require collaboration within the legal system. The authors of this chapter encourage you to expand your knowledge of these topics, especially in relation to multicultural competence.

Case Study Summary

One of this chapter's case studies reviewed the behaviors of John. As you process the story and examine possible diagnostic criteria, take a few minutes to answer the following questions:

1. What would be the correct diagnosis for John?

2. What are the specific symptoms or criteria that led you to this diagnosis?

3. What other possible disorders might you diagnose John with and why?

4. Briefly discuss what types of treatment may be beneficial for John. Could you see using a certain counseling theory and/or medication?

Guided Practice Exercises

Scenario 1

Martin

Martin, 29, lives alone in a third-story apartment in a small city. Marin at first thought that his obsession with long black boots was normal, but now the fetish is beginning to negatively affect his life. He needs to have shoes nearby to feel aroused. If the shoes are not present, then Martin will not become "turned on," even when watching porn. After Martin sees long black boots or a women in long black boots, he feels strong sexual arousal. He will then typically masturbate afterward. Martin has only had one serious relationship. His girlfriend was at first aroused when Martin asked her to wear black boots before they had sex, but then she became creeped out when she realized Martin needed the boots to be able to have an orgasm. Martin keeps a large collection of tall black leather boots in his apartment. He missed work last week because there was a boot sale going on at a local store during his work hours. He has even begun trying to touch women wearing black leather boots on the street. Martin does not know who will be able to help him with his problem.

What would be the correct disorder? What are the specific symptoms or criteria that led you to this diagnosis?

_____
_____
_____

What specific behaviors caused you to diagnose the disorder?

_____
_____
_____

What other possible disorders might you consider and why?

_____
_____
_____

Do you believe that different colored boots would also arouse Martin (i.e., brown boots, tan boots)? Explain your reasoning.

_____
_____
_____

Scenario 2

Gabriella

Gabriella, 34, is married with two children. Her husband is the only one who knows her shameful secret. Gabriella is extremely aroused by touching and kissing feet. If she is unable to do this, then she cannot reach orgasm. This started during Gabriella's teen years when one of her earliest boyfriends gave her a foot massage before they had sex. Since then, Gabriella has been increasingly turned on by feet. This issue is beginning to affect Gabriella's day-to-day life. She is being plagued at work by the thought of others' feet. She is aroused when she sees someone take off their shoes in public and has had to swallow the urge to touch them. Her boss has almost fired her for a lack of productivity. Gabriella cannot focus, especially with other feet in the room.

What would be the correct disorder? What are the specific symptoms or criteria that led you to this diagnosis?

_____
_____
_____

What specific behaviors caused you to diagnose the disorder?

_____
_____
_____

What other possible disorders might you consider and why?

_____

_____

_____

Explain how conditioning can lead to the development of a fetish.

_____

_____

_____

Do you believe that conditioning is always involved in fetishes? What is another way a fetish may develop?

_____

_____

_____

Scenario 3

George Michael, 34, has become increasingly involved in the sadism and masochism community because of its connections to a bar. He works as a bartender and often goes home with women who come to the bar for drinks. For years, it has sexually aroused George Michael to tie women up and "punish" them. He used to be able to reach an orgasm after roughly spanking women and then penetrating them. Now his preferences have become more violent. The part of sex that George Michael enjoys the most is seeing the other person suffer. It makes George Michael feel in control of them and of his life. The last sexual encounter that George Michael was involved in almost ended in an arrest. He had tied the woman to his bedpost and beat her roughly with a belt. She pleaded for him to stop to no avail and ended up leaving the house bloody and bruised. Now George Michael makes sure that the women he takes home are masochists. A friend of George's suggested that he get help for his "deviant" behavior, but George does not believe he has a problem.

What would be the correct disorder? What are the specific symptoms or criteria that led you to this diagnosis?

_____

_____

_____

What specific behaviors caused you to diagnose the disorder?

_____

_____

_____

What other possible disorders might you consider and why?

_____

_____

_____

Why do you think that George Michael is hesitant in coming to counseling?

_____

_____

_____

Is the desire for dominance in the bedroom something you believe is a learned behavior or genetic?

_____

_____

_____

Web-Based and Literature-Based Resources

Mayo Clinic: https://www.mayoclinic.org/diseases-conditions/erectile-dysfunction/diagnosis-treatment/drc-20355782

Mount Sinai: https://www.mountsinai.org/health-library/condition/sexual-dysfunction

References

Abdel-Hamid, I., & Ali, O. (2018). Delayed ejaculation: Pathophysiology, diagnosis, and treatment. *World Journal of Men's Health*, 36(1), 22–40. https://doi.org/10.5534/wjmh.17051

Allan, C. A., Forbes, E. A., Strauss, B. J. G., & McLachlan, R. I. (2008). Testosterone therapy increases sexual desire in ageing men with low-normal testosterone levels and symptoms of androgen deficiency. *International Journal of Impotence Research*, 20(4), 369–401. https://doi.org/10.1038/ijir.2008.22

Alper, M., &. Durose, M. R. (2019). *Recidivism of sex offenders released from state prison: A 9-year follow-up (2005-2014)*. *Prepared by the Bureau of Justice Statistics of the U.S. Department of Justice* (NCJ 251773). U.S. Department of Justice. https://www.bjs.gov/content/pub/pdf/rsorsp9yfu0514.pdf

Ashley, F. (2019). The misuse of gender dysphoria: Toward greater conceptual clarity in transgender health. *Perspectives on Psychological Science*. https://doi.org/10.1177/1745691619872987

Basson, R. (2014). On the definition of female sexual interest/arousal disorder. *Archives of Sexual Behavior*, 43(7), 1225–1226. https://doi.org/10.1007/s10508-014-0324-0

Biography. (2018, November 01). *Caitlyn Jenner*. https://www.biography.com/people/caitlyn-jenner-307180

Brewer, G. & Tidy, P. (2017). Premature ejaculation: Therapist perspectives. *Sexual and Relationship Therapy*, 32(1), 22–35. https://doi.org/10.1080/14681994.2016.1188200

Caldeano, A. R., Nunes, J., & Da Costa, P. (2016). Paraphilic disorder in the 21st century. *European Psychiatry*, 33(S1), S591–S591. https://doi.org/10.1016/j.eurpsy.2016.01.2203

Clark, S. K., Jelgic, E. L., Calkins, C., & Tartar, J. R. (2016). More than a nuisance: The prevalence and consequences of frotteurism and exhibitionism. *Sexual Abuse: A Journal of Research and Treatment*, 28(1), 3–19. https://doi.org/10.1177/1079063214525643

Cleveland Clinic. (2015). *Sexual dysfunction and disease*. https://my.clevelandclinic.org/health/diseases/9125-sexual-dysfunction-and-disease

Coluccia, A., Gabbrielli, M., Gualtieri, G., Ferretti, F., Pozza, A., & Fagiolini, A. (2016). Sexual masochism disorder with asphyxiophilia: A deadly yet underrecognized disease. *Case Reports in Psychiatry*, 2016, 1–4. https://doi.org/10.1155/2016/5474862

Conforti, C. (2017). Genito-pelvic pain/penetration disorder (GPPPD): An overview of current terminology, etiology, and treatment. *University of Ottawa Journal of Medicine*, 7(2), 48–53. https://doi.org/10.18192/uojm.v7i2.2198

Corona, G., Rastrelli, G., Limocin, E., Sforza, A., Jannini, E. A., & Maggi, M. (2015). Interplay between premature ejaculation and erectile dysfunction: A systematic review and meta-analysis. *Journal of Sexual Medicine*, 12(12), 2291–2300. https://doi.org/10.1111/jsm.13041

Dahan, O. (2019). Submission, pain, and pleasure: Considering an evolutionary hypothesis concerning sexual masochism. *Psychology of Consciousness: Theory, Research, and Practice*, 6(4), 386–403. https://doi.org/10.1037/cns0000202

Di Sante, S., Mollaioli, D., Gravia, G. L., Ciocca, G., Limoncin, E., Carosa, E., Lenzi, A., & Jannini, E. A. (2016). Epidemiology of delayed ejaculation. *Translational Andrology and Urology*, 5(4), 541–548. http://doi.org/10.21037/tau.2016.05.10

Downing, L. (2015). Heternormativity and repronormativity in sexological "perversion theory" and the DSM-5's "paraphilic disorder" diagnosis. *Archives of Sexual Behavior, 44*, 1139–1145. https://doi.org/10.1007/s10508-015-0536-y

Garcia, F. D., Delavenne, H. G., Assumpcao, A. D., & Thibaut, F. (2013). Pharmacologic treatment of sex offenders with disorders. *Current Psychiatry Reports, 15*(5), 1–6. https://doi.org/10.1007/s11920-013-0356-5

Hopkins, T. A., Green, B. A., Carnes, P. J., & Campling, S. (2016). Varieties of intrusion: Exhibitionism and voyeurism. *Sexual Addiction & Compulsivity, 23*(1), 4–33. https://doi.org/10.1080/10720162.2015.1095138

James, S. E., Herman, J. L., Rankin, S., Keisling, M., Mottet, L., & Anafi, M. (2016). *The Report of the 2015 U.S. Transgender Survey*. Washington, DC: National Center for Transgender Equality.

Jordan, K., Wild, T. S. N., Fromberger, P., Müller, I., Müller, J. L. (2020). Are there any biomarkers for pedophilia and sexual child abuse? A review. *Frontiers in Psychiatry, 10*, 940. https://doi.org/10.3389/fpsyt.2019.00940

Kurt, H., & Ronel, N. (2017). Addicted to pain: A preliminary model of sexual masochism as addiction. *International Journal of Offender Therapy and Comparative Criminology, 61*(15), 1760–1774. https://doi.org/10.1177/0306624X15627804

Kuyper, L. & Wijsen, C. (2014). Gender identities and gender dysphoria in the Netherlands. *Archive of Sexual Behavior, 43*, 377–385. https://doi.org/10.1007/s10508-013=0140-y

Laan, E., & Rellini, A. H. (2011). Can we treat anorgasmia in women? The challenge to experiencing pleasure. *Sexual and Relationship Therapy, 26*(4), 329–341. https://doi.org/10.1080/14681994.2011.649691

Laumann, E. O., Glasser, D. B., Neves, R. C., & Morira, E. D. (2009). A population-based survey of sexual activity, sexual problems and associated help-seeking behavior patterns in mature adults in the United States of America. *International Journal of Impotence Research, 21*(3), 171–178. https://doi.org/10.1038/ijir.2009.7

Lavie-Ajayi, M. (2005). "Because all real women do": The construction and deconstruction of "female orgasmic disorder." *Sexualities, Evolution and Gender, 7*(1), 57–72. https://doi.org/10.1080/14616660500123664

Longhofer, J. L. (2013). Shame in the Clinical Process with LGBTQ Clients. *Clinical Social Work Journal, 41*, 297–301. https://doi.org/10.1007/s10615-013-0455-0

Longpré, N., Guay, J., Knight, R. A., & Benbouriche, M. (2018). Sadistic offender or sexual sadism? Taxometric evidence for a dimensional structure of sexual sadism. *Archives of Sexual Behavior, 47*, 403–416. https://doi.org/10.1007/s10508-017-1068-4

McCarthy, B., & Ginsber, R. L. (2007). Male hypoactive sexual desire disorder: A conceptual model and case study. *Journal of Family Psychotherapy, 18*(4), 29–42. https://doi.org/10.1300/J085v18n04_03

McCarthy, B., Koman, C. A., & Cohn, D. (2017). A psychobiosocial model for assessment, treatment, and relapse prevention for female sexual interest/arousal disorder. *Sexual and Relationship Therapy, 33*(3), 353–363. https://doi.org/10.1080/14681994.2018.1462492

McCarthy, B., & McDonald, D. (2009). Assessment, treatment, and relapse prevention: Male hypoactive sexual desire disorder. *Journal of Sex & Marital Therapy, 35*(1), 58–67. https://doi.org/10.1080/00926230802525653

McNally, M. R., & Fremouw, W. J. (2014). Examining risk of escalation: A critical review of the exhibitionistic behavior literature. *Aggression and Violent Behavior, 19*(5), 474–485. https://doi.org/10.1016/j.avb.2014.07.001

Meana, M., & Steiner, E. (2014). Hidden disorder/hidden desire: Presentations of low sexual desire in men. In Y. M. Blink & K. S. K. Hall (Eds.), *Principles and practice of sex therapy* (pp. 42–60). Guilford Press.

Millner, V., & Ullery, E. (2002). A holistic treatment approach to male erectile disorder. *Family Journal, 10*(4), 443–447. https://doi.org/10.1177/106648002236768

Moreau, C., Kågesten, A. E., & Blum, R. W. (2016). Sexual dysfunction among youth: An overlooked sexual health concern. *BMC Public Health, 16*(1), 1170. https://doi.org/10.1186/s12889-016-3835-x

Muhall, J. P., Giraldi, A., Hackett, G., Hellstrom, W., Jannini, E. A., Rubio-Aurioles, E., Trost, L., & Hassan, T. A. (2018). The 2018 revision to the process of care model for management of erectile dysfunction. *Journal of Sexual Medicine, 15*(9), 1434–1445. https://doi.org/10.1016/j.jsxm.2018.06.005

Music, G. (2016). Angels and devils: Sadism and violence in children. *Journal of Child Psychotherapy, 42*(3), 302–317. https://doi.org/10.1080/0075417X.2016.1238142

Najari, B. B. & Kashanian, J. A. (2016). Erectile dysfunction. *JAMA, 316*(17), 1838.

National Institute of Justice. (2019). *Recidivism*. https://nij.ojp.gov/topics/corrections/recidivism

Newman, V. (2018, May 11). *Caitlyn Jenner opens up about harrowing suicidal thoughts and almost ending it*. Mirror. https://www.mirror.co.uk/3am/celebrity-news/ive-gun-caitlyn-jenner-opens-12518211

Nitschke, J., Osterheider, M., & Mokros, A. (2009). A cumulative scale of severe sexual sadism. *Sexual Abuse: Journal of Research and Treatment, 21*(3), 262–278. https://doi-org.libproxy.clemson.edu/10.1177/1079063209342074

Özen, B., Özdemir, Y. Ö., & Beştepe, E. E. (2019). Childhood trauma and dissociation among women with genito-pelvic pain/penetration disorder. *Neuropsychiatric Disease and Treatment, 14*, 641–646. https://doi.org/10.2147/NDT.S151920

Parish, S., Shahpurwala, Z., Athavale, A., Ravindranath, R., Hadker, N., & Lim-Watson, M. (2019). Describing the clinical approach to diagnosis and treatment of patients with hypoactive sexual desire disorder. *Journal of Sexual Medicine*, 16(6, S3), S32–S33. https://doi.org/10.1016/j.jsxm.2019.03.527

Potik, D., & Rozenberg, G. (2018). Self psychology, risk assessment of individuals with exhibitionistic disorder and the good lives model—more than meets the eye. Journal of Aggression, Maltreatment & Trauma. https://doi-org.libproxy.clemson.edu/10.1080/10926771.2018.1530714

Russell, T. D., Doan, C. M., & King, A. R. (2017). Sexually violent women: The PID-5, everyday sadism, and adversarial sexual attitudes predict female sexual aggression and coercion against male victims. *Personality and Individual Differences*, 111, 242–249. https://doi.org/10.1016/j.paid.2017.02.019

Salmani, Z., Zargham-Boroujeni, A., Salehi, M., Killeen, T. K., & Merghati-Khoei, E. (2015). The existing therapeutic interventions for orgasmic disorders: Recommendations for culturally competent services, narrative review. *Iranian Journal of Reproductive Medicine*, 13(7), 403–412.

Setoodeh, R. (2018, August 07). How Caitlyn Jenner is secretly fighting Trump's White House on transgender rights. *Variety*. https://variety.com/2018/politics/features/caitlyn-jenner-trans-rights-advocate-1202896320/

Tenbergen, G., Wittfoth, M., Frieling, H., Ponseti, J., Walter, M., Walter, H., Beier, K. M., Schiffer, B., & Kruger, T. H. (2015). The Neurobiology and Psychology of Pedophilia: Recent Advances and Challenges. *Frontiers in human neuroscience*, 9, 344. https://doi.org/10.3389/fnhum.2015.00344

Thrower, E., Bretherton, I., Pang, K. C., Zajac, J. D., & Cheung, A. S. (2019). Prevalence of autism spectrum disorder and attention-deficit hyperactivity disorder amongst individuals with gender dysphoria: A systematic review. *Journal of Autism and Developmental Disorders*, 50, 695–706. https://doi.org/10.1007/s10803-019-04298-1

Ventriglio, A., Bhat, P. S., Torales, J., & Bhugra, D. (2019). Sexuality in the 21st century: Leather or rubber? Fetishism explained. *Medical journal, Armed Forces India*, 75(2), 121–124. https://doi.org/10.1016/j.mjafi.2018.09.009

World Health Organization (WHO). (2016). *International statistical classification of diseases and related health problems, 10th revision (ICD-10)*.

Zietsch, B. P., Miller, G. F., Bailey, J. M., & Martin, N. G. (2011). Female orgasm rates are largely independent of other traits: Implications for "female orgasmic disorder" and evolutionary theories of orgasm. *Journal of Sexual Medicine*, 8(8), 2305–2316. https://doi.org/10.1111/j.1743-6109.2011.02300.x

Zion Market Research. (2019). Global Erectile Dysfunction Drugs Market Set For Rapid Growth, To Reach Value Around USD 7.10 Billion by 2024. https://www.zionmarketresearch.com/news/erectile-dysfunction-drugs-market

Credits

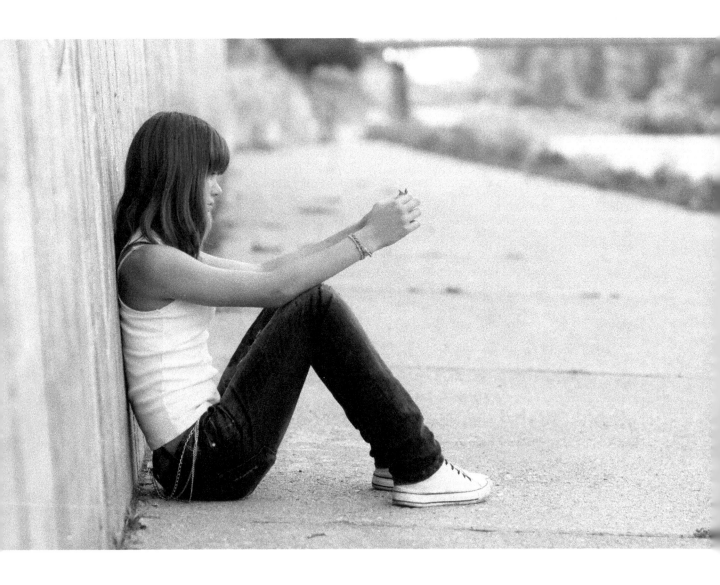

CHAPTER TWELVE

DISRUPTIVE, IMPULSE-CONTROL, AND CONDUCT DISORDERS

Robin Moody, Theresa C. Allen, and David A. Scott

CASE STUDY 12.1 Christopher, 16, looks harmless, but in reality, he has a pending assault charge against him and has been expelled from three different schools. He has seen many counselors and psychiatrists, few of whom made any progress with his volatile moods or violent and inappropriate behavior. Christopher has always been the bully of his class. He was expelled this year after hitting a classmate in the face with a brick during an outdoor gym class. The prior year, he was expelled for threatening to kill a teacher and bringing a knife to school after being denied recess for bad behavior. Christopher recently horrified his neighbors by stealing a small dog and setting it on fire. When asked why he did this, Christopher replied, "It was funny, and I wanted to see how it [the dog] would react." Christopher hardly speaks to counselors. When he does, he will say things such as, "I can't wait to get out of here and get high." His elderly grandparents are raising Christopher. They have little energy for his exploits. They began caring for Christopher around the time he was 3 months old. His mother was trying to pawn Christopher off to another addict in exchange for drugs. Nobody knows who Christopher's father is.

Did You Know?

- In the United States, 2% to 16% of youth are diagnosed with oppositional defiant disorder (Cleveland Clinic, 2019).

- Pyromania is not a response to a hallucination or impaired judgment (Grohol, 2019).

- All adolescents diagnosed with oppositional defiant disorder *do not* go on to develop conduct disorder.

- White males between the ages of 18 and 35 have the highest rates of fire setting (Merrick et al., 2013).

Overview

Infancy, childhood, and adolescence are periods of development that include exponential growth, rapid learning, and boundary testing. It is not uncommon for children to test or push back against authority figures with hostile behaviors, such as angry outbursts or temperamental crying. However, in approximately 1%–11% of the preschool population, a more severe pattern of oppositional behaviors occurs (American Psychiatric Association [APA], 2013). Symptoms include lack of temper control and emotional overreaction (Cavanagh et al., 2017), excessively argumentative, easily annoyed, and persistently defiant (Mikolajewski et al., 2019). These deficiencies in emotional self-regulation in childhood may be predictive of lifelong antisocial behaviors that develop into other forms of psychopathology (Burnette, 2013; Mikolajewski et al., 2019). Subsequently, such disruptive and antisocial behaviors can lead to criminal activity and legal ramifications (Grant & Leppink, 2015).

Table 12.1 provides a brief comparison between the *International Statistical Classification of Diseases (ICD-10)* and *Diagnostic and Statistical Manual of Mental Disorders, 5th*

Edition (DSM-5) codes to give you a quick view of some of the most prevalent disorders discussed in this chapter.

TABLE 12.1 *ICD-DSM* Comparison

ICD-10	DSM-5 CODES
Behavioral Disorders (F91.x)	*Disruptive, Impulse-Control, and Conduct Disorders*
Oppositional defiant disorder (F91.3) Listed under conduct disorders	**Oppositional defiant disorder** (313.81)
Other habit and impulse disorders (F63.81) This disorder is listed within the disorders of adult personality and behaviors under habit and impulse disorders	**Intermittent explosive disorder** (312.34)
Conduct disorders (F91.x)	**Conduct disorder** (312.8x)
Listed several locations: **Dissocial personality disorder (F60.2) Mixed and other personality disorders (F61) Other problems related to lifestyle (Z72.8)**	**Antisocial disorder** (301.7) Grouped within the personality disorders (Cluster B).
Pathological fire setting (pyromania; F63.1) This disorder is listed within the disorders of adult personality and behaviors under habit and impulse disorders	**Pyromania** (312.33)
Pathological stealing (kleptomania; F63.2) This disorder is listed within the disorders of adult personality and behaviors under habit and impulse disorders	**Kleptomania** (312.32)
Other conduct disorders (F91.8)	**Other disorders** (312.89)

Note: Adapted from ICD-10 (WHO, 2016); DSM-5 (APA, 2013)

Oppositional Defiant Disorder (F91.3) (313.81)

It is common for children to display aggressive behavior at times. One toddler may snatch a toy from another toddler. A child may cry or melt into a tantrum when they are denied their desire of the moment. As children mature, most learn how to manage their aggressive impulses (Schoorl et al., 2016). This is accomplished to a great extent through social interactions, such as learning to share or bargaining for a compromised resolve to situations. These "others-regarding" behaviors become increasingly normative between the ages of 3 and 8 years old as a child learns to meet their own needs and maintain prosocial behaviors (Steinbeis et al., 2012).

Some people, however, do not develop these strategic social behaviors and instead find themselves on an antisocial continuum (Steinbeis et al., 2012). Various studies have explored the reasons for this. One such study examined how brain structure in children affects behavior and discovered that greater cortical thickness of the left dorsolateral prefrontal cortex is positively related to increased prosocial behaviors and impulse control (Steinbeis et al., 2012). Another study that focused on the autonomic nervous system suggested that a malfunctioning of the vagus nerve, which is the main nerve of the parasympathetic nervous system and responsible for helping to instigate calm in times of stress, may trigger emotional dysregulation and poor management of hostility (Schoorl et al., 2016).

Oppositional defiant disorder (ODD) is a potential outcome of sustained negative patterns of aggression. This disorder is typically more prevalent in prepubescent males, with most diagnoses occurring around the age of 8 years old (Burnette, 2013). The essence of oppositional defiant disorder is a repetitive pattern of poorly controlled behaviors—such as angry/irritable mood, argumentative/defiant behavior, or vindictiveness—that deviate from social norms and often manifest as physical or verbal injury to self, others, or objects (WHO, 2016).

CASE STUDY 12.2 The parents of Hiroshi, age 5, do not know how they went wrong in raising their child. Hiroshi has always been the problem child in his class. He throws tantrums, deliberately annoys his classmates, and can be downright spiteful. When confronted, Hiroshi will often lose his temper and blame everyone else for his problems. In his most recent outburst, Hiroshi told the teacher, "I hate you, and I hate this school! All you do is tell me what to do! The reason I do bad is because I sit next to Collin. He makes me more stupid!" Hisoshi will not listen to his parents at home. He will always do the opposite of what they ask. They have given up asking him to pick up his toys or clear his plate because it only results in an angry outburst. Hiroshi often knocks things off of other students' desks or punches and kicks his classmates. His parents are not sure where to turn for help.

To meet the diagnostic criteria for oppositional defiant disorder, these behaviors must last at least 6 months, as evidenced by at least four of the symptoms listed in Box 12.2, and the symptoms must occur with at least one person who is not a sibling.

Box 12.2 Oppositional Defiant Disorder Symptoms

- Easily loses temper
- Argues with or defies the authority of adults
- Deliberately annoys others
- Places blame on others for their mistakes
- Easily annoyed with people or circumstances
- Resentful of others

Risk Factors

PERSONALITY TRAITS

Individuals have unique patterns of thoughts, feelings, and behaviors, which are commonly referred to as personality traits. Subsequently, personality is believed to be a strong predictor of psychological adjustment in a person (Wang et al., 2017). The five-factor model of personality, developed by Robert McCrae and Paul Costa, is a well-established model that identifies five basic personality traits: (1) neuroticism, (2) openness, (3) conscientiousness, (4) extraversion, and (5) agreeableness. Studies on children with oppositional defiant disorder have discovered similar personality traits consisting of higher levels of neuroticism and lower levels of agreeableness and conscientiousness (Herzhoff et al., 2016; Tackett et al., 2013; Zastrow et al., 2018).

Neuroticism

Neuroticism is most related to experiences of distress and poor well-being (Sobol-Kwapinska, 2016). Neuroticism is considered to be the outcome of hyperreactivity in the limbic system. The result is that people with a high degree of neuroticism experience fear, depression, shame, or other negative emotional or environmental stimuli with a greater intensity than people without this trait (Sobel-Kwapinska, 2016). This often manifests in maladaptive behaviors, such as anger, hostility, defiance, and impulsiveness.

Agreeableness

Agreeableness is associated with effortful control. It reflects the degree to which one is willing to be cooperative and to inhibit negative thoughts and impulses to maintain prosocial behaviors and interpersonal relationships (Want et al., 2017). Conversely, low agreeableness is reflective of poor self-regulation and adjustment difficulties. This often manifests in negative emotionality, aggressive behaviors, and rejection sensitivity in a person.

Conscientiousness

Conscientiousness is the personality trait associated with reliability, organization, and productivity (Akram et al., 2019). Studies show that individuals with lower levels of conscientiousness are at greater risk of reduced emotional stability; mental health difficulty, such as anxiety, depression, and sleep disorders; and an increased risk of mortality (Akram et al., 2019).

Subsequently, each of these prevalent personality traits may account for oppositional defiant disorder comorbidity with both internalizing and externalizing disorders (Herzhoff et al., 2016; Tackett et al., 2013).

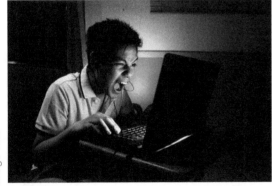

Image 12.2

TEMPERAMENT TRAITS

Temperament is conceptualized as one's ability to self-regulate and manage reactivity (Zastrow et al., 2018). High levels of negative emotions and low levels of inhibitory control have been predictive of oppositional defiant disorder (APA, 2013; Zastrow et al., 2018).

OTHER FACTORS

Other risk factors for the development of oppositional defiant disorder in children include harsh, inconsistent, or neglectful environments and genetic and physiological markers, such as reduced gray matter volume in the prefrontal cortex, amygdala, temporal lobes, and anterior insula, as well as other basal cortisol reactivity abnormalities (Ogundele, 2018).

Oppositional defiant disorder is frequently comorbid with attention deficit hyperactivity disorder and conduct disorder. It has also been associated with an increased risk of self-harm and suicide. Would you diagnose Christopher with oppositional defiant disorder?

Intermittent Explosive Disorder (F63.81) (312.34)

Intermittent explosive disorder typically occurs in late childhood—early adolescence—and is more common in males than females. It is characterized by anger-based or impulsive outbursts that are commonly triggered by a perceived social threat or low frustration tolerance that is disproportionate to the situation (Coccaro, 2015). These behaviors have no premeditation or planning. Instead, outbursts have a spontaneous onset and last for 30 minutes or less (APA, 2013). The *ICD-10* (WHO, 2016) diagnostic criteria for the disorder include the following:

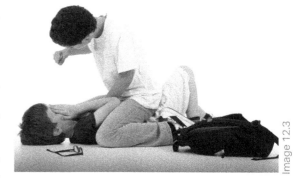

Image 12.3

- Recurrent verbal aggressions or assaultive acts
- Impulsive, destruction of property
- Emotional response is grossly disproportionate to the perceived provocation
- The outbursts are not the etiological factors of another disorder or medical condition

The duration of intermittent explosive disorder ranges from approximately 10 years to the entirety of one's life span (Coccaro, 2015).

Risk Factors

ENVIRONMENTAL

Individuals who have experienced physical or emotional trauma in childhood or early adulthood are at an increased risk for intermittent explosive disorder. Consequently, these individuals often experience severe difficulties in relational, social, and occupational functioning and incur financial and legal problems throughout their lives because of their aggressive behaviors (Fahlgren et al., 2019).

OTHER FACTORS

There is a strong genetic predisposition for intermittent explosive disorder. In fact, individuals with first-degree relatives who have this disorder are highly likely to experience the condition.

Furthermore, physiological studies have shown that individuals with intermittent explosive disorder may have serotonergic abnormalities in the anterior cingulate and orbitofrontal cortex areas of the brain (APA, 2013). In addition, deficits in the limbic and paralimbic systems reduce alexithymia and empathy, which may contribute to the inability of individuals with impulsive aggression symptoms to accurately interpret nonverbal cues in others, such as facial expressions (Coccaro et al., 2007; Fahlgren et al., 2019). Subsequently, intermittent explosive disorder is frequently comorbid with mood disorders (Coccaro et al., 2016).

Also important to note is the frequent association between aggressive behavior and substance use disorder (Coccaro et al., 2016). Studies have shown that the presence of intermittent explosive disorder may increase the likelihood of substance use and abuse; although, a substance use disorder does not cause intermittent explosive disorder (Coccaro et al., 2016).

CLINICIAN'S CORNER 12.1

Disruptive, Impulse-Control, and Conduct Disorders

Working with children and adolescents who demonstrate disruptive, impulse-control, and conduct disorders can be challenging for a clinician since it is not only the client but also the family system and beyond that need to be educated and trained. However, there is hope for achieving success in the home, success in the school, and success in interpersonal relationships for struggling juveniles.

Through empirically based treatments, a child or adolescent experiencing these types of maladaptive behaviors can learn to manage racing thoughts and impulsive urges and reclaim a sense of balance in life. From a clinician's standpoint, it is important to understand that increasing executive skills functioning and emotion regulation in young clients is a time-based process. Nevertheless, victorious living is an attainable goal for many.

~Theresa C. Allen, PhD, LPC, NCC

Conduct Disorder (F91-)

Impulse control and self-regulation are learned throughout the normal developmental stages of childhood. Children who do not develop self-control and continue to display a pervasive pattern of hostility in emotional and behavioral functioning are at greater risk for "delinquency, unemployment, depression, anxiety, and other psychiatric problems" (Schoorl et al., 2016, p. 821). As such, oppositional defiant disorder is considered an early stage of conduct disorder since the criteria for oppositional defiant disorder is satisfied among the many symptoms of conduct disorder (Cavanagh et al., 2017; Rowe et al., 2010). It is important to note, however, that "most children with oppositional defiant disorder do not eventually develop conduct disorder" (APA, 2013, p. 461).

While conduct disorder may be diagnosed in adults, onset after the age of 16 years old is rare. Instead, this disorder primarily develops in childhood or early adolescence and is more prevalent in males, who demonstrate both physical and relational aggression, than females, who primarily demonstrate relational aggression. The development and course of the disorder vary, but symptomatic behaviors tend to increase in severity with age (APA, 2013).

The *DSM-5* (APA, 2013) and *ICD-10* (WHO, 2013) diagnostic criteria for conduct disorder include repetitive and persistent patterns of behavior that violate social norms, as well as the basic rights of others. At least three types of behaviors from the following categories must have occurred within the past 12 months with at least one of the behaviors occurring in the past 6 months:

1. Aggression to people and animals (excessive levels of fighting and cruelty to people and animals)
2. Severe destructiveness to property (fire setting, property damage)
3. Repeated lying and stealing
4. Truancy, running away from home, breaking curfew

The *DSM-V* (APA, 2013) also included a callous-unemotional (CU) specifier to its diagnostic criteria for conduct disorder. The purpose of this limited prosocial emotions specifier is to identify a subgroup of the conduct disorder population with high levels of CU traits, such as lack of remorse or guilt, lack of empathy, shallow affect, and no concern about performance (Vanwoerden et al., 2016). CU traits are associated with heightened levels of aggression and depressive symptoms in both males and females. In addition, the CU specifier has been shown to predict the severity of offenses and antisocial behavior in youth, as well as predict psychopathy in adulthood (Vanwoerden et al., 2016).

Risk Factors

TEMPERAMENTAL

Temperament can be an early predictor of conduct disorder. Low frustration tolerance, as well as lower than average IQ have been identified as risk factors for the development of conduct disorder (APA, 2013).

ENVIRONMENTAL

Individuals who experience rejection by parents, insecure attachments, physical or sexual abuse, neglect, or lack of supervision are at risk for the development of conduct disorder. Likewise, delinquent peer groups and exposure to violence or criminal behaviors are also risk factors for the disorder (Rowe et al., 2010).

OTHER FACTORS

Hereditable factors also influence the development of conduct disorder. There is a substantial genetic predisposition for children with a first-degree relative who has conduct disorder, depressive or bipolar disorder, schizophrenia, attention deficit hyperactivity disorder, or alcohol use disorders (APA, 2013; Rowe, 2010). In addition, neurobiological studies have shown morphometric brain abnormalities, such as reduced gray matter volume in the left the orbitofrontal cortex, the temporal lobes, and the limbic system in the brain, may correlate with the development of impulsive and aggressive behavior disorders (Huebner et al., 2008).

Would Christopher be diagnosed with conduct disorder?

TRUE LIFE 12.1

David Berkowitz

David Berkowitz, famously named "Son of Sam," was not only diagnosed as antisocial but also with pyromania. Even before his killing sprees in New York City, he was setting fires to hundreds of buildings in efforts to vent his internal anger (Fire Line School, n.d.). Berkowitz struggled as a teenager after the death of his adopted mother when he was 14. Even at an

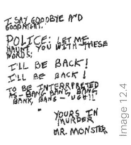

early age, Berkowitz was involved in pyromania and petty larceny. He was also described as above-average in intelligence (Crime Library, 2020). He served in the military and was known as an excellent marksman (Biography. com, 2020). After returning home, he worked as a postal service employee. Berkowitz claimed that his neighbor's Labrador retriever named "Harvey" was demon-possessed and ordered him to set over 1,500 fires and kill six people. He also described hearing other voices telling him to commit the murders. Despite numerous psychological evaluations, Berkowitz was declared competent to stand trial. Upon hearing of his guilty verdict, he tried to jump out of a seventh-floor window (Biography.com, 2020). Berkowitz was given six 25-years-to-life sentences for his crimes.

Antisocial Personality Disorder (F60.2) 301.7

Antisocial personality disorder begins to manifest in childhood or adolescence as chronic defiance of authority or purposeful harmful actions to the physical, psychological, or material well-being of others (Leedom et al., 2013). The injurious actions, such as lying, stealing, or bullying, occur without a sense of remorse or loyalty to anyone (WHO, 2016). While initially the incidence of deviant behaviors may not be criminal, there is a continuum of behavior severity that could lead to criminal activities (Leedom et al., 2013). According to a study of prisons worldwide, antisocial personality disorder is a common personality disorder found among the prison population, averaging about 50% of men and about 20% of women (Fazel & Danesh, 2002; Sher et al., 2015). This makes sense in light of the definition of the disorder, as most crimes include a disregard for the rights of others (stealing, falsifying information, assault, and murder, etc.).

To assign the diagnosis of antisocial personality disorder, the individual must be at least 18 years old with prior evidence of a conduct disorder since the age of 15 (APA, 2013). Other diagnostic features are listed in Box 12.3.

Box 12.3 Diagnostic Features of Antisocial Personality Disorder

1   Frequent conflict with others
2   Inability to tolerate stressful situations or unpleasant feelings
3   Impulsivity and reckless behaviors
4   Rejection of authority
5   Rejection of discipline
6   Lack of self-awareness (WHO, 2016)

These malignant behaviors cannot be evident only during the natural sequence of bipolar disorder or schizophrenia (APA, 2013). In addition, gender studies have shown that there is a slightly higher percentage of males who are diagnosed with antisocial personality disorder than females (Sher et al., 2015). This may be due to the fact that men with this disorder are more likely to be involved with the police or because of the fact that men with borderline personality may be misdiagnosed as having antisocial personality disorder (Sher et al., 2015).

Individuals with antisocial personality disorder tend to be very charming, manipulative, and exciting. However, they also tend to lack empathy and can be quite indifferent in regard to others' feelings and emotions. They may also have difficulty maintaining employment, taking care of their child, sustaining a home, and otherwise being responsible citizens. Drugs and alcohol may also be a factor in the life of someone with antisocial personality disorder, as they tend to take risks and may also engage in multiple sexual partners.

Yang et al. (2008) found that brain imaging of individuals with antisocial personality disorders found impairment in the areas of the prefrontal cortex, superior temporal gyrus, amygdale-hippocampal complex, and anterior cingulated cortex. The prefrontal cortex affects concentration, judgment, decision making, and impulsivity. Therefore, someone who has damage to the prefrontal cortex may be prone to making bad decisions, have impulsive risk-taking behavior, and have difficulty maintaining attention in the workplace or school. The anterior cingulated cortex functions similarly in that it affects attention, morality, and personal ethics. Damage to the superior temporal gyrus and amygdale-hippocampal may cause someone to fail to follow social rules and standards, have a poor moral code, and impose on the rights of others, which could result in a diagnosis of antisocial personality disorder (Yang et al., 2008). Therefore, these individuals with this disorder could have a biological reason for their behavior. Learning more about brain function and how it affects psychological disorders will no doubt help in the formulation of treatment.

Risk Factors

GENETIC AND PHYSIOLOGICAL

Antisocial personality disorder is more prevalent among first-degree relatives who also have the disorder. If the individual has a female relative with the disorder, they are more likely to also have the diagnosis than those with a male relative. Males tend to have substance abuse issues in addition to the personality disorder, whereas females tend to have somatic complaints. Adoptive parents, as well as biological parents, with the disorder increase the chances of the child developing antisocial personality disorder (APA, 2013).

Pyromania (F63.1) 312.33

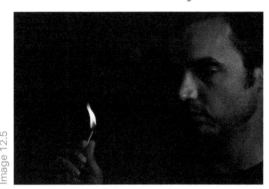

Image 12.5

Pyromania has been a controversial disorder over the years. The argument over how to address deliberate fire-setting perpetrators has followed a pendulum-like movement, vacillating between legal culpability to medical excusability (Dalhuisen, 2018). The term pyromania was first introduced in 1833 by Marc to describe a fire-perversion based on instinctive madness and irresistible impulse that is devoid of motive (Dalhusien, 2018; Johnson & Netherton, 2016). As early as 1932, however, Freud categorized the condition as a psychosexual disorder, whereby the fire setter experienced an affective arousal and irresistible draw when watching a fire (Palermo, 2015).

Pyromania is a rare and specific psychiatric condition. Only about 3%–6% of fire setting offenders meet the full criteria for the diagnosis (APA, 2013; Palermo, 2015). The diagnostic criteria for pyromania include the following:

1. Compulsive fire setting
2. Fascination with fires and repeated fire setting preceded by tension or arousal and followed by pleasure or gratification
3. The fire setting is not done with ulterior motives, as the result of other disorders, such as antisocial personality disorder, conduct disorder, schizophrenia, or as a result of alcohol or substance intoxication (WHO, 2016)

The *DSM-5* (APA, 2013) described individuals with the disorder as having voyeur-like behavior and deriving pleasure not only from the fire itself but also from things affiliated with fires, such as fire departments, firemen, and fire paraphernalia (Johnson & Netherton, 2016).

Risk Factors

Pyromania is not diagnosed until the age of 18 years old, although the symptoms of the disorder typically manifest during adolescence and continue through adulthood (John & Netherton, 2016). The exact causes of the disorder are unknown, but it is prevalent in males, especially in those who lack social skills or who have learning disabilities (Doymaz et al., 2018). Comorbidity considerations and differential diagnoses should include curious fire-setting behavior (primarily in children), attention deficit hyperactivity disorder, conduct disorder, antisocial personality disorder, mood disorders, or response to hallucinations or delusions, such as experienced in schizophrenia or substance use disorders (Doymaz et al., 2018; Johnson & Netherton, 2016).

Kleptomania (F63.3) 312.32

Kleptomania is a rare compulsive disorder that occurs in less than 1% of the general population and is more prevalent in females than males (APA, 2013). The term *kleptomania*, which refers to the relentless involuntary urges to steal, was first introduced by Equirol and Marc in the 19th century (Shinkar et al., 2016). The term suggested that a person was compelled to steal because of mental distress and not because of a lack of moral restraint (Shinkar et al., 2016).

Kleptomania is classified by some as a behavioral addiction and shares some of the same diagnostic features, such as internal tension and intense cravings associated with the activation of specific reward centers of the brain (Black, 2013; Mangot, 2014a; Mangot, 2014b); repetitive compulsive behaviors even in the face of negative consequences; and lack of self-control over the maladaptive behavior (Black, 2013). Research on the pathogenesis of the disorder has linked unstable levels of dopamine and serotonin to its development (Mangot, 2014a; Mangot, 2014b).

Diagnostic criteria for kleptomania include the following:

1. Failure to resist the urge to steal
2. Items taken have no essential value to the person
3. Mounting internal tension prior to stealing
4. A sense of gratification, often followed by guilt, after stealing
5. Stealing is not a result of another disorder or medical condition (WHO, 2016)

Risk Factors

GENETIC AND PHYSIOLOGICAL

There is a higher rate of drug and alcohol use disorders in relatives of those with kleptomania than the general public. In addition, first-degree relatives of individuals with kleptomania have higher rates of obsessive-compulsive disorder (APA, 2013).

Treatment Interventions

Disruptive, impulse control, and conduct disorders are often comorbid with other mental disorders. Mood disorders, such as depression and anxiety, have been found to coexist with oppositional defiant disorder, intermittent explosive disorder, and conduct disorder. In fact, a study using data from the National Comorbidity Survey–Adolescent Supplement found that more than half of adolescents with intermittent explosive disorder interviewed also had an anxiety disorder in comparison to only 22.88% of adolescents without intermittent explosive disorder (Galbraith et al., 2018). Interestingly, the study also reported that adolescents with intermittent explosive disorder and comorbid anxiety disorder were more likely to be female than male and were more likely to have three or more co-occurring diagnoses, including depressive or substance abuse disorders (Galbraith et al., 2018).

Attention deficit hyperactivity disorder is another diagnosis that is frequently comorbid with oppositional defiant disorder, intermittent explosive disorder, conduct disorder, and antisocial personality disorder. Subsequently, many of the documented treatment interventions are based on meta-analysis of this comorbidity. While the core symptoms of these behavioral disorders are not amenable to psychopharmacology, medication may help with the comorbid attention deficit hyperactivity disorder symptom of poor impulse control and may be used as an adjunctive treatment with evidence-based behavior modification therapies (Hood et al., 2015).

In addition, substance use has been highly comorbid with the disruptive, impulse control, and conduct disorders. Antisocial personality disorder is a group highly susceptible to substance use. Consequently, homelessness, sexual risk behavior, increased criminal activity, and severity of drug dependency are found to be the potential by-products of antisocial personality disorder (Mueser et al., 2006). Studies have shown that having a history of recurring, impulsively aggressive behavior is a risk factor for the development of a substance use disorder (Coccaro et al., 2016). One study found that intermittent explosive disorder preceded substance use disorder in 80% of the comorbid cases, which suggested that early treatment of impulse aggression might decrease the likelihood of developing a substance disorder in adolescents with intermittent explosive disorder (Coccaro et al., 2016).

Pharmacotherapy Treatments

OPPOSITIONAL DEFIANT DISORDER

While no medications have been FDA approved specifically for oppositional defiant disorder, stimulants such as methylphenidate and d-amphetamine have been found to be effective in managing oppositional defiant disorder because of the high comorbidity with attention deficit hyperactivity disorder (Grant & Leppink, 2015). Other attention deficit hyperactivity disorder medications, such as the antipsychotic risperidone and the alpha-2 agonist clonidine, have also shown some efficacy in treating that disorder in conjunction with oppositional defiant disorder, but there are limited studies on treating oppositional defiant disorder alone (Grant & Leppink, 2015).

INTERMITTENT EXPLOSIVE DISORDER

Studies on drug treatment for intermittent explosive disorder are limited. However, fluoxetine and oxcarbazepine reduced intermittent explosive disorder symptom severity, such as impulsive aggressive behaviors, in some studies (Grant & Leppink, 2015).

CONDUCT DISORDER

Likewise, there is currently no FDA-approved medication for conduct disorder. However, in treatment trials, lithium and haloperidol have shown promising results for symptom management (Grant & Leppink, 2015).

ANTISOCIAL PERSONALITY DISORDER

Evidence-based psychopharmacology treatment for antisocial personality disorder is primarily focused on decreasing impulsive aggression because of the repeated violent and criminally based acts frequently associated with the disorder (Ripoll et al., 2011). Research with prisoners diagnosed with antisocial personality disorder involving treating them with lithium demonstrated a decrease in aggressive acts, as well as diminished anxiety-related behaviors and depression (Ripoll et al., 2011). In addition, research with male prisoners reported phenytoin outperformed placebos in decreasing impulsive acts of aggression but not premeditated acts (Khalifa et al., 2010).

PYROMANIA

Treatment for pyromania has included a number of pharmacological medications. One study found a patient to have a left inferior frontal perfusion deficit (Grant, 2006). When treated with 3 weeks of cognitive behavioral therapy (CBT) and 1 week of topiramate, the individual reported a remission in his urges to set fires (Grant, 2006; Johnson & Netherton, 2017). This study suggested that the anticonvulsant topiramate combined with CBT helped to control the cortico-mesolimbic dopamine function, which plays a role in regulating incentive salience (Grant, 2006). Other studies have demonstrated abatement in pyromania by using selective serotonin reuptake inhibitors (SSRIs), lithium, antiandrogens, and antiepileptic medications (Johnson & Netherton, 2017).

KLEPTOMANIA

Some studies with SSRIs, such as fluoxetine, paroxetine, fluvoxamine, and sertraline, have demonstrated positive results in reducing the thoughts and cravings associated with kleptomania (Mangot 2014a; Mangot, 2014b). Likewise, mood stabilizers, such as lithium; antiseizure medication, such as topiramate and valproic acid; and addiction medications, such as naltrexone have produced some favorable outcomes in helping to manage the impulsive urges of kleptomania (Mangot, 2014a; Shinkar et al., 2016). Treatment of the disorder, however, can be complicated because of the comorbidity of other psychiatric disorders or because of compromises in functional anatomy, such as in head trauma (Mangot, 2014a).

Psychological Treatments

CBT is the standard therapy-based treatment for disruptive, impulse-control, and conduct disorders in both individual and group formats. The goal of therapy is to help a person identify irrational thoughts and learn to reframe those thoughts to become a better manager of emotional and behavioral outcomes.

Early treatment interventions hold potential for managing the severity of conduct disorder and may help to stymie the development of antisocial personality disorder in severely antisocial children (Scott et al., 2014). Multisystemic therapy, which includes partnerships among family, school, community resources, and criminal justice systems, and functional family therapy, which includes the immediate family environment, are two evidence-based models for treating adolescents with conduct disorder (British Psychological Society, 2010).

A long-term, follow-up of two randomized controlled studies found that a multi-method of intervention including individual and family therapy; a telephone helpline for parents; and parent and teacher training may help to improve the academic performance of children with antisocial behaviors in the short term and interrupt the progression of impairment in the long term (Scott et al., 2014).

Family-based and school-based therapies have also proven beneficial in helping support systems better cope with the disorder of a loved one and to limit positive reinforcement of impulsive and oppositional behaviors (Grant & Leppink, 2015). One such support-system-based approach to treatment is parent management training. This model is an operant conditioning approach to behavior management that uses a rewards and punishment model to reduce negative behaviors and increase positive parent/child relationships (Hood et al., 2015).

Another support-system-based approach to treatment is the collaborative problem solving model. This approach is an intervention designed to increase executive skills functioning in children and adolescents, which can enable them to better regulate their emotions and problem solve more constructively (Hood et al., 2015). Parents and teachers are trained to use the model in whatever circumstances their youths may be struggling (Hood et al., 2015).

Case Study Summary

One of this chapter's case studies reviewed the behaviors of Christopher. As you process the story and examine possible diagnostic criteria, take a few minutes to answer the following questions:

1. What would be the correct diagnosis for Christopher?

    _____

    _____

2. What are the specific symptoms or criteria that led you to this diagnosis?

    _____

    _____

3. What other possible disorders might you diagnose Christopher with and why?

    _____

    _____

4. Briefly discuss what types of treatment may be beneficial for Christopher. Could you see using a certain counseling theory and/or medication?

    _____

    _____

Guided Practice Exercises

Scenario 1

Paisley, 7, has always had an issue with authority figures. She seems to be unable to follow any instructions given to her by an adult, especially a teacher. Paisley prides herself on knocking everything off of a table in the cafeteria or the teacher's desk. She has been suspended multiple times. Unfortunately, her parents are both extremely busy doctors and do not have much time or concern for Paisley's behavior. Once, a classmate named Jill told Paisley that she didn't have to be so loud all of the time. Paisley reacted vindictively, by pushing everything off of Jill's desk and kicking her. Paisley still seems bent on revenge, often calling Jill names and pushing her. Paisley has an extremely low tolerance for any annoyance and will lose her temper easily. She is a nightmare for any teacher.

What would be the correct disorder? What are the specific symptoms or criteria that led you to this diagnosis?

_____

_____

_____

_____

What specific behaviors caused you to diagnose the disorder?

_____

_____

_____

_____

What other possible disorders might you diagnose Paisley with and why?

_____

_____

_____

_____

Often, oppositional defiant disorder presents with attention deficit hyperactivity disorder. Why do think this is?

_____

_____

_____

_____

Scenario 2

Aaliyah, 6, is an African American girl whose time is split between an uncle's house and a foster family home. Aaliyah's parents died in an auto accident soon after she was born. Her uncle brings her to the clinic as a condition for her not being expelled from her school. Aaliyah is manipulative of both other students and teachers. Almost daily, Aaliyah tries to steal things from the classroom. The teacher has started searching Aaliyah and her book bag when the girl is on the way out of the classroom. Her uncle confides that she often tries to sneak out of her window at night, and he has nailed boards over the window to prevent her escapes. The foster parents are so stretched thin that they do not notice Aaliyah's comings and goings at night when she stays with them. Aaliyah is pending expulsion from the school because she hit another student with a baseball bat during gym class. The student got a concussion, and his parents are considering pressing charges against Aaliyah. Last week, Aaliyah's uncle found her behind their house with a tub of water, drowning newborn bunnies. Aaliyah's uncle does not know how to help her.

What would be the correct disorder? What are the specific symptoms or criteria that led you to this diagnosis?

_____

_____

_____

_____

What specific behaviors caused you to diagnose the disorder?

_____

_____

_____

_____

What other possible disorders might you diagnose Aaliyah with and why?

_____

_____

_____

_____

Scenario 3

Graham, 11, is fascinated by everything about fire: the way it looks, the way it sounds, the way it consumes everything it touches. Graham has several burns on his carpet at home from setting small fires in his room and then putting them out. His parents tell the therapist that their shed burned down a few years ago, and the fire marshal believed it to be arson. No suspects have been arrested, but they both suspect that Graham was behind the fire. Graham's mother tells the therapist that other small fires in sheds and garages have occurred in the neighborhood, and they are worried that Graham may also be involved with those fires. His dad caught him walking through the yard trying to conceal a gasoline can a few weeks earlier. When asked about his obsession with fire, Graham does not express a desire to harm anybody. Instead, he is obsessed with the flames and the way that fire burns. He discloses to the therapist that after setting a fire, he will often regret the damage it creates, but the thrill beforehand makes it worth it.

What would be the correct disorder? What are the specific symptoms or criteria that led you to this diagnosis?

_____

_____

_____

_____

What specific behaviors caused you to diagnose the disorder?

_____

_____

_____

_____

What other possible disorders might you diagnose Graham with and why?

_____

_____

_____

_____

Web-Based and Literature-Based Resources

Child Mind Institute: https://childmind.org/guide/oppositional-defiant-disorder/

Mayo Clinic: https://www.mayoclinic.org/diseases-conditions/intermittent-explosive-disorder/diagnosis-treatment/drc-20373926

Mental Health America: https://www.mentalhealthamerica.net/conditions/conduct-disorder

Minnesota Association for Children's Mental Health: https://www.macmh.org/oppositional-defiant-disorder-odd-resources/

Society for Adolescent Health and Medicine: https://www.adolescenthealth.org/Topics-in-Adolescent-Health/Mental-Health/Resources/Disruptive,-Impulse-Control-and-Conduct-Disorders.aspx

References

Akram, U., Gardani, M., Akram, A., & Allen, S. (2019). Anxiety and depression mediate the relationship between insomnia symptoms and the personality traits of conscientiousness and emotional stability. *Heliyon*, 5(6), e01939. https://doi-org.libproxy.clemson.edu/10.1016/j.heliyon.2019.e01939

American Psychiatric Association (APA). (2013). *Diagnostic and statistical manual of mental disorders* (5th ed.).

Biography.com. (2020). *David Berkowitz*. A&E Television Networks. https://www.biography.com/crime-figure/david-berkowitz

Black, D. W. (2013). Behavioral addictions as a way to classify behaviors. *Canadian Journal of Psychiatry*, 58(5), 249–251. https://doi.org/10.1177/070674371305800501

British Psychological Society. (2010). Antisocial personality disorder: Treatment, management and prevention. *National Collaborating Centre for Mental Health (UK) NICE Clinical Guidelines*, 77(5). https://www.ncbi.nlm.nih.gov/books/NBK55328/

Burnett, M. L. (2013). Gender and the development of oppositional defiant disorder: Contributions of physical abuse and early family environment. *Child Maltreatment*, 18(3), 195–204. https://doi.org/10.1177/1077559513478144

Cavanagh, M., Quinn, D., Duncan, D., Graham, T., & Balbuena, L. (2017). Oppositional defiant disorder is better conceptualized as a disorder of emotional regulation. *Journal of Attention Disorders*, 21(5), 381–389. https://doi.org/10.1177/1087054713520221

Cleveland Clinic. (2019). *Oppositional defiant disorder*. https://my.clevelandclinic.org/health/diseases/9905-oppositional-defiant-disorder

Coccaro, E. F. (2015). Intermittent explosive disorder. *Psychiatric Times*, 32(3), https://link-galegroup-com.ezproxy.liberty.edu/apps/doc/A405023795/HRCA?u=vic_liberty&sid=HRCA&xid=36c2254f

Coccaro, E. F., Fridberg, D. J., Fanning, J. R., Grant, J. E., King, A. C., & Lee, R. (2016). Substance use disorders: Relationship with intermittent explosive disorder and with aggression, anger, and impulsivity. *Journal of Psychiatric Research*, 81, 127–132. https://doi.org/10.1016/j.jpsychires.2016.06.011

Coccaro, E., McCloskey, M., Fitzgerald, D., & Phan, K. L. (2007). Amygdala and orbitofrontal reactivity to social threat in individuals with impulsive aggression. *Biological Psychiatry*, 62, 168–178. https://doi.org/10.1016/j.biopsych.2006.08.024

Crime Library. (2020). *David Berkowitz: Son of Sam killer*. https://www.crimemuseum.org/crime-library/serial-killers/david-berkowitz/

Dalhuisen, L. (2108). Pyromania in court: Legal insanity verses culpability in Western Europe and the Netherlands (1800–1950). *International Journal of Law and Psychiatry*, 58, 36–47. https://doi.org/10.1016/j.ijlp.2018.02.009

Doymaz, Y., Ayyıldız, E., Baltacıoğlu, M., & Hocaoğlu, Ç. (2018). A rare known topic 'pyromania': A case report. *Klinik Psikofarmakoloji Bulteni*, 28, 248. http://ezproxy.liberty.edu/login?url=https://search-proquest-com.ezproxy.liberty.edu/docview/2072274500?accountid=12085

Fahlgren, M. K., Puhalla, A. A., Sorgi, K. M., & McCloskey, M. S. (2019). Emotion processing in intermittent explosive disorder. *Psychiatry Research*, 273, 544–550. https://doi.org/10.1016/j.psychres.2019.01.046

Fazel, S., & Danesh, J. (2002). Serious mental disorder in 23,000 prisoners: A systematic review of 62 surveys. *Lancet*, 359, 545–550.

Fire Line School. (n.d.). *10 famous arsonists and why*. https://www.firelineschool.com/student_files/10%20Famous%20Arsonists%20and%20Why.pdf

Galbraith, T., Carliner, H., Keyes, K. M. N., McLaughlin, K. A., McCloskey, M. S., & Heimberg, R. G. (2018). The co-occurrence and correlates of anxiety disorders among adolescents with intermittent explosive disorder. *Aggressive Behavior*, 44(6), 581–590. https://doi.org/10.1002/ab.21783

Grant, J. E. (2006). SPECT imaging and treatment of pyromania. *Journal of Clinical Psychiatry*, 67(6), 998–998. https://www.psychiatrist.com/JCP/article/_layouts/ppp.psych.controls/BinaryViewer.ashx?Article=/JCP/article/Pages/2006/v67n06/v67n0619e.aspx&Type=Article

Grant, J. E, & Leppink, E. W. (2015). Choosing a treatment for disruptive, impulse-control, and conduct disorders: Limited evidence, no approved drugs to guide treatment. *Current Psychiatry, 14* (1), 28–36.

Grohol, J. (2019). *Pyromania symptoms.* Psych Central. Retrieved on February 18, 2020, from https://psychcentral.com/disorders/pyromania-symptoms/

Herzhoff, K., Smack, A. J., Reardon, K. W., Martel, M. M., & Tackett, J. L. (2016). Child personality accounts for oppositional defiant disorder comorbidity patterns. *Journal of Abnormal Child Psychology, 45,* 327–335. https://doi.org/10.1007/s10802-016-0162-8

Hood, B. S., Elrod, M. G., & DeWine, D. B. (2015). Treatment of childhood oppositional defiant disorder. *Current Treatment Options in Pediatrics, 1*(2), 155–167. https://doi.org/10.1007/s40746-015-0015-7

Huebner, T., Violet, T. D., Marx, I., Konrad, K., Fink, G. R., Herpertz, S. C., & Herpertz-Dahlmamm, B. (2008). Morphometric brain abnormalities in boys with conduct disorder. *Journal of the American Academy of Child & Adolescent Psychiatry, 47*(5), 540–547. https://doi.org/10.1097/CHI.0b013e3181676545

Johnson, R. S., & Netherton, E. (2016). Fire setting and the impulse-control of pyromania. *American Journal of Psychiatry Residents' Journal, 11*(7), 14–16.

Khalifa, N., Duggan, C., Stoffers, J., Huband, N., Völlm, B. A., Ferriter, M., & Lieb, K. (2010). Pharmacological interventions for antisocial personality disorder. *Cochrane Database of Systematic Reviews, 8,* (CD007667). https://doi.org/10.1002/14651858.CD007667.pub2

Leedom, L., Bass, A., & Almas, L. (2013). The problem of parental psychopathy. *Journal of Child Custody, 10*(2), 154–184. https://doi.org/10.1080/15379418.2013.796268

Mangot A. G. (2014a). Kleptomania: Beyond serotonin. *Journal of Neurosciences in Rural Practice, 5*(Suppl 1), S105–S106. https://doi.org/10.4103/0976-3147.145244

Mangot, A. G. (2014b). Neurobiology of kleptomania: An overview. *Sri Lanka Journal of Psychiatry, 5.* https://doi.org/10.4038/sljpsyc.v5i2.7305.

Merrick, J., Howell Bowling, C., & Omar, H. A. (2013). Firesetting in childhood and adolescence. *Frontiers in Public Health, 1,* 40. https://doi.org/10.3389/fpubh.2013.00040

Mikolajewski, A. J., Hart, S. A., & Taylor, J. (2019). The developmental propensity model extends to oppositional defiant disorder: A twin study. *Journal of Abnormal Child Psychology.* https://doi.org/10.1007/s10802-019-00556-z

Mueser, K. T., Crocker, A. G., Frisman, L. B., Drake, R. E., Covell, N. H., & Essock, S. M. (2006). Conduct disorder and antisocial personality disorder in persons with severe psychiatric and substance use disorders. *Schizophrenia Bulletin, 32*(4), 626–636. https://doi.org/10.1093/schbul/sbj068

Ogundele, M. O. (2018). Behavioural and emotional disorders in childhood: A brief overview for paediatricians. *World Journal of Clinical Pediatrics, 7*(1), 9–26. https://doi.org/10.5409/wjcp.v7.i1.9

Palermo, G. B. (2015). A look at firesetting, arson, and pyromania. *International Journal of Offender Therapy and Comparative Criminology, 59*(7), 683–684. https://doi.org/10.1177/0306624X15586217

Ripoll, L. H., Triebwasser, J., & Siever, L. J. (2011). Evidence-based pharmacotherapy for personality disorders. *International Journal of Neuropsychopharmacology, 14*(9), 1257–1288. http://dx.doi.org.ezproxy.liberty.edu/10.1017/S1461145711000071

Rowe, R., Costello, E. J., Angold, A., Copeland, W. E., & Maughan, B. (2010). Developmental pathways in oppositional defiant disorder and conduct disorder. *Journal of Abnormal Psychology, 119*(4), 726–738. https://doi.org/10.1037/a0020798

Schoorl, J., Van Rijn, S., De Wied, M., Van Goozen, S. H. M., & Swaab, H. (2016). Variability in emotional/behavioral problems in boys with oppositional defiant disorder or conduct disorder: The role of arousal. *European Child & Adolescent Psychiatry, 25*(8), 821–830. https://doi.org/10.1007/s00787-015-0790-5

Scott, S., Briskman, J., & O'Connor, T. G. (2014). Early prevention of antisocial personality: Long-term follow-up of two randomized controlled trials comparing indicated and selective approaches. *American Journal of Psychiatry, 171*(6), 649–657, https://doi.org/10.1176/appi.ajp.2014.13050697

Sher, L., Siever, L. J., Goodman, M., McNamara, M., Hazlett, E. A., Koenigsburg, H. W., & New, A. S. (2015). Gender differences in the clinical characteristics and psychiatric comorbidity in patients with antisocial personality disorder. *Psychiatry Research, 229,* 685–589. https://doi.org/10.1016/j.psychres.2015.08.022

Shinkar, D. M., Pandya, D. B., & Saudagar, R. B. (2016). Kleptomania: An overview. *Asian Journal of Pharmacy and Technology, 6*(2), 127–130. https://doi.org/10.5958/2231-5713.2016.00017.9

Sobol-Kwapinska, M. (2016). Calm down—it's only neuroticism. Time perspectives as moderators and mediators of the relationship between neuroticism and well-being. *Personality and Individual Differences, 94,* 64–71. http://dx.doi.org/10.1016/j.paid.2016.01.004

Steinbeis, N., Bernhardt, B. C., & Singer, T. (2012). Impulse control and underlying functions of the left DLPFC mediate age-related and age-independent individual differences in strategic social behavior. *Neuron, 73*(5), 1040–1051. https://doi.org/10.1016/j.neuron.2011.12.027

Tackett, J. L., Daoud, S. L. S. B., De Bolle, M., & Burt, S. A. (2013). Is relational aggression part of the externalizing spectrum? A bifactor model of youth antisocial behavior. *Aggressive Behavior, 39,* 149–159. https://doi.org/10.1002/ab.21466.

Vanwoerden, S., Reuter, T., & Sharp, C. (2016). Exploring the clinical utility of the *DSM-5* conduct disorder specifier of 'with limited prosocial emotions' in an adolescent inpatient sample. *Comprehensive Psychiatry, 69,* 116–131. https://doi.org/10.1016/j.comppsych.2016.05.012

Wang, J. M., Hartl, A. C., Laursen, B., & Rubin, K. H. (2017). The high costs of low agreeableness: Low agreeableness exacerbates interpersonal consequences of rejection sensitivity in U.S. and Chinese adolescents. *Journal of Research in Personality, 67,* 36–43. https://doi.org/10.1016/j.jrp.2016.02.005

World Health Organization (WHO). (2016). *International statistical classification of diseases and related health problems, 10th revision (ICD-10).*

Yang, Y., Glenn, A., & Raine, A. (2008). Brain abnormalities in antisocial individuals: Implications for the law. *Behavioral Sciences and the Law, 26*(1), 65.

Zastrow, B. L., Martel, M. M., & Widiger, T. A. (2018). Preschool oppositional defiant disorder: A disorder of negative affect, surgency, and disagreeableness. *Journal of Clinical Child & Adolescent Psychology, 47*(6), 967-977. https://doi.org/10.1080/15374416.2016.1225504

Credits

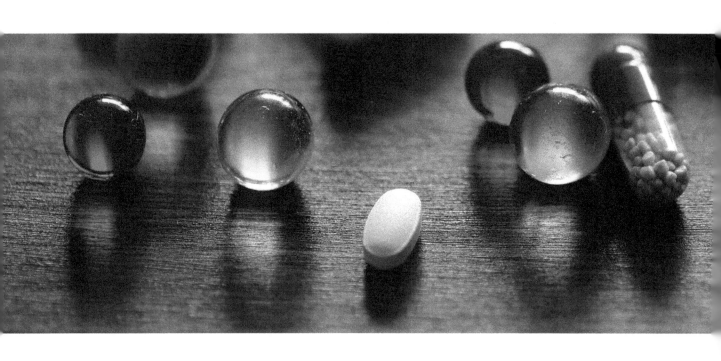

CHAPTER THIRTEEN

SUBSTANCE-RELATED AND ADDICTIVE DISORDERS

Andy J. Flaherty, David A. Scott, and Michelle Grant Scott

CASE STUDY 13.1 *Substance-Related Disorders Example* Austin is a 17-year-old African American boy. His mother brought him to you after she noticed a change in his personality and his group of friends. When you were doing your intake session, you noticed that he seemed disinterested, that he struggled to pay attention to what you were talking about, and that he fidgeted constantly. When you asked about previous injuries, you found out that he is still in recovery from an anterior cruciate ligament tear that occurred during basketball season. You're still worried about his behaviors, so you asked if he was taking any medications. He mentioned that his prescription for Vicodin had run out, but he was still taking it without his mother knowing.

Basketball is Austin's life. He has been playing since he was 5 years old. All of his friends play basketball and now he can no longer play. He could no longer bare to go to practices or games because he couldn't play. He believed his dreams of playing Division I college basketball were crushed. He could not even stand to be around his friends anymore, so he became withdrawn.

At physical therapy, he made some new friends who were in college. They invited him to go out with them. He thought he had nothing to lose anymore, so it couldn't hurt to go. They went to a house party that Friday night where Austin experimented with alcohol for the first time. There was also a bowl of pills in the middle of the table. His friends were all grabbing three, so he did too. He recognized one of them as the Vicodin that he had been taking. The next morning, he was sicker than he'd ever been, but he remembered the guy who had brought those pills had lived in the house where his new friends were staying. He found the guy in the morning and made a deal with him to continue to buy the pills.

Although Austin's knee was no longer in pain, he disclosed that the pills took away the pain of not being able to play basketball anymore. He could not survive without them. One day when he ran out of pills, he found himself feeling sick, getting cold sweats, and being restless until he could get more later that day.

Overview

Substance use has become a severe public health crisis in the United States (Madras et al., 2009). Specifically, Substance Abuse and Mental Health Services Administration (SAMHSA, 2016) reported that approximately 25% of adults in the United States engaged in at least one day of heavy drinking (defined as five or more drinks for men under 65 and four or more drinks for women) in the past month, and more than 27 million

Did You Know?

- Substance use is a huge cost to society; illicit drug use costs the United States approximately $181 billion annually, and excessive alcohol use costs the country approximately $235 billion annually (Substance Abuse and Mental Health Services Administration [SAMHSA], 2018).

- Twenty-four million Americans aged 12 and older have used illegal drugs (SAMHSA, 2018).

- Marijuana is still the most frequently abused drug, with more than 20 million Americans citing the use of marijuana within the last 30 days (SAMHSA, 2018).

- One hundred people die every day from drug overdoses. This rate has tripled in the past 20 years (SAMHSA, 2018).

- Less than half of the population (38.3%) drinks alcohol; this means that those who do drink consume on average 17 liters of pure alcohol annually (SAMHSA, 2018).

Americans, age 12 or older, engaged in current (past month) drug use. In the research base, it is well established that individuals with unaddressed substance use disorders are likely to experience a broad range of complex health and psychiatric challenges across several biopsychosocial domains, including physical health complications and premature death, comorbidity with other mental health challenges, and other relational and interpersonal impacts (Babor et al., 2007; Ginzer et al., 2007).

Many people do not use substances for reasons other than personal and social enjoyment. However, for a significant number of people, somewhere between 5% and 7% of the population, substance use becomes problematic, and they may find themselves dependent on a substance. Within the *Diagnostic and Statistical Manual of Mental Disorders, 5th Edition* (*DSM-5;* American Psychiatric Association [APA], 2013), substance use disorder is the diagnostic classification that encompasses specific substance use, dependence, and addictive behavior.

DSM-5 Model of Substance Use Disorders

The *DSM-5* (APA, 2013) presents a model for understanding substance use that focuses on an individual's level of impairment. This definition of substance use disorder is concerned with how a person is affected by their use of a specific substance. Specifically, it addresses the question, how does the use of this substance impact their functioning? In diagnosing and understanding substance use disorder within the *DSM-5* framework, it is essential for a clinician to be able to understand how addiction and dependence develop and affect those who are using substances. Therefore, the current conceptualization of substance use disorders is a much more streamlined approach to understanding, assessing, and diagnosing clients than in previous editions of the *DSM* because now substance use disorder is an overall diagnostic heading that captures common patterns of use and impairment across substances.

Model of Substance Use in the *ICD-10* (11)

Unlike the *DSM-5, the International Statistical Classification of Diseases* (ICD-10; World Health Organization [WHO], 2016) definition of substance use still includes the concepts of substance abuse and substance dependence. Substance abuse is defined as a pattern of maladaptive drug taking, which includes impacts to social functioning, to physical well-being, and to mental health in patients who have not yet reached a state of dependence. Substance dependence is defined as a chronic mental or physical condition related to the patient's pattern of drug taking and characterized by both physiological and psychological responses. These responses include the following: compulsion to take the drug to experience its psychic effects or to avoid the discomfort associated with its absence, lack of ability to stop using the substance despite strong incentives to do so, and symptoms of physical dependence.

When documenting substance use disorders within the *ICD-10* (WHO, 2016), the following information is included regardless of the type of substance: (1) severity—mild, moderate, severe; (2) pattern of use—continuous use, in remission, relapsed; (3) substance-induced mood/psychotic symptoms—depression, hallucinations, anxiety; (4) current presentation—intoxication, drunkenness, withdrawal; and (5) treatment plan—rehabilitation, maintenance therapy (specify drug), referral to talk therapy.

CLINICIAN'S CORNER 13.1

As a clinician, I have learned so much from working with clients in substance use recovery. The most important lesson being that recovery happens! Although it is seldom a linear process, I have seen repeatedly that for those clients who make long-term life changes, profound levels of recovery are possible. It has been a joy to repeatedly see people learn new coping skills and new ways of living first in sobriety but then to begin the fulfilling but difficult journey of addressing the traumas and other intrapsychic conflicts that play into and negatively affect their substance use patterns. The old adage in recovery circles is "one day at a time," and I find that it is important to remember myself and to remind clients that recovery happens in the present and that lasting change is made often through doing small new things over and over. Live in the day and measure change in the decade.

Andy J. Flaherty, MSW

Person-First Substance Use Treatment

It is essential that clinicians view substance use disorder and the pathology of addiction in an accurate manner. People who are challenged with this disorder deserve our empathy and support, just as if they were suffering from any other form of psychopathology. However, regarding substance use disorder, it is easy for clinicians to inadvertently slip into moralistic and judgmental thinking and perceive people who use substances as being weak, having little character, or merely being in the "habit" of making wrong or choices. Moralistic and judgmental thinking about substance use disorder has no place in the approach of the modern clinician.

Substance use disorder should rightly be understood as the "hijacking" of the brain's pleasure-seeking system. Specifically, it is a chronic impairment to the brain's pleasure-seeking system that keeps people caught in a severe challenge to re-regulate this system. As substance use disorders often bring other social consequences, such as legal or criminal justice involvement, as well as other social and economic problems, the process of recovery and the challenge to re-regulate the brain's pleasure-seeking system can be difficult. Therefore, it is vital that as clinicians we do not lose sight of the person in the midst of problems and consequences associated with the disorder they are facing.

Understanding Substance Use and Addiction

The precise and complex neurological process of addiction is involved, and addiction science is an ever-expanding area of research. The field of the brain and addiction science is a rapidly evolving and specialized field/area, which cannot be comprehensively covered in this chapter. We, therefore, encourage you to spend time with relevant research and literature, building a greater appreciation and insight into the way the brain is affected by chronic and persistent substance use. This chapter offers a much more generic description of the development of substance use disorder in individuals with high levels of substance use.

Within the *DSM-5*, addiction is understood as the repeated use of substances, which leads to gross impairment to the brain's dopamine (and other pleasure neurochemicals) regulation system. Essentially, this is the brain's reward and pleasure system, and dysfunctional activation of this system is central to how addiction and substance use disorders develop. The "high" that people feel when they are using substances is in part because of excessive amounts of dopamine and other chemicals in the brain. Dopamine is a hormone that is strongly associated with feelings of euphoria and bliss, and most importantly, in excess, it manifests within people as an intense feeling of reward and pleasure. However, and with regard to substance use, the increase in dopamine is so profound that people may begin to neglect other normal activities in favor of using their substance of choice. Repeated use of a substance, in this manner, begins to cause the brain to stop or significantly reduce its production of dopamine. The consequences of diminished production of dopamine are that the person using the substance begins to experience an intense need for the substance. They need a certain amount of the substance just for their levels of neurochemicals to be at their previous baseline or average level, which is essential for keeping the symptoms of withdrawal at bay. It is at this point that people who are excessively using substances must continue to use them to feel any sense of pleasure reward or well-being and in cases of severe dependency, any sense of normal functioning.

It is important to note that while the precise pharmacological mechanisms for each class of substance are different and distinct and that different substances affect the brain in distinct ways, the most common feature of substance use disorder is that the repeated activation of the brain's reward system produces feelings of euphoria and pleasure. However, eventually, with all substances, the individual becomes dependent on using for the ongoing regulation of the pleasure and reward system. A chronically impaired reward and pleasure center results in symptoms of impairment across many domains. Therefore, as the *DSM-5* states, a "substance use disorder describes a problematic pattern of using alcohol or another substance that results in impairment in daily life and noticeable distress."

Diagnostic Overview

Substance use disorders are present when the repeated use of alcohol, drugs, or other substances causes an individual significant clinical and functional impairment. This impairment may take several forms, such as health problems, disability, impaired social functioning, and failure to meet significant responsibilities at work, school, or home. According to the *DSM-5*, a diagnosis of substance use disorder is based on evidence of 11 criteria across four domains. The domains of substance use disorder are impaired control, social impairment, risky use, and pharmacological criteria. Specifically, the assignment of a diagnosis of substance use disorder requires the identification of two out of 11 criteria during the previous 12-month period. Table 13.1 provides an overview of the 11 criteria.

Substance Use Disorder Domains

A. IMPAIRED CONTROL

Impaired control describes the increasing lack of control that the individual has over their pattern of substance use. Impaired control is evident and observable through several different behavioral symptoms:

TABLE 13.1 The 11 Criteria of Substance Use (APA, 2013)

IMPAIRED CONTROL
1. *Using for extended periods of time*
2. *Persistently thinking about using*
3. *Investing excessive time into getting the drug*
4. *Intense craving for the substance*

SOCIAL IMPAIRMENT
5. *Continuation of use in spite of functional impairments*
6. *Intrapersonal problems*
7. *Giving up meaningful activities*

RISKY USE
8. *Using in physically dangerous situations*
9. *Continuing to use in spite of worsening health*

TOLERANCE AND WITHDRAWAL
10. *Needing more of the substance (tolerance)*
11. *Symptoms of withdrawal (vary from substance to substance)*

Note: Adapted from DSM-5 (APA, 2013)

1. Using for more extended periods than the individual intended and/or using more substantial amounts than initially intended
2. Persistent mental preoccupation with wanting to reduce use while being consistently unsuccessful in reducing substance use
3. Investing excessive time procuring, using, and recovering from the use of substances
4. Intense psychological "craving" for the substance, with the effect that for the individual, it is painful to think about anything else

B. SOCIAL IMPAIRMENT

The social impairment criteria encapsulate the reality that substance use disorder influences and frequently directly harms/threatens the social functioning and social relationships of an individual.

1. Continuation of the pattern of substance use despite problems with functioning. Functional impairments may manifest at work, in an employment setting, school, or in meeting family and other social obligations. Examples of these criteria include repeated work absences, poor academic performance, neglect of children and/or dependents, and chronic failure to meet household responsibilities
2. Contributing to interpersonal problems. Examples of interpersonal problems could include conflict with family members or the neglect of previously meaningful relationships and friendships

3. Giving up on relevant and meaningful activities. As it is difficult to maintain previous interests and social activities, individuals suffering from substance use disorders may abandon and give up previously pleasurable social and recreation activities

C. RISKY USE

The critical issue in the criterion of risky use is the failure of the individual to refrain from using the substance, despite the overt harm it causes or may potentially cause.

1. Repeatedly using substances in physically dangerous and perilous situations. Evidence would include driving or operating other heavy machinery while intoxicated by alcohol or other drugs
2. The continuation of the pattern of substance use despite the individual being aware that the pattern is contributing to or even worsening physical health and psychological conditions. Evidence for this criterion would include the person who continues to smoke cigarettes despite having a respiratory disorder such as throat cancer or chronic obstructive pulmonary disease.

D. PHARMACOLOGICAL INDICATORS: TOLERANCE AND WITHDRAWAL

In many cases, tolerance and withdrawal are the classic indicators of advanced and severe addiction. These criteria indicate the physiological adjustments made by an individual's body as it adjusts to the ongoing use of the substance.

1. Increased tolerance to a substance develops as people have a physiological need to increase the amount of a substance to achieve the same (or usual) desired effect. People experience tolerance differently, and it is important to remember that several individual factors and variables influence an individual's sensitivities to specific substances. In addition, specific substances vary regarding how quickly tolerance develops and the associated doses needed for an increase in tolerance to develop
2. Symptoms of withdrawal are the body's response to not receiving a sufficient dosage of the substance once tolerance has been developed. Withdrawal is usually seen as a cluster of complicated and problematic symptoms that are unique to the substance that is being used. In many instances withdrawal is a very unpleasant and potentially hazardous experience. (Note: If a person presents with withdrawal symptoms during a comprehensive assessment and evaluation, they should be diagnosed concurrently with substance use disorder and substance withdrawal.)

Severity of Substance Use Disorder

It should be noted that the *DSM-5* does not use the term *substance abuse* and *substance dependence*. Preferably, substance use disorders are defined as mild, moderate, or severe to indicate a level of severity. The level of severity is determined by the number of diagnostic criteria that are met by the individual client. *DSM-5* uses a symptom count-based severity index in which one or two symptoms are classed as mild, four to five symptoms classified as moderate, and six or more symptoms are classified as severe.

Think about our case study for Austin. Is Austin exhibiting some of these symptoms? How do you know that Austin has an addiction?

Classes of Substances

The *DSM-5* recognizes substance-related disorders resulting from the use of 10 separate classes of drugs, which are as follows: (1) alcohol; (2) caffeine; (3) cannabis; (4) hallucinogens (phencyclidine or similarly acting arylcyclohexylamines and other hallucinogens, such as LSD); (5) inhalants; (6) opioids; (7) sedatives, hypnotics, or anxiolytics; (8) stimulants (including amphetamine-type substances, cocaine, and other stimulants); (9) tobacco; and (10) other or unknown substances.

The *DSM-5* recognizes that vulnerability to developing substance-related disorders is not the same across all people and that there is variability in why and how some people are at risk of developing substance use disorders.

CASE STUDY 13.2 Sike, 57, is a retired carpenter who lives on an Indian reservation. He has a wife, Maria, and three children. Maria gives Sike an ultimatum to go to counseling, or she and the children will leave. Sike has struggled with alcohol since he was young. His father was an alcoholic, and Sike always remembers alcohol being a part of day-to-day life. On the reservation, men usually begin drinking around age 15, if not younger. Sike found himself craving more and more alcohol. During high school, it was socially acceptable to get drunk on the weekends. As Sike got older, he never "grew out" of drinking like his friends did. In fact, he began drinking increasingly more alone than with others. Now Sike drinks a pint of whiskey in the morning just to be able to mentally function throughout the day. In the afternoon, he usually goes to the grocery and spends a large amount of the family's small income on cases of beer and bottles of whiskey and vodka. Around five, Sike will begin to work his way through a couple of six packs. He has tried to no avail to "cut back" on alcohol. It seems that money or marital issues or depression always drive him back to drinking. The withdrawal symptoms are almost unbearable as well. Sike cannot stand the insomnia, vomiting, headaches, and hallucinations.

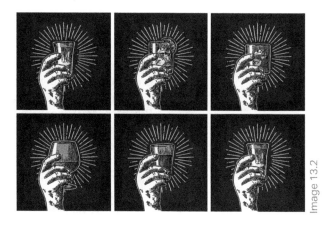

Image 13.2

Alcohol-Related Disorder F10.10 (Mild) F10.20 (Moderate and Severe)

Excessive alcohol use and or dependence increases a person's risk of developing serious health and psychiatric problems and complications, in addition to issues associated with intoxication and alcohol withdrawal symptoms.

Alcohol Use Rates

Alcohol use is widespread, as evidenced by the fact that according to the 2015 National Survey on Drug Use and Health, 86.4% of people ages 18 or older reported that they drank alcohol at some point in their lifetime. The past year and past month figures indicate that 70.1% of people reported that they drank in the past year and 56.0% reported that they drank in the past month. Binge drinking and heavy alcohol use are a little less common than social use but still frequently occurs. In 2015, 26.9% of people ages 18 or older reported that they engaged in binge drinking in the past month, and 7.0% reported that they engaged in heavy alcohol use in the past month.

Alcohol Use Definitions from the National Institute on Alcohol Abuse and Alcoholism (NIAAA)

BINGE DRINKING

- NIAAA (2004) defines binge drinking as a pattern of drinking that brings blood alcohol concentration (BAC) levels to 0.08 g/dL. This typically occurs after four drinks for women and five drinks for men—in about 2 hours.
- The Substance Abuse and Mental Health Services Administration (SAMHSA, 2016), which conducts the annual National Survey on Drug Use and Health, defines binge drinking as five or more alcoholic drinks for males or four or more alcoholic drinks for females on the same occasion (i.e., at the same time or within a couple of hours of each other) on at least 1 day in the past month.

HEAVY ALCOHOL USE

The Substance Abuse and Mental Health Services Administration defines heavy alcohol use as binge drinking on 5 or more days in the past month.

NIAAA's (2016) Definition of Drinking at Low Risk for Developing Alcohol Use Disorder (AUD). For women, low-risk drinking is defined as no more than three drinks on any single day and no more than seven drinks per week. For men, it is defined as no more than four drinks on any single day and no more than 14 drinks per week. NIAAA (2016) research shows that only about two in 100 people who drink within these limits have AUD.

Identifying problematic alcohol use is a complex task in large part because patterns of use vary significantly over time, and many individuals who use alcohol lack insight into their pattern of use. Many people who drink excessively and fall in the at-risk category of alcohol use do not consider themselves "alcoholics" and, therefore, do not pay attention to their pattern of use; this is in part why the *DSM-5* does not use the word alcoholic.

The NIAAA (2016) moderation guidelines are helpful when assessing for AUD. Alcohol consumption guidelines are based on the number of standard drinks consumed per day. A standard drink is defined as a 12 oz beer, a 5 oz glass of wine, or a 1.5 oz shot of liquor. For men, the maximum limits are no more than three drinks per day and no more than 14 drinks in a week. For women, the maximum limits are no more than two drinks per day and no more than seven drinks per week. Moderate drinking is defined as up to one drink per day for women and up to two drinks per day for men.

The Substance Abuse and Mental Health Services Administration (SAMHSA, 2013) defines heavy drinking as a pattern of use in which five or more drinks are consumed on the same occasion on each of 5 or more days in the past 30 days.

Most people who develop AUD do so by their late 30s. However, AUD can develop at any time during the life span. In addition, genetics play an essential role in its development.

Alcohol Withdrawal F10.239 (Without Perceptual Disturbances) F10.232 (With Perceptual Disturbances)

Typically, alcohol withdrawal begins four to 12 hours after stopping or significantly reducing heavy use. Symptoms of alcohol withdrawal are often very unpleasant, specifically delirium tremors (DTs). DTs take the form of extreme hyperactivity of the autonomic nervous system, along with hallucinations, which are also referred to as perceptual disturbances. DTs must be treated by appropriate medical intervention and supervision. Additional symptoms of concern of alcohol withdrawal include extreme sweating, insomnia, nausea, vomiting, hallucinations, agitation, anxiety, and even seizures. Alcohol withdrawal can result in death because of complications such as convulsions, seizures, and cardiac arrhythmia.

Alcohol Intoxication F10.129 (Mild) F10.229 (Moderate or Severe) F10.929 (Without Substance Use Disorder)

Alcohol intoxication can be recognized through physiological and behavioral symptoms. The most common behavioral symptoms of alcohol intoxication are impaired judgment and antisocial behavior. In addition, some people may engage in risky sexual behavior and/or interpersonal aggression. Regarding physical symptoms, alcohol intoxication causes slurred speech, unsteady gait, impaired coordination, and impaired memory; in extreme cases, it has been known to induce a comma.

Would Austin be diagnosed with alcohol use disorder?

CASE STUDY 13.3 David, 17, is a junior in high school. He has always struggled with "finding his crowd" since he started high school in the ninth grade. Previously, he had been homeschooled. The only one who has been friendly to David is Kevin. Thus David spends most of his time after school with Kevin. At first, they would just talk about sports, girls, and the school, but now it is different. Each time David goes to Kevin's, they smoke pot in the basement. Kevin's parents work long hours and do not usually check in on them. David was at first apprehensive about using but now finds it difficult to make it through the day without smoking. David got Kevin to introduce him to his dealer, and now David spends most of his money and some stolen money from his parents on marijuana. He goes to school high often and has been sent home several times. He ignores his parents' lectures and gets high again later in the day. The few times he attempted to quit, Kevin experienced the unpleasant withdrawal symptoms and went back to using. David finally decides to go to a drug abuse center after being caught with weed by the police.

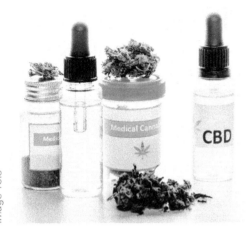

Cannabis Use Disorder F12.10 (Mild) F12.20 (Moderate and Severe)

Cannabis is commonly known as marijuana, and other names include pot, hash, grass, dope, herb, and reefer. Cannabis contains tetrahydrocannabinol (THC). It occurs in organic form as the buds of a plant that contain this psychoactive chemical. THC produces an almost immediate high through rapidly entering the bloodstream through the lungs when it is inhaled or smoked. It can also be eaten/ingested.

Presently in the United States, laws, attitudes, and widespread perception of marijuana use are rapidly changing. Twenty-three states now have medical marijuana laws, and marijuana use is higher in states with legal use laws than in other states. In addition, four of these states have also legalized marijuana for recreational use. More Americans now favor legalization of marijuana than in previous years, and far fewer Americans view marijuana use as risky (Motel, 2015). The result of this shift in attitude toward marijuana is that more people are using it than ever before; the previous stereotype about marijuana being a substance used by adolescent males is defunct.

Marijuana is the most-used drug after alcohol and tobacco in the United States. According to the Substance Abuse and Mental Health Services Administration data: in 2014, about 22.2 million people ages 12 and up reported using marijuana during the past month; in 2014, there were 2.6 million people in that age range who had used marijuana for the first time within the past 12 months. People between the ages of 12 and 49 report first using the drug at an average age of 18.5.

Cannabis disorders are more prevalent in males than in females, and approximately 5% of people over the age of 12 meet the criteria for cannabis use disorder, which illustrates that many people first use cannabis as teenagers. Cannabis dependence develops gradually, usually beginning with infrequent, casual, and perhaps even social use. However, over time, patterns of use increase, becoming more frequent, as people begin to use marijuana regardless of the time of day. Cannabis dependence is often detectable through people complaining about the emergence of symptoms associated with withdrawal and or a reduction of use. These symptoms include mood and sleep disturbance, impaired appetite, craving cannabis, psychomotor agitation, and physical discomfort.

A common misconception about the risk of cannabis use dependence among users is that it is sporadic. As Hasin (2017) pointed out, this assumption is based on findings from 25 years ago that few cannabis users developed dependence (Anthony et al., 1994; Joy et al., 2017). However, this assumption does not bear out in more recent U.S. national data, as three out of 10 cannabis users developed *DSM-IV* cannabis use dependence (Hasin et al., 2015). Moreover, extending analyses of the *DSM-5* diagnoses of cannabis use dependence (Hasin et al., 2016), 19.5% of lifetime users met criteria for the disorder, of whom 23% were symptomatically severe (>6 criteria). Of these, 48% were not functioning in any occupational or social major role. Thus cannabis use dependence is not rare and can be severe; it is much more common than previously thought (Hasin et al., 2017). Cannabis use interferes with an individual's ability to carry out daily routines and is strongly associated with amotivational syndrome (Lynskey & Hall, 2000). This condition has been posited/put forward as an explanation of poor educational and social performance connected to cannabis use characterized by a lack of ambition, malaise, motivation, and desire to accomplish things. Even in young users, ongoing cannabis consumption interferes with the dopamine centers in the brain that are linked to motivation, reward, and a sense of accomplishment.

The Effects of Cannabis

Cannabis intoxication has a rapid onset, initially producing feelings of a euphoric "high" and altered perceptions; however, this can quickly fade into a state of anxiety. Other symptoms include a lack of coordination, reduced judgment, memory problems, decreased alertness, and difficulties engaging in social interaction. People with cannabis intoxication quickly lose the flow of their thoughts and may have difficulty following a conversation and engaging in rational discussion. Therefore, attempts at conversation and social engagement can be nonsensical. Additional physiological symptoms of cannabis intoxication include increased appetite, colloquially known as the munchies; dry mouth; persistent cough; and reduced heart rate.

Would Austin be considered for cannabis use disorder?

CASE STUDY 13.4 Mia, 18, is a senior at a large public high school. She is one of the top students in her class and competing for the valedictorian spot. Mia would do anything to score well on her school exams and the advanced placement tests. She studies for hours every day and forgoes many social events to be the best. After scoring a "B+" on a major exam, Mia is afraid she has put herself in jeopardy. One of her best friends tells her that if she takes Ritalin before exams, it will help her to concentrate better. Mia first obtains the stimulant from her friend. The drug works and helps Mia to score high on her advanced placement biology exam. At first, Mia only uses the drug to concentrate on important exams. Soon, she begins using it for all exams and even just assignments. She feels that it helps her to focus and lets her forget about her parent's divorce. Slowly, Mia works up to taking the Ritalin every day and sometimes takes five or six tablets. After her friend runs out of medication, Mia goes to her doctor and fakes the symptoms of attention deficit hyperactivity disorder to be prescribed more medication. To celebrate the end of the school year, Mia goes over to a friend's house and snorts a large number of pills to get high.

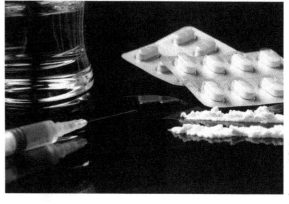

Image 13.4

Stimulant Use Disorder (Including Cocaine Use Disorder) 305.70 (F15.10)

Stimulants increase alertness, attention, and energy, and a wide range of stimulant drugs have historically been used to treat conditions, such as obesity; attention deficit hyperactivity disorder; and occasionally/historically depression. However, like medications, stimulants can be diverted for illegal use. The most commonly abused stimulants are amphetamines, methamphetamine, and cocaine. Stimulants can be synthetic (such as amphetamines) or plant-derived (such as cocaine). Stimulants can be taken several ways: orally, snorted, or intravenously.

Stimulants are sometimes prescribed for a variety of legitimate health conditions. When used correctly, the use of stimulants does not meet diagnostic criteria; however, if someone begins to exceed the dose and frequency, then a diagnosis of substance use disorder, amphetamine-type use may be used. However, those prescribed stimulants open themselves up to the possibility of abuse. According to Compton et al. (2018), among U.S. adults, 6.6% (annual average) used prescription stimulants overall, 4.5% used without misuse, 1.9% misused without use disorders, and 0.2% had use disorders. The most commonly reported motivations for misuse were to help with alertness or concentration (56.3%), and the most likely source of misused prescription stimulants was obtaining them for free from friends or relatives (56.9%). Frequent prescription stimulant misuse and use disorder is associated with an increased likelihood of obtaining medications from physicians or drug dealers or strangers and the reduced likelihood of obtaining them from friends or relatives (Compton et al., 2018).

Stimulant use may be either chronic or episodic; periods of continued use without periods of abstinence are defined as chronic use. Episodic use refers to periods of heavy use interspersed with periods of reduced use or even abstinence. For example, some people choose to use stimulants on the weekend and then may not use during the week.

Effects of Stimulants

A range of psychological and behavioral symptoms indicates stimulant intoxication. Stimulant intoxication produces feelings of extreme euphoria, well-being, and confidence. However, dramatic changes in behavior and mood may also occur, with people possibly becoming highly paranoid, extremely irritable, anxious, angry, or depressed. In addition to these negative psychological symptoms, dramatic mood swings can also occur. These psychological symptoms can add to the dangers associated with people exhibiting poor judgment and aggression because of stimulant intoxication. Besides, in some cases, people may also become delusional and experience tactile or auditory hallucinations. Hypervigilance, hyperactive activity, confusion, and talkativeness are also common.

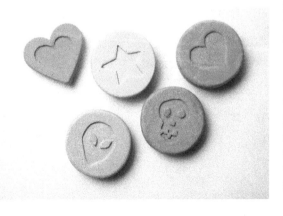

Image 13.5

Physical changes that indicate stimulant intoxication include pupil dilation, altered body temperature, nausea or vomiting, weight loss, psychomotor changes, muscular weakness, chest pain, and elevated or lowered blood pressure.

Stimulant Withdrawal Symptoms

Withdrawal usually begins several days after the last use. It includes symptoms of depressed mood, fatigue, vivid dreams, sleep difficulties, psychomotor slowing or agitation, and powerful cravings. It is essential to monitor stimulant withdrawal, as psychiatric symptoms and/or complications may develop.

Hallucinogen Use Disorder

A decades-long trend is the significant rise in the use of hallucinogens and accompanying changes of attitude from young people toward their use. In a recent study of hallucinogen use disorder, one in five (20%) MDMA (methylenedioxymethamphetamine, ecstasy) users and about one in six (16%) other hallucinogen users reported at least one clinical feature of the disorder. In the United States, MDMA is classified as a hallucinogen, a category comprising LSD (lysergic acid diethylamide), PCP (phencyclidine, or angel dust), peyote, mescaline, and psilocybin (mushrooms; Wu et al., 2008). Among MDMA users, the prevalence of hallucinogen abuse, subthreshold dependence, and dependence was 4.9%, 11.9%, and 3.6%, respectively. It is not surprising, therefore, that the use of MDMA has come to be conceptualized as a growing public health concern (Wu et al., 2008).

Hallucinogens can be chemically synthesized (for example, LSD) or may occur naturally (such as psilocybin mushrooms, peyote). The hallucinogen-related disorder has two subtypes: (1) PCP and (2) other hallucinogens. Most hallucinogens are taken orally, with only one very small subtype being smoked. The use of these drugs is marked by visual and auditory hallucinations, in addition to feelings of detachment from one's environment and oneself and distortions in time and other sensory perceptions.

Effects of PCP

PCP intoxication produces extreme behavior changes, which may include impulsivity and belligerence, hallucinations, and impaired social functioning. Troubling, violent behavior can also occur, as PCP users may believe they are being attacked and/or in danger/peril. The fact that an increase in the pain threshold often accompanies these perceptual distortions can severely magnify potentially dangerous behavior and situations.

Effects of Other Hallucinogens

Use of generic hallucinogens may also create extreme behavior and psychological symptoms. Positive psychological symptoms include hallucinations and perceptual disturbances. Negative psychological and behavioral symptoms may include severe anxiety, depression, paranoia or fearfulness, poor judgment and relational disturbance, panic, and perceptual distortions. Physical symptoms and side effects include sweating, slow heart rate, dilated pupils, blurred vision, tremors, and lack of coordination.

Hallucinogen Withdrawal

There are no documented withdrawal symptoms for hallucinogen use. However, some people who use them report that even after the first effects have long subsided, vivid flashbacks and perceptual disturbances can continue for many months and even occur years later.

CASE STUDY 13.5 Adair, 43, works in a plant that produces interior car parts. A few years ago, Adair hurt her back at work while lifting a heavy box. Worker's compensation paid for her to have time off and for her medical bills. Her pain was intense and long lasting. Adair could not sleep at night because of her back pain. The doctor first

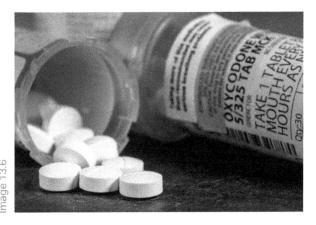

prescribed a mild pain reliever, but Adair was still visibly in a lot of pain. The doctor decided to prescribe Percocet to Adair to ease her pain. Adair found that the painkiller not only eased her pain but also made her feel extremely happy and able to better manage life. Adair had been through a recent divorce and the family drama that surrounded it. When she was on the painkillers, she was able to forget her pain. Adair began faking and exaggerating her pain symptoms to keep her doctor prescribing the medication. When he finally discontinued her prescription, she began seeking out the medications from others. She called a relative whom she knew had chronic hip pain to try to buy her pain medications. Adair began asking coworkers and friends for pain medications as well. When one friend confronted Adair and told her she needed help, Adair denied the allegation and instead decided to use the internet and go to other doctors to obtain more pills.

Opioid Use Disorder

Opioid misuse in the United States has become a significant public health crisis, with nonmedically prescribed opioid use (NMPOU) being a significant cause of health and social impairment. Drug poisoning death rates more than tripled between 1999 and 2012; the quarterly abuse rates associated with opioids reported by U.S. poison centers increased from 0.20/100,000 population to 0.56/100,000 population in 2012, and emergency department visits increased by 153% from 2004 to 2011. Drug treatment admission rates for non-heroin opiates increased 236% from 2002 to 2012 (Saha et al., 2016). Additional adverse health consequences of NMPOU include transitions to injection drugs or heroin use with resultant infection (e.g., hepatitis C, human immunodeficiency virus), risk, falls and fractures among older adults, neonatal opioid withdrawal syndrome, cognitive impairment, and drug interactions. Societal costs of NMPOU are estimated at $53 to $72 billion annually (Saha et al., 2016).

The *DSM-5* uses *opioid use disorder* as an umbrella term that captures both opiate drugs, which are those naturally derived from the opium poppy plant, and synthetic opioids. Common varieties of opioids are opium, morphine, heroin, codeine, methadone, oxycodone, and fentanyl. Fentanyl is a particularly problematic opioid, as it is a synthetic analgesic similar to morphine, except with up to 100 times the potency. This intense potency greatly increases the risk of overdose. Originally, fentanyl was approved for the treatment of severe pain; however, the advent of large-scale illegal production has made this opioid particularly deadly.

People may misuse opioids as prescription pain medications, such as Oxycontin and Vicodin. In many instances, people have legitimate medical prescriptions for using opioid drugs. However, they may begin to use them more frequently or in larger doses than initially prescribed by their primary/attending physician. Therefore, opioid dependence develops very quickly, and as tolerance increases, larger dosages are needed to avoid the impending development of withdrawal symptoms.

One recent development that has contributed to the rise of the opioid epidemic has been the phenomena of people becoming addicted to painkillers prescribed by physicians, which in turn leads to them becoming dependent on opiates and then beginning to use heroin, as it is much cheaper and regularly available on the street in contrast to prescription painkillers.

Opioids can be taken orally or injected. However, they can also in some cases be smoked or snorted. Opioids reduce the perception of pain but can also produce drowsiness, mental confusion, euphoria, nausea, constipation, and, depending on the amount of drug taken, depress respiration. Often, people experience an intense euphoric response to opioid medications and substances, and it is common that people misusing opioids try to intensify the "high" they experience by snorting or injecting them. These methods of use increase the risk for serious medical complications, including overdose. Many people who begin misusing their prescription for painkillers can quickly switch from prescription opiates to heroin because of the greater availability and lower price of heroin. This, however, is extremely dangerous because of inconsistencies with the purity of heroin and the reality that other drugs are mixed in dramatically increases the risk of drug overdose.

Effects of Opioid Intoxication

Opioid toxification is extremely dangerous, and it is evidenced by symptoms of elevated mood followed by a severely flattened demeanor. Impairments also accompany the initial effect of opioids on memory, judgment, and attention. Physiological changes including pupil size, slurred speech, and drowsiness are also present.

Opioid intoxication can result in a coma because of the way in which it the substances depresses the central nervous system. The danger of a depressed central nervous system is that essential functioning begins to slow and shut down. Additional symptoms include the track marks that affect people who use opioids intravenously. Also, as needles require a prescription, people using opioids illegally are at risk of several health complications from reusing and sharing needles.

Opioid Withdrawal

Opioid withdrawal occurs quickly after the cessation of heavy or prolonged use. It is important to note that opioids are designed to be both short acting and long acting. Short-acting drugs are those that quickly pass through the bloodstream, whereas long-lasting opioids take much longer to leave the body and bloodstream.

In the case of short-acting opioids, such as heroin, intense withdrawal symptoms begin just 6–12 hours after the last dose and can last between 5 and 7 days. However, long-lasting opioid withdrawal symptoms may take several days to emerge, and the symptoms may be present for several weeks, with withdrawal taking place over a more extended period but with significantly less intense symptoms.

Opioid withdrawal is extremely uncomfortable and may include symptoms of anxiety, restlessness, irritability, muscle aches, depressed mood, nausea, vomiting, diarrhea, sweating fever, intense cravings for the substance, and sleep disturbances.

TRUE LIFE 13.1

Robert Downey Jr.

Robert Downey Jr. is an American actor who is most famous for his role as Iron Man in the Marvel world. However, there is more than meets the eye when it comes to Downey. When his family became the topic of discussion during an interview with *People* magazine, Downey shared, "There was always a lot of pot and coke around." Drugs became an emotional bond. "When my dad and I would do drugs together," explained Downey, "it was like him trying to express his love for me in the only way he knew how" (Gliatto, 1996). A long and tough road to sobriety would be ahead of one of America's most renowned actors.

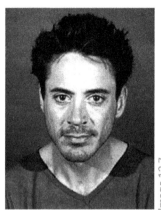

Image 13.7

Downey was brought up in New York City, and at age 5, he premiered in his father's (Robert Downey Sr.) film *Pound*. Through the '70s and '80s, Downey would take on roles that would build his portfolio as an actor, but it wasn't until 1987 that Downey finally received recognition for his acting (Empire, n.d.). Downey took a role on *Saturday Night Live* that would foreshadow a

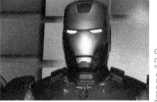

Image 13.8

dark future to come. Downey starred in Marek Kanievska's *Less Than Zero* as a young man addicted to drugs. Despite the Academy Award nominations and apparent success, Downey found a way to be in trouble with the law because of his continuous substance abuse.

Downey appeared in films such as *The Singing Detective* (2003), *Kiss Bang Bang* (2005), *A Scanner Darkly* (2006), *Gothika* (2003), and *Zodiac* (2007; Empire). These productions were ones that he was able to hold on to later in his career because of his newfound relationship with sobriety. However, before he reached a drug-free state, there were numerous run-ins with the law. Early on in his acting career, he was "court-ordered to a 45-day treatment program for cocaine and heroin addiction, had entered a plea of not guilty to two felony charges and three misdemeanors, including possession of heroin and cocaine, driving under the influence of alcohol and drugs, and carrying an unloaded .357 Magnum handgun in his truck" (Gliatto, 1996). Another time, Downey broke into the home of his neighbors and went to sleep in their 11-year-old son's bed (Bull, 2015). Downey claimed this to be uncommon of him, but as more and more incidents occurred with him as the center of attention, this became hard to believe. Downey thought it was normal that at some point in a person's life, they would become addicted to something, and cocaine and heroin just so happened to be his addictions.

Researcher for the RAND Institute of Santa Monica Jonathan Caulkins said, "Heroin becomes part of [an addict's] self-definition," and "to give up the habit amounts to giving up one's identity. It's like a death." How was Downey expected to let go of a piece of his identity?

People close to Downey have claimed that he suffers from depression and has received a diagnosis of bipolar, but Downey refutes these claims (Bull, 2015). Despite the many obstacles Downey has encountered, he continues to be an inspiration to a number of people across America. Although he faced many struggles with his drug addiction, he lives by the motto, "I swear to God. I am not my story" (Vanity Fair, 2014). He has proven to live by this motto during a 16-year stretch of sobriety and has refused to let drugs negatively affect his career again. Downey credits his drug-free state to the "support of his friends and family, meditation, yoga, therapy and a twelve-step recovery program" (Bull, 2015). Currently, Downey is working to end the vicious cycle drugs has had over his family, for his son also suffers from drug addiction.

Downey remarked in an issue of *Playboy*, "Not having done drugs for literally five or six years is a lifetime." "I think of myself as someone who has no desire, use for or conscious memory of that life. And yet I don't shut the door on it, and I don't pretend it didn't happen." "To me, here's the only thing: You take responsibility, whether you're outraged by the results or not, that you in some way participate in and create what you're experiencing" (Manor, 2010).

Sedative Use Disorders

Goodwin and Hasan (2002) discovered that the lifetime prevalence of self-perceived sedative dependence was 0.5%, with 7.1% reporting nonprescribed sedative use and 17.0% being prescribed sedatives and denying misuse. Individuals who used sedatives without a prescription were more likely to be male, have lower incomes, more education than a general high school diploma, high incidence of major depression, and agoraphobia.

The *DSM-5* recognizes three classes of sedatives: (1) anxiolytics (anti-anxiety) drugs, such as benzodiazepines (e.g., Valium, Klonopin, and Rohypnol); (2) barbiturates (e.g., Amytal, Nembutal Seconal, and Phenobarbital); and (3) other anti-anxiety medications.

Sedatives act in a way that severely depresses the central nervous and respiratory system. As a result of this effect on the central nervous system, they can be dangerous and even deadly when taken in high doses. Sedative addiction is often co-occurrent with the use of other drugs, which is usually reflective of an effort on the part of the person using the substance to counteract the effects of other drugs such as stimulants with the effects of sedatives. For example, people may use sedatives when looking to come down from cocaine use.

Sedative Withdrawal

Withdrawal symptoms occur after the sudden end of prolonged use and may be quite uncomfortable and particularly dangerous; specifically, because longer term use of sedatives at higher doses leads to a more intense period of withdrawal. A range of symptoms of withdrawal may include sweating, increased heart rate, insomnia, anxiety, seizures, hallucinations, and nausea and vomiting. Because of the nature of these symptoms, medical consultation and supervision for withdrawal are critical.

Sedative Intoxication

Sedative use is evident by signs of significant behavior change, with the most prominent changes including altered mood and impaired judgment. Sedatives also have a disinhibiting effect that is much like alcohol. Physiological signs of intoxication include slurred speech, lack of coordination, impaired memory, decreased blood pressure and pulse, and possibly coma. Because of the severity of these symptoms, both behavioral and physiological, it is not uncommon for serious injuries because of accidents and overdoses to occur with people with substance use disorder.

Inhalant Use Disorder

More than 22 million Americans age 12 and older have used inhalants, and every year, more than 750,000 use inhalants for the first time. Despite the substantial prevalence and severe inhalant toxicities use, it has been termed "the forgotten epidemic." Inhalant abuse remains the least-studied form of substance abuse, although research on its epidemiology, neurobiology, treatment, and prevention has accelerated in recent years (Howard et al., 2011).

The most prominent characteristic of inhalant use disorder is the practice of inhaling a wide variety of household items. Users inhale or "huff" products, such as glue, gasoline, paint thinners, certain types of cleansers, and various aerosols. Inhalants reach the bloodstream very quickly, and this results in significant psychoactive effects. Because they are so cheap and readily available, inhalants are one of the first drugs used by young people.

Inhalant use among males during adolescence and young adult years occurs more than any other demographic. In can be detected through a residue, odor, and, occasionally, burns on the skin. Sometimes those people who are using may attempt to conceal this odor with various types of fresheners. Those individuals may also present with a rash near the nose and mouth, and their eyes may appear to be reddened and irritated.

Effects of Inhalants: Inhalant Intoxication

Inhalants produce various behavioral and psychological changes, which may include aggressiveness, impaired judgment, anxiety, poor social functioning, and even delusions and hallucinations. Inhalants produce a variety of physical effects; common symptoms include dizziness, headaches, poor coordination, slurred speech, coughing, lack of balance, sleepiness, poor reflexes, slowed movements and tremors, muscle weakness, poor vision, and even coma. Because of the toxic nature of inhalant products, inhalant use can be fatal, and death does not appear to be related to dose.

Treatment for Substance Use Disorder
Detoxification

For clients with multiple symptoms of withdrawal and a diagnosis of substance use disorder, treatment should include substance use rehabilitation and medically supervised detoxification. Detoxification may take place at an inpatient facility or within an outpatient facility with regularly scheduled medical supervision. Certain medications can be used to assist with the detoxification process and work to minimize the symptoms of withdrawal. Medically supervised detoxification dramatically reduces the chance of developing health complications from the negative effect of withdrawal symptoms.

Psychotherapy

Talk-based therapies have been shown to be effective in addressing patterns of substance use, as well as some of the underlying causes of an individual's substance use disorder. Therefore, it is common to include some form of psychotherapy within most treatment plans for those with a substance use disorder. A broad range of talk therapies can address underlying issues connected to the onset of a substance-related disorder, such as trauma, adverse childhood experiences, and interpersonal and family relationships. Talk therapy can also equip individuals with substance use disorders to develop healthy coping mechanisms and assist them in developing new ways of dealing with stressful situations in their lives.

Therapy can help clients to develop increased insight into their cognitive processes, trauma histories, and personality traits.

Medication-Assisted Treatment (MAT)

In addition to any drugs that are used to treat withdrawal symptoms in the detoxification process, extensive evidence has shown that some substance use disorders can be managed with long-term MATs. Specifically, MAT is used to treat a range of substance use disorders, and there are currently medications that are used in the treatment of alcohol, opioid, and tobacco use.

Dependence on opioids can be treated with methadone, buprenorphine, and naltrexone. Methadone and buprenorphine work in a very similar way to each other by reducing the cravings for opioids and providing relief from the symptoms of opioid withdrawal. In contrast, naltrexone works on the principle of blocking the euphoric and sedative effects of other opioid drugs if the patient experiences a relapse and uses an opioid again. Alcohol can be treated with disulfiram, which is suitable for people who have already gone through detoxification; acamprosate, which is suitable for those in recovery who have already stopped drinking; and naltrexone, which blocks the effects of intoxication, allowing for a reduction in drinking behaviors. Tobacco dependence is commonly treated with a number of drugs. Two of the most common are varenicline (brand name Chantix), which reduces withdrawal symptoms and lessens the pleasure from use and bupropion (brand name Zyban/Wellbutrin), which reduces cravings and reduces withdrawal symptoms.

Peer Support Services and Recovery Groups

Peer support services have been shown to be very useful in helping people to recover from substance use. These services can be informal and may take the form of support groups, such as the 12 step groups (i.e., Alcoholics Anonymous [AA] and Narcotics Anonymous). While AA is a popular choice for many people in substance use recovery, there is only limited scientific evidence about the success of AA in helping people in recovery; for instance, such groups have very high dropout rates; about 40% of people who attend AA do so for less than a year (Lilienfeld & Arkowitz, 2011). In addition,

Kaskutas (2009) concluded that the evidence for AA's effectiveness is mixed at best after conducting a meta-review of the available information on the program. However, some have criticized AA as being overly focused on days of sobriety, which can in some cases lead to challenges with relapse prevention and management.

Other peer support groups may use self-management and recovery training recovery approaches. Many substance use agencies use peer support specialists, as these workers can provide support through the paradigm of lived experience, which is proving to be increasingly active support for those individuals with substance use disorder.

Case Study Summary

One of this chapter's case studies reviewed the behaviors of Austin. As you process the story and examine possible diagnostic criteria, take a few minutes to answer the following questions:

1. What would be the correct diagnosis for Austin?

_____

_____

2. What are the specific symptoms or criteria that led you to this diagnosis?

_____

_____

3. What other possible disorders might you diagnose Austin with and why?

_____

_____

4. Briefly discuss what types of treatment may be beneficial for Austin. Could you see using a certain counseling theory and/or medication?

_____

_____

Guided Practice Exercises

Scenario 1

Marlisa, 35, knows that she has a problem, but she is hesitant in getting help. For the last 5 years, she has been drinking heavily. After her divorce, alcohol was the only thing that seemed to dull the pain. Now Marlisa lives alone and feels even more alone. She works at a local restaurant as a bartender. The owner is lenient, and Marlisa often drinks on the job. By the time the bar closes, she stumbles back to her apartment and will often continue drinking until 4 or 5 a.m. Marlisa needs increasingly more alcohol to dull her emotional pain. She sleeps for most of the day and then goes back to work. Lately, she has not had time for family because of her nocturnal schedule and drinking habits. Marlisa does not hang out with anyone outside of the bar. She has almost missed work the last 2 days because of severe depression, making it difficult for her to get out of bed, let alone work. At her latest checkup, the doctor told Marlisa she was at risk for anemia, cirrhosis, and pancreatitis. Subsequently, Marlisa tried to cut down unsuccessfully. She has been in and out of AA for years. She is now considering checking into an inpatient alcohol facility.

What would be the correct disorder? What are the specific symptoms or criteria that led you to this diagnosis?

_____
_____
_____
_____

What specific behaviors caused you to diagnose the disorder?

_____
_____
_____
_____

What other possible disorders might you diagnose Marlisa with and why?

_____
_____
_____
_____

Scenario 2

Astrid, 26, moved from Singapore to the United States with her parents at age 16. She is now attending Stanford University and pursuing a degree in economics. The pressure of trying to maintain good grades and make friends is overwhelming for Astrid. She has always found it difficult to connect with people, especially those in the United States. Astrid has found a secret weapon: marijuana. When she gets high, she is able to spend time with people and talk openly. Although she can get suspicious sometimes, she is usually friendly and outgoing when high. Astrid has noticed that the occasional weekend buzz of the drug no longer seems to be sufficient. She has been getting high during the week. This has caused a drop in her grades because she has been missing assignments and classes. Astrid knows her parents will disown her if she drops out of school. After all, they came to America to give her more opportunities. Astrid has tried and failed to quit using several times. She feels like she has no place to go and is contemplating suicide.

What would be the correct disorder? What are the specific symptoms or criteria that led you to this diagnosis?

_____
_____
_____
_____

What specific behaviors caused you to diagnose the disorder?

_____
_____
_____
_____

What other possible disorders might you diagnose Astrid with and why?

_____

_____

_____

_____

What are some of the withdrawal symptoms of marijuana use?

_____

_____

_____

_____

Some people argue that there is no proof of cannabis addiction. Look at the research and respond to this statement.

_____

_____

_____

_____

How would you address culture in the treatment of Astrid?

_____

_____

_____

_____

Scenario 3

Edward, 25, is a third-year medical student. For years, Edward has used alcohol and marijuana, but he has never gotten into the "heavy stuff." At a party, some of his friends introduced him to cocaine. Edward figured that like alcohol and marijuana, he would be able to quit using cocaine whenever he wanted to. Unfortunately, his recreational use quickly turned into a daily habit, costing him about $100 a day. To offset the expense of his use, Edward became a dealer. He found that he studied better when high. That high become harder and harder to get though as Edward's use continued. Edward finally hit the reality that he had a problem when he began missing classes to buy and sell cocaine. He was put on academic probation and would be kicked out of medical school if he did not get his grades up. Edward decided to drop out of school and check into a drug rehab facility.

Describe what happens physiologically when a person uses stimulants.

_____

_____

_____

_____

Attention deficit hyperactivity disorder medication abuse is becoming more popular in high school, and college students use it for both weight loss and help with concentration. Describe why this medication might be attractive to a college student.

_____

_____

_____

_____

What are the withdrawal symptoms for cocaine use?

_____

_____

_____

_____

Scenario 4

Aria, 23, dropped out of college a few years ago because of low grades. It was not that she couldn't handle the schoolwork but rather she had a difficult time stopping her partying long enough to get her grades up. Aria loved going out with friends on Fridays and getting stoned or drunk. Afterward, she always fell into a bit of a depression and was unable to do much for a few days. She knew that during the times she was intoxicated, guys would take advantage of her, but she couldn't remember who she had sex with the next day. After nights like that, Aria wouldn't eat and just opted to sleep all day. Now, she works at a department store in the mall, and her drug use has increased. One of her coworkers introduced her to LSD, and Aria feels like she cannot stop using it. She loves the hallucinations it gives her. The problem is that she will fall into a deep depression after using it and will be unable to work for a few days. She has almost gotten fired because of this behavior. Aria has also started to withdraw from others besides when she is getting high. She feels that she could stop using but does not want to, even after "bad trips."

Do you think Aria is experiencing depression as a result of using drugs or is it its own separate entity?

_____

_____

_____

_____

LSD is not typically physically addictive, but some people like Aria become psychologically addicted (they believe they cannot stop). How would you go about treating someone like Aria?

_____

_____

_____

_____

During a session, Aria tells a counselor that she is contemplating suicide. When the counselor informs her that he needs to call 911, Aria becomes agitated. How would you deal with a situation like this?

_____

_____

_____

_____

What are the withdrawal symptoms of hallucinogens?

_____

_____

_____

_____

How might you tell if someone is using a hallucinogen?

_____

_____

_____

_____

Scenario 5

Nick, 32, first got into heroin when convinced to try it by one of his girlfriends, Eve. She told him that it would give him a high that was better than any food or sex or other drugs he had ever had. Nick was quickly caught up in the calming effects of the drug. He did not understand how people got addicted to heroin. It just helped him to feel "chill." Nick felt he did his job as the human resource manager at a large store better when intoxicated. Problems that arose just didn't provoke as much anxiety anymore. Soon he was contacting Eve's dealer every day. Even though he was not comfortable with it, the dealer carried a gun and insisted on meeting in the "bad" part of town. Slowly, Nick began needing more heroin to feel calm. His mind revolved around getting the next fix. He fell out of contact with his friends and family. He didn't spend time with others unless it was to get high. He began missing work and was fired by the store manager. This finally prompted Nick to get treatment.

Describe signs of both painkiller and heroin abuse.

_____

_____

_____

_____

Describe the withdrawal symptoms of painkillers and heroin abuse.

_____

_____

_____

_____

How do you think doctors and therapists can work holistically to prevent painkiller abuse?

_____

_____

_____

_____

Scenario 6

Connor, 28, has felt "on edge" for as long as he can remember. He has always experienced some anxiety, but it has worsened with the pressure of his job. Connor is a fire fighter but was put on probation when he had an anxiety attack on the job. His boss wanted him to take some time to "sort things out." First, Connor's doctor prescribed an

SSRI for his anxiety, but Connor still experienced anxiety, even when on high dosages. The doctor subsequently prescribed Xanax. This helped Connor substantially, and he was able to go back to work. Unfortunately, Connor has found it difficult to function without the Xanax. After witnessing the death of a child in a fire, Connor began using more of the Xanax. Now he has to use twice as much as he previously did to feel the same relaxed state. When Connor runs out of his medication early, the doctor suspects that he is addicted and tries to taper back the dosage. Connor finds that a lower dosage produces insomnia and racing thoughts. He fears that this will affect his work performance and goes to another doctor in an effort to obtain more drugs.

What steps would you take if you believed that a relative or friend was abusing anti-anxiety medication?

_____
_____
_____
_____

What are the withdrawal symptoms of sedative, hypnotic, or anxiolytic drug abuse?

_____
_____
_____
_____

Describe what tolerance is and how it can be seen in Connor's story.

_____
_____
_____
_____

Scenario 7

Abel, 13, is one of the most popular boys in his class at school. He has already dated and had sexual contact with several of his peers. He is always at the most exclusive parties and is known for stealing alcohol from his parents for parties. Abel flaunts the fact that he regularly inhales turpentine fumes to get high. He has also used bath salts, glues, and other substances to get high. Abel would never admit this to anyone, but he believes he has a problem with the inhalants. Although he has tried to stop using, the nausea, headaches, and abdominal cramping he experiences when trying not to use thwart his efforts. Abel now uses a turpentine rag every day to get high. His mom has questioned the burn marks that have appeared under Abel's nose. Finally, his parents take him to the hospital one day when they find Abel in a delirious state. He is happy but also confused. The doctors notice the burns on his nose and mouth and his elevated pulse and vital signs. They recommend that Abel's parents take him to a treatment clinic.

How might you know that someone is high on inhalants?

_____
_____
_____
_____

What are the withdrawal symptoms?

_____
_____
_____
_____

In the last few years, the use of bath salts to get high has increased. Many stores regulate items like salts, glues, and paint thinners by not selling them to minors. Do you think this strategy will help to lessen abuse?

_____
_____
_____
_____

Why do you think that a huge number of adolescents abuse inhalants over other drugs?

_____
_____
_____
_____

Web-Based and Literature-Based Resources

Substance Abuse and Mental Health Services Administration. Alcohol, tobacco and other drugs website: https://www.samhsa.gov/find-help/atod

National Institute on Drug Abuse: https://www.drugabuse.gov/publications/drugfacts/treatment-approaches-drug-addiction

USA government website on mental health and substance abuse: https://www.usa.gov/mental-health-substance-abuse

U.S. Department of Veterans Affairs. Alcohol and drug misuse: https://www.mentalhealth.va.gov/substance-abuse/index.asp

References

Anthony, J. C., Warner, L. A., & Kessler, R. C. (1994). Comparative epidemiology of dependence on tobacco, alcohol, controlled substances, and inhalants: basic findings from the National Comorbidity Survey. *Experimental and Clinical Psychopharmacology, 2*, 244–268.

American Psychiatric Association (APA). (2013). *Diagnostic and statistical manual of mental disorders* (5th ed.).

Babor, T. F., McRee, B. G., Kassebaum, P. A., Grimaldi, P. L., Ahmed, K., & Bray, J. (2007). Screening, brief intervention, and referral to treatment (SBIRT) toward a public health approach to the management of substance abuse. *Substance Abuse, 28*(3), 7–30.

Bull, A. (2015, July 01). *Robert Downey Jr. – Actor, Alcohol Abuse, Drug Abuse and Mental Illness.* http://www.abconsultation.com.au/news/robert-downey-jr-actor-drug-abuse-mental-illness

Compton, W. M., Han, B., Blanco, C., Johnson, K., & Jones, C. M. (2018). Prevalence and Correlates of Prescription Stimulant Use, Misuse, Use Disorders, and Motivations for Misuse Among Adults in the United States. *The American Journal of Psychiatry, 175*(8), 741–755. https://doi.org/10.1176/appi.ajp.2018.17091048

Empire. (n.d.). *Robert Downey Jr.* https://www.empireonline.com/people/robert-downey-jr/

Gliatto, T. (1996). *Hitting Bottom.* https://people.com/archive/hitting-bottom-vol-46-no-8/

Goodwin, R. D., & Hasin, D. S. (2002). Sedative use and misuse in the United States. *Addiction, 97*(5), 555–562.

Joy, J. E., Watson, S. J., & Benson, J. A. (2017). *Marijuana and medicine: Assessing the science base.* National Academies Press.

Hasin, D. S., Saha, T. D., Kerridge, B. T., Goldstein, R. B., Chou, S. P., Zhang, H., Jung, J., Pickering, R. P., Ruan, W. J., Smith, S. M., Huang, B., & Grant, B. F. (2015). Prevalence of marijuana use disorders in the United States between 2001-2002 and 2012-2013. *JAMA Psychiatry, 72*(12), 1235-1242. https://doi-org.libproxy.clemson.edu/10.1001/jamapsychiatry.2015.1858

Hasin, D. S., Kerridge, B. T., Saha, T. D., Huang, B., Pickering, R., Smith, S. M., Jung, J., Zhang, H., & Grant, B. F. (2016). Prevalence and correlates of DSM-5 cannabis use disorder, 2012-2013: Findings from the National Epidemiologic Survey on Alcohol and Related Conditions–III. *The American Journal of Psychiatry, 173*(6), 588–599. https://doi-org.libproxy.clemson.edu/10.1176/appi.ajp.2015.15070907

Hasin, D. S., Sarvet, A. L., Cerdá, M., Keyes, K. M., Stohl, M., Galea, S., & Wall, M. M. (2017). US Adult Illicit Cannabis Use, Cannabis Use Disorder, and Medical Marijuana Laws: 1991-1992 to 2012-2013. *JAMA psychiatry, 74*(6), 579–588. https://doi.org/10.1001/jamapsychiatry.2017.0724

Howard, M. O., Bowen, S. E., Garland, E. L., Perron, B. E., & Vaughn, M. G. (2011). Inhalant use and inhalant use disorders in the United States. *Addiction Science & Clinical Practice, 6*(1), 18.

Lynskey, M., & Hall, W. (2000). The effects of adolescent cannabis use on educational attainment: A review. *Addiction, 95*(11), 1621–1630.

Lilienfeld, S., & Arkowitz, H. (2011). Does Alcoholics Anonymous work? *Scientific American Mind, 22*(1), 64–65. https://doi.org/10.1038/scientificamericanmind0311-64

Kaskutas, L. A. (2009). Alcoholics Anonymous effectiveness: Faith meets science. *Journal of Addictive Diseases, 28*(2), 145–157.

Madras, B. K., Compton, W. M., Avula, D., Stegbauer, T., Stein, J. B., & Clark, H. W. (2009). Screening, brief interventions, referral to treatment (SBIRT) for illicit drug and alcohol use at multiple healthcare sites: Comparison at intake and 6 months later. *Drug and Alcohol Dependence, 99*(1–3), 280–295.

Manor, W. (2010, October 14). *Robert Downey Jr. Talks About Sobriety.* http://blog.whitesidemanor.com/2010/10/robert-downey-jr-sobriety.html

Motel, S. (2015). *6 facts about marijuana.* Pew Research Center.

National Institute on Alcohol Abuse and Alcoholism. (2004). NIAAA Council approves definition of binge drinking. *NIAAA Newsletter,* (3).

Saha, T. D., Kerridge, B. T., Goldstein, R. B., Chou, S. P., Zhang, H., Jung, J., Pickering, R. P., Ruan, W. J., Smith, S. M., Huang, B., Hasin, D. S., & Grant, B. F. (2016). Nonmedical Prescription Opioid Use and DSM-5 Nonmedical Prescription Opioid Use Disorder in the United States. *The Journal of Clinical Psychiatry, 77*(6), 772–780. https://doi-org.libproxy.clemson.edu/10.4088/JCP.15m10386

Substance Abuse and Mental Health Services Administration. (2018). *Find help: ATOD.* https://www.samhsa.gov/find-help/atod

Substance Abuse and Mental Health Services Administration (SAMHSA). (2013). *Systems-Level Implementation of Screening, Brief Intervention, and Referral to Treatment.* Technical Assistance Publication (TAP) Series 33. HHS Publication No. (SMA)13-4741. Rockville, MD: Substance Abuse and Mental Health Services Administration.

Substance Abuse Mental Health Services Administration (SAMHSA). (2016). *SBIRT: Screening, brief intervention, and referral to treatment.*

Vanity Fair. (2014, September 23). *Robert Downey Jr. Speaks About His Addictions.* https://www.vanityfair.com/hollywood/2014/09/robert-downey-jr-cover

World Health Organization (WHO). (2016). *International statistical classification of diseases and related health problems, 10th revision (ICD-10).*

Wu, L. T., Ringwalt, C. L., Mannelli, P., & Patkar, A. A. (2008). Hallucinogen use disorders among adult users of MDMA and other hallucinogens. *American Journal on Addictions, 17*(5), 354–363.

Credits

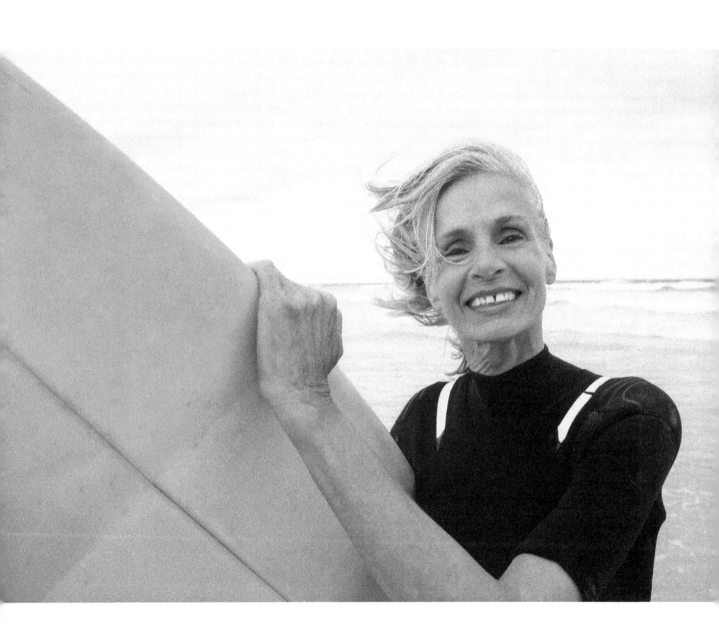

CHAPTER FOURTEEN

NEUROCOGNITIVE DISORDERS

David A. Scott, Michelle Grant Scott, and Robin L. Moody

CASE STUDY 14.1 Daniel is a 65-year-old Latino male from Augusta, Georgia. His wife, Norma, has brought Daniel into the clinic after noticing significant changes in his cognitive functioning. Norma has begun to notice that Daniel has become increasingly forgetful. Norma reports that she first noticed his memory declining a year prior but did not think much about it. She believed it was normal aging until recently when his symptoms worsened, and their three children began to question why. Norma reports that Daniel has difficulty remembering names of individuals, including friends and family, Bible verses, and locations of household items that previously he had no difficulty remembering. She also states that Daniel often neglects to take his arthritis medication, as well as his daily vitamin and can no longer recall their home phone number. Daniel is very agitated to be at the clinic and does not believe he has any memory concerns. He states that his wife and children are overreacting and that receiving help is a waste of time. Although he is clearly agitated, during the initial assessment, Daniel is alert and engaged. Family history reveals that Daniel's grandfather suffered from memory concerns in his later years, but the client reports that this was normal for his age and no diagnosis was ever given. With this, it is reported that Daniel's brother suffered from depressive symptoms throughout much of his life, but like Daniel, he did not see the value in seeking help. Although Daniel is suffering from memory lapses, according to his self-report, he has not exhibited any behavioral or mood concerns.

Did You Know?

- The elderly population in the United States is growing faster than the total population in the United States (Werner, 2011).

- The world's population of people over 60 years old will double (12% to 22%) between 2015 and 2050 (World Health Organization [WHO], 2015).

- The "baby boomer" generation is retiring in record numbers. By 2030, 20% of the population will be over 65 (Ortman et al., 2014).

- End of life care costs are some of the most expensive, with estimates around 3 times more than an average working-age adult earns.

Overview

When you think of an elderly person, how old is old? The older we get, the more we try to push back our definition of old. Many people fear getting old because of the mental and health complications that can present in old age. Mental health professionals will need to have knowledge and resources to help the growing elderly population in the United States. Neurocognitive disorders are not just specific to aging. Many people may experience neurocognitive issues related to traumatic brain injury, exposure to toxic substances, or even chronic substance abuse. Table 14.1 provides a list of the most common neurodevelopmental disorders found in both the *International Statistical Classification of Diseases (ICD-10)* and *Diagnostic and Statistical Manual of Mental Disorders, 5th Edition (DSM-5)*.

A neurocognitive disorder is a condition in which the brain function has become impaired and functioning is distinguished from the premorbid condition. The brain

TABLE 14.1 *ICD-10-DSM-5* Neurocognitive Comparisons

ICD-10 Disorders	*DSM-5* Disorders
Organic, including symptomatic, mental disorders (F00-F09)	*Neurocognitive disorders*
Dementia (F00-F03)	Delirium (291.xx-292.xx)
Organic amnesic syndrome (F04)	Major (294.1x) and Mild (331.83) Neurocognitive disorders with these Specifiers:
Other mental disorders because of brain damage and dysfunction and to physical disease (F06)	Alzheimer's disease
	Another medical condition
Personality and behavioral disorders because of a brain disease, damage, and dysfunction (F07)	Frontotemporal lobar degeneration
	HIV infection
	Huntington's disease
	Lewy body disease
	Parkinson's disease
	Prion disease
	Substance/medication use
	Traumatic brain injury
	Vascular disease
	Another medical condition
	Multiple etiologies
	Unspecified
Unspecified organic or symptomatic mental disorder (F09)	
Diseases of the nervous system Other degenerative diseases of the nervous system (G30-G32)	
Alzheimer's disease (G30.x)	
Other degenerative diseases of nervous system, not elsewhere classified (G31.x)	
Other degenerative disorders of nervous system in diseases classified elsewhere (G32.x*)	

Note: Adapted from ICD-10 (WHO, 2016); DSM-5 (APA, 2013)

is involved in everything that we do. It controls our ability to remember, maintain attention, learn, comprehend, speak, move, reason, and draw conclusions. Disease, injuries, substances and medications, strokes, and other insults are often the etiology for neurocognitive disorders. However, sometimes it is difficult to identify the exact origin.

Clinicians diagnose a neurocognitive disorder by conducting an interview with the client, family member, or friend; through direct observation; and by conducting neuropsychologist testing. Neuropsychological testing is used to determine the extent of the impairment and often evaluates many factors, such as auditory and visual memory, concentration/attention, processing speed, mental flexibility, verbal abilities, language, executive functioning, learning ability, and visual perceptual processing.

To fully understand the various types of cognitive impairments, it is necessary to define the aforementioned factors. One of the most obvious deficits in most individuals with a neurocognitive disorder is processing speed. *Processing speed* is the ability to process routine information quickly and without error. An example of processing speed may be a timed typing exercise. Most individuals with impairment in processing speed have extreme difficulty completing simple tasks within an allotted time frame. This can affect all areas of their lives negatively. Other impairments associated with processing speed deficits include difficulty with handwriting and motor skills. When testing an individual's processing speed, they are often asked to visually identify particular colored shapes within a specific time. This task also involves focused attention, which is the second cognitive factor we will discuss.

Concentration and attention abilities are necessary for all aspects of life, including learning and daily living activities (managing medication, cleaning the house, and cooking dinner). Attention and concentration are also required for learning and work related tasks. Imagine driving a car with limited focus. You may not see the traffic light turn red, or the pedestrian in the road, or the oncoming truck that failed to yield. Limited concentration is not only problematic but also dangerous. Fortunately, this is one factor of brain functioning that can often be easily treated with medication. Individuals with neurocognitive disorders are often unaware of how much their attention has declined. It is not until they have overdrawn their checking account or failed to turn off the eye on the stove that it comes to their attention.

Mental flexibility is the cognitive ability to rapidly and easily transition from one topic to another or one task to another. Individuals diagnosed with autism spectrum disorder often have this problem. They become rigid in their thinking and struggle to change both their mindsets and their behaviors.

Verbal abilities and *language* often change when damage to the brain has transpired. Frequently, when working with a client who has suffered a traumatic brain injury, we notice their speech is different. The individual may struggle to find the words they want to use in conversation; this is called anomia. When the individual's ability to produce language is affected, it is called aphasia. This is also frequently seen in patients with a dementia or Alzheimer's diagnosis.

Executive functioning is a broad term that encompasses the individual's ability to make decisions and plan but also includes the use of memory, concentration, and mental flexibility. *Learning* ability is another factor that is often associated with traumatic brain injury. Learning ability is associated with processing speed because it is the rate at which a person can mentally process information correctly. When a processing speed deficit is noted it is assumed this individual is a slow learner and would require more time to comprehend information. *Visual perceptual processing* is the ability to recognize and abstract meaningful relationships or concepts from spatial objects or visual information. For instance, the ability to pick up a grapefruit and understand it is the same shape as a basketball.

Are any of these issues a factor in Daniel's life?

Major and Mild Neurocognitive Disorders

The different types of neurocognitive disorders, as described in the *DSM-5*, include two major categories: mild and major. The easiest way to understand the differences between a mild and major neurocognitive disorder is to ask the question, "Does this affect independent living?" An individual with a major neurocognitive disorder may need assistance with banking, managing medication, managing their health care, and completing daily activities, such as chores, cooking, or bathing. A mild neurocognitive disorder is a decline from previous functioning that is noticeable and requires some accommodations. For instance, a person may need to make a list before going to the grocery store for three items, whereas prior to their condition, they would be capable of recalling the three items by memory.

While the authors of the *DSM-5* made the decision to bring together many of the neurocognitive disorders under the term *major and mild neurocognitive disorders*, the *ICD-10* lists many of these disorders under *diseases of the nervous system* (G00-G99) and within the chapter on *mental and behavioral disorders* (F00-F09).

The Dementias

Dementia is the term used to describe common symptoms (listed earlier and in Box 14.1) caused by several neurocognitive disorders. The Alzheimer's Association (2016) estimated that there were 47 million people worldwide with dementia. Figure 14.1 provides information on the global impact of dementia. They went on to state that this number will *double* every 20 years and reach 115.4 million in 2050. The cost of care for

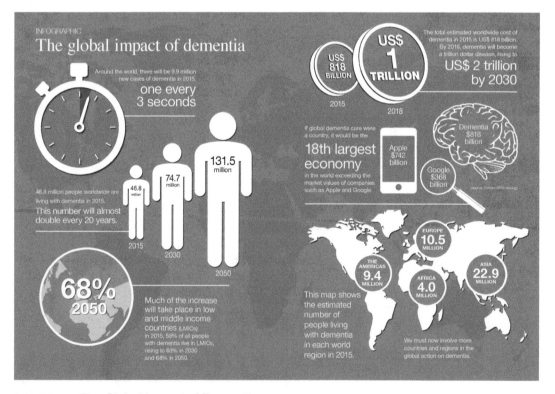

FIGURE 14.1 The Global Impact of Dementia

dementia is staggering. The World Health Organization (WHO, 2015) reported that the cost of care for people with dementia is around 604 billion dollars per year. This cost is also expected to continue to rise exponentially around the world. The WHO declared dementia as a *priority condition* because of the rising numbers of people with the diagnosis. Included in the web-based resources is a link to a video discussing dementia created by the Alzheimer's Society.

Box 14.1 Common Dementia Symptoms

- Memory loss
- Difficulty in thinking
- Problems with comprehension, calculation, language (aphasia), and judgment
- Possible deterioration in social behavior and emotional control

The most common of these mental disorders include Alzheimer's disease, frontotemporal dementia (formerly Pick's disease), Huntington disease, and Parkinson disease. The National Institute of Neurological Disorders and Stroke (NINDS, 2016a) pointed out that while many people believe that dementia is a normal part of aging, it is not necessarily true and more of a misperception. While age can be a risk factor, there are several other common risk factors. Alexander and Larson (2016) listed that age, family history (genetics, first-degree family member), and some physical issues (smoking, high blood pressure, substance abuse) can possibly play a role in dementia. They went on to say that people who are physically and mentally active and maintain personal relationships have a greater chance of developing dementia later (if at all) than those who do not engage in these activities.

Dementia is typically broken down into two or three stages with various symptoms at each stage. Table 14.2 provides a more detailed description of the symptoms related to dementia in each stage.

Think about our case study of Daniel. Is Daniel exhibiting some of the symptoms listed in Table 14.2?

TABLE 14.2 Stages of Dementia

EARLY STAGE (YEARS 1 & 2)	MIDDLE STAGE (YEARS 2–5)	LATE STAGE (5 AND AFTER)
• Forgetting things that happened recently • Difficulty with keeping up with time (hour, day, etc.) • Increased need for help in keeping up with finances and making decisions • Changes in mood that are noticed by family	• Increase in forgetting recent events • Speech and comprehension issues • Behaviors become more inappropriate • Unable to complete routine daily activities	• Unable to recognize family or friends • Incontinence • Needs assistance for most activities • Dramatic increases in aggressive behaviors and mood swings

Adapted from Duthey (2013)

Alzheimer's Disease

Probably the most well-known neurocognitive disorder is Alzheimer's disease. Most of us will have, or have had, a family member or acquaintance who has been diagnosed with Alzheimer's disease. Alexander and Larson (2016) reported that 60%–80% of all cases of dementia are caused by Alzheimer's disease. The National Institute on Aging (NIA, 2016) suggested that there are around five million people in the United States diagnosed with Alzheimer's.

In 1906, Dr. Alois Alzheimer was treating Auguste D. for significant memory loss, hallucinations, and unexplained changes in her mood and behaviors. It was not until an autopsy on Auguste D. revealed abnormal clumps around nerve cells and severe brain degeneration that Dr. Alzheimer and his colleagues began to think about these types of symptoms as markers for a specific brain disease. One of Dr. Alzheimer's colleagues, Dr. Emil Kraepelin, actually coined the term "Alzheimer's disease" in 1910 (Alzheimer's Association, 2016).

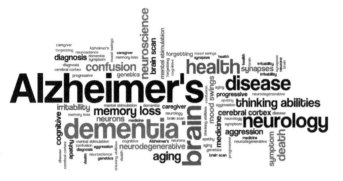

Image 14.2

Dr. Alzheimer was instrumental in creating guidelines for diagnosing and examining this mental disorder.

What we do know about Alzheimer's disease is that it is a progressive disorder that destroys neurons, starting in the hippocampus, and then affects the entire brain. Alzheimer's disease impacts the brain in several ways: (a) ventricles enlarge, (b) severe hippocampus shrinkage, (c) reduction in the size of the cortex (see Image 14.3), (d) clumps of a protein called *beta-amyloid* build up between nerve cells, and (e) dying nerve cells contain *tangles*, which inhibit movement of essential supplies to the brain.

As with dementia, researchers are discovering possible links between Alzheimer's disease and our genetics, health, environment, and lifestyle. A specific gene that could cause Alzheimer's has yet to be discovered, but current research has suggested that having

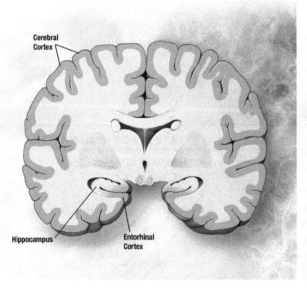

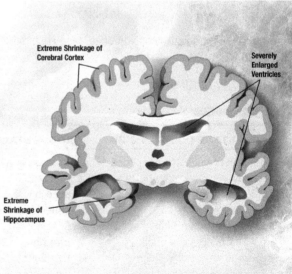

Image 14.3

one form of the *apolipoprotein E* (APOE ε4) gene on chromosome 19 will increase the risk of developing Alzheimer's disease (NIA, 2015a). The researchers were quick to point out that people with this APOE ε4 gene does increase the risk but does not guarantee a person with this gene will develop Alzheimer's. There is also a category of Alzheimer's disease that affects people who are 30 to 60 named *early onset familial Alzheimer's disease*. The NIA (2016) contended that people with a biological father or mother who carries the specific genetic mutations on chromosomes 21, 14, and 1 are at about a 50% chance of developing early onset familial Alzheimer's disease. Our health, environment, and lifestyle also play an important role in the possible development of Alzheimer's disease. As mentioned earlier, health issues related to the vascular system, obesity, and diabetes may also play a role in either increasing or reducing the risk of developing Alzheimer's.

The most common early symptom of Alzheimer's disease is memory problems, but this can vary from person to person. The NIA (2016) reported that there continues to be improvements in early detection, but more research in this area is needed to strengthen these early detection techniques. The current advances in brain imaging techniques are allowing researchers to explore how inflammation, brain atrophy, and free radicals play a possible role in the development of Alzheimer's disease.

Currently, there are no known cures, and most medications try to slow the progress of the disease or relieve the symptoms associated with the disease. Current drugs used in the treatment of symptoms of Alzheimer's disease include Aricept, Namenda, Razadyne, and Exelon. Most of the medications focus on trying to regulate neurotransmitters. A discussion on treatment options can be found later in this chapter.

When It's Not Alzheimer's

With all of the advances in the study of Alzheimer's disease, the actual evaluation and diagnosing has not seen significant changes in criteria since 1984 (Beach et al., 2012). The researchers went on to say that the rates of correctly diagnosing Alzheimer's ranged from 71%–87% for sensitivity and only 44%–71% for specificity. This wide range of diagnosing strongly suggests the use of additional testing to accurately provide a true diagnosis. Proper diagnosis can mean the difference in a person being placed on an Alzheimer's treatment plan (including a bleak prognosis) verses an appropriate diagnosis that could lead to treatment to actually improve the person's symptoms.

Normal pressure hydrocephalus (NPH) is when an abnormal amount of cerebrospinal fluid builds up in the brain's ventricles and actually pushes the brain against the skull and puts pressure on brain tissue. The symptoms of NPH are very similar to Alzheimer's (difficulty walking, problems with thought processing, changes in behavior) and can go misdiagnosed for years, if not for the rest of the person's life. A more extensive evaluation and magnetic resonance imaging (MRI) can help doctors determine the correct diagnosis. If the patient is diagnosed with NPH, the insertion of a shunt to drain the excess fluid can increase the chances of a successful treatment and improve the quality of life.

Frontotemporal dementia is the new name associated with **Pick's disease**. This new classification includes Pick's disease, primary progressive aphasia, and semantic dementia. The common brain markers include frontal and temporal anterior lobe shrinkage. The typical symptoms include changes in behavior (impulsive, inappropriate social skills, decreased energy) or problems with language (difficulty with speech; NINDS, 2016b). Unfortunately, there is no known treatment at this time. Medications can help decrease some maladaptive behaviors, and antidepressants show promise with some symptoms.

TABLE 14.3 Symptoms of Frontotemporal Disorders

TYPE	SYMPTOMS
Progressive motor decline	Muscle rigidity Frequent falls Poor coordination
Progressive behavior/personality decline	Inappropriate behaviors Noticeable changes in personality *Memory mostly intact*
Progressive language decline	Noticeable changes in speaking Can't understand words Trouble finding the correct words

Source: National Institute on Aging (NIA, 2015b)

Huntington's disease (HD) is a genetic disorder that appears in people between 30 and 50 years old. There is a form of the disease (juvenile Huntington's disease) that can begin as early as before 20 years old. The disease is inherited and affects both the brain and muscle control. Studies have found that those with African, Chinese, and Japanese ancestry have lower occurrences of HD (U.S. National Library of Medicine, 2016). The Huntington's Disease Society of America (2016) reported, "Many describe the symptoms of HD as having ALS, Parkinson's and Alzheimer's—simultaneously." Children of parents with HD have a 50% chance of developing HD. A child cannot pass down the HD gene if they did not inherit the gene from a parent who did have the HD gene. HD causes loss of control of muscles (walking, speech problems, involuntary movements) and cognitive and personality changes (including depression). HD typically follows three stages (early, middle, and late), with those in the late stage requiring extensive help by caregivers. While genetic testing can confirm the presence of the HD, there are no known cures at this time. There are medications that can help treat the involuntary movements and several drugs that are in the "clinical development" stages that may provide future treatment options.

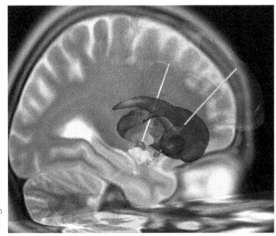

Image 14.4

Vascular dementia (VaD) is caused by blocked or reduced blood flow to the brain. VD is the second-leading cause of dementia (around 30% of all cases) behind Alzheimer's, and it impairs both memory and cognitive functioning (Lee, 2011). Symptoms of VaD include memory loss, disorientation, trouble with walking, and weakness in a person's limbs. Although there is no cure for VaD, a focused effort on eliminating/reducing risk factors associated with heart disease and strokes can help protect the brain and reduce the chances of having VaD.

Parkinson's disease (PD) is the result of the loss of brain cells that produce dopamine. The actor Michael J. Fox has played a public role in supporting treatment for PD since he was diagnosed in 1991 at the early age of 30 (www.michaeljfox.org). People diagnosed with PD have symptoms of trembling/shaking in their arms and legs, trouble with coordination, and a slowing of motor activity (bradykinesia). As the disease progresses, the symptoms will increase to the point of interfering

CLINICIAN'S CORNER 14.1

I work as a psychologist on an acute brain injury rehabilitation unit in a large hospital. I see both survivors and their families with the overall goal of helping them understand and begin to come to terms with the effect of the injury. Traumatic brain injury is an interesting phenomenon in that every brain is different, so every outcome is different. Typically, the first things family members want to know are how much progress the survivor will make and how long that will take. Unfortunately, those are two questions professionals in the field are at a loss to answer.

What I've observed is that when someone sustains a traumatic brain injury, there is a precise moment in time when the past, present, and future collide. Family members grieve the loss of what was, as well as the loss of what could have been. As such, the survivor and their family are challenged to establish a "new normal." And that's often a tough job. More than 50% of our patients and their families report adjustment problems in the months following hospital discharge. Those might include emotional issues, such as depression and frustration; or behavioral issues, such as impulsivity, disinhibition, and anger management problems; or daily challenges caused by poor memory or communication deficits. Not surprisingly, social isolation is the number one concern brain injury survivors report over time.

Recovery from traumatic brain injury is an arduous process that takes time—often, a lot of time. I know survivors who report they are still making functional gains years after their injury occurred, and I find this encouraging. Our program has an annual reunion party for former patients that is very well attended. For our staff, seeing the progress these survivors have made since leaving the hospital makes it all worthwhile.

Beth Mumford MA, LPA

with their daily activities and require a need for more and more direct care (NINDS, 2016c). Although there is no cure for PD, advances in research have produced several medications (examples are Levodopa and Carbidopa) to help the brain replenish its level of dopamine and anticholinergics to help with the body tremors. Another promising treatment technique is the use of deep brain stimulation. With deep brain stimulation, a patient has electrodes (connected to an external device) implanted in their brain that help to reduce the multitude of symptoms associated with PD.

Traumatic Brain Injury

One of the most common types of neurocognitive disorders is traumatic brain injury. Brain injuries occur suddenly and often include loss of consciousness, amnesia, and disorientation. Although in most instances of a traumatic brain injury (TBI) there may be a loss of consciousness, this is not required for the diagnosis.

There are two types of traumatic brain injuries: *open* and *closed*. A closed head injury occurs when there has been an impact to the brain that does not result in any open wound; for example, if you were to accidently bump your head on the cabinet door. When a closed head injury occurs, the brain shifts within the skull. While the brain itself is like silicone or Jell-O® in consistency, the underside of the skull is rigid and sharp. When the brain is thrust forward and backward or side to side, the soft brain is damaged by the impact of the hard, sharp skull. Often, individuals are unaware that they have suffered such an injury until they begin to notice a decline in functioning. Recently, this has become more apparent within the National Football League (NFL) and sports industry as football players are suffering cognitive declines years after they experienced similar injuries (Flaskerud, 2015; Greenhow & East, 2015). Closed head injuries are often difficult to diagnose, as they are sometimes not found through brain imagery. Therefore, neuropsychological testing is required to establish premorbid condition and cognitive decline.

An open head injury is one in which there is an open wound, whether it be to the tissue outside the brain, cracked skull, or damage to the brain itself. These are often common in car accidents. Upon impact, the driver is thrust forward in the seat and hit's their head on the windshield. They begin to bleed, feel dizzy, or even lose consciousness. In the military service, men and women are often in combat and become victims of an open head wound as they are hit with shrapnel.

Treatment for traumatic brain injury can range from X-rays to checking for any bone or spinal injuries to lengthy treatment protocols, including various types of therapy, such as physical, speech/language, occupational, and mental health therapies (NINDS,

TRUE LIFE 14.1

Junior Seau

Tiaina "Junior" Seau Jr. began his professional football career after being drafted by the San Diego Chargers in the 1990 NFL draft. Seau played 20 seasons, was selected eight times as an All-Pro and made the Pro-Bowl 12 times (National Football Hall of Fame [NFHF], 2016). Seau was considered one of the best linebackers and amassed hundreds of tackles during his stellar career. Seau committed suicide on May 2, 2012. His autopsy revealed that he suffered from the degenerative brain disease chronic trau-

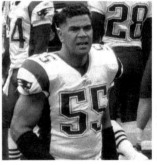

Image 14.5

matic encephalopathy, commonly known as CTE. CTE is typically the result of numerous blows to the head and is a major issue in the NFL. The NFL is currently being sued by former players for their alleged negligence in their knowledge and handling of players (and former players) with possible CTE. Seau's family members reported an increase in mood swings, depression, and detachment during the final years of his life (Fainaru-Wada et al., 2013). As more research is completed on the connection between concussions and CTE, concern will continue to grow as to the safety of children and young people playing football and the long-term effects of multiple concussions. Currently, programs (junior, college, and professional) are increasing their awareness and instituting "concussion guidelines" to increase the safety of their players.

2016d). The main focus of treatment is to stabilize the client, prevent any further injury, and make sure that blood flow to the brain and body is at an adequate level.

Is Daniel suffering from a traumatic brain injury?

Delirium

Delirium is characterized by a sudden onset of symptoms affecting mental abilities occurring within days or even hours. It is not chronic in nature and is typically temporary and treatable. A person can have both dementia and delirium at the same time. Delirium is diagnosed when a person experiences sudden changes in mental abilities, confusion, and possible memory loss. These symptoms can be accompanied by hallucinations, irritability or personality changes, social withdrawal, difficulty communicating, and overall disorientation to person, place, and time. Symptoms may fluctuate throughout the day and worsen in the evening hours or when it is dark outside (i.e., "sundowning").

There are varying causes of delirium, including physical illness, infection, sodium deficiency, substance or medication induced, or combined etiologies. All cases are somehow related to a physiological change in the client. The three major types of delirium are (1) hyperactive type (restlessness, agitation, possible hallucinations), (2) hypoactive (drowsiness or slowed motor functions), and (3) mixed (client may fluctuate quickly between the first two types). A person may experience symptoms of delirium for a few hours to a few days or in more persistent cases, weeks or months. Caregivers can help a person with delirium by reducing external stimuli (bright lights, television, excessive noise) and letting the person know that they are not alone (many are frightened by their confused mental state). Many cases of delirium are treatable, but people nearing death may experience delirium because of organ failure (U.S. National Library of Medicine, n.d.). Typically, nonpharmacological treatment approaches are the primary treatment options. Medications are usually only used if behaviors and/or anxiety are so severe that they can't be controlled by other treatment options.

Although delirium and dementia share some common symptoms, there are some distinct differences in the two disorders, as noted in Table 14.4.

TABLE 14.4 Differences Between Delirium and Dementia

SYMPTOMS	DELIRIUM	DEMENTIA
Changes in intellect and memory	Can take place very quickly	Usually gradual
Fluctuation issues (i.e., confusion or alertness)	Can significantly fluctuate throughout the day	Symptoms stay mostly consistent. Can have some fluctuation at different times of the day (i.e., "sundowning" issues)
Attention	Significantly impaired	Can remain stable and alert in early stages

Source: Mayo Clinic (2015)

Treatment Options

As stated earlier, there is no known cure for most of the dementias. Most of the treatments available now focus on trying to slow down the symptoms of dementia. One key aspect of treatment is early diagnosing. The sooner a correct diagnosis can be provided, the sooner the client can be placed on appropriate medications and any lifestyle changes that are needed can be made. The most common medications are as follows:

- *Cholinesterase Inhibitors.* These drugs target memory and thinking. Common drug names are Aricept, Razadyne, and Exelon.
- *NMDA Receptor Agonists.* These focus on learning and memory by blocking NMDA receptors. Common drug names are Namenda and Axura.
- *Antibody-Based Immunotherapy.* A recent study showed promise in the use of the antibody named Aducanumab. This antibody can help clear the amyloid plaques out of the brain, leading to improved brain communication between neurons (Sevigny et al., 2016).
- *Antidepressants.* Many times, depression is an associated symptom of dementia. Along with mental health therapy, antidepressants may help with reducing the client's depression. Common antidepressants include Prozac, Zoloft, Paxil, and Celexa.
- *Antianxiety Medications.* These medications can help if the client with dementia exhibits aggression or anxiety.

Addressing one's lifestyle, predementia could have an effect on the rate of mental decline in the elderly and those diagnosed with dementia. Research is now suggesting that people who engage in *mentally stimulating leisure activities* can possibly reduce

TABLE 14.5 Reversible Dementias

CONDITION	SYMPTOMS	TREATMENT
Cerebral vasculitis inflammation and death of blood vessel walls in the brain	Forgetfulness Confusion Weakness	Immune suppressants and steroids
Metabolic disorders of the nervous system (mitochondrial disorders, leukodystrophies)	Muscle weakness Problems with balance	Medications to relieve symptoms (Coenzyme, Creatine, and L-Arginine), changes in diet and exercise
Nutritional deficiencies (B1 and B12) caused by chronic alcoholism	Confusion Weakness	Vitamin supplements Balanced diet
Normal pressure hydrocephalus	Trouble walking Changes in thinking and behavior	Implanting a shunt to remove the excess fluid from the brain
Endocrine abnormalities (Thyroid problems)	Muscle weakness Irritability Anxiety	Treatment of correcting hormone imbalance

Source: National Institute of Neurological Disorders and Stroke (2015)

the risk of dementia and cognitive impairment (Yates et al., 2016). Lifestyle changes can include routine exercise, quitting smoking, eating properly, taking care of your mental health, maintaining relationships, and challenging your brain (puzzles, brain game activities) as much as possible (Sauer, 2016).

While the diagnosis of a dementia-related disorder can be life changing, there are several conditions that can potentially be reversed with proper treatment. Table 14.5 describes some of the reversible dementias.

As the elderly population continues to grow worldwide, the rates of dementia-related disorders will also continue to rise. Many times, the focus is on treating the client, but there is a large number of people who are overlooked in the treatment of dementia: the caregivers. Caregivers are typically assigned the task of taking care of the family member or loved one as their ability to take care of themselves diminishes. Caregivers can see a rise in their emotional stress, neglect their own needs (health, family time, work), and quickly become overwhelmed. This can put an enormous strain on the caregivers. Caregivers may need to be provided with resources of their own, including mental health services, community resources, and community support. Letting caregivers know that they do not have to do this alone and that there are resources available can make the difference between successful treatment or not for both the caregiver and the patient.

Case Study Summary

This chapter's case study reviewed the symptoms of Daniel. As you process the story and examine possible diagnostic criteria, take a few minutes to answer the following questions:

1. What would be the correct diagnosis for Daniel?

2. What are the specific symptoms or criteria that led you to this diagnosis?

3. What other possible disorders might you diagnose Daniel with and why?

4. Briefly discuss what types of treatment may be beneficial for Daniel. Could you see using a certain counseling theory and/or medication?

5. What kinds of support can be offered for the caregiver?

Guided Practice Exercises

Scenario 1

Ashley is a successful, 32-year-old chef. She has just achieved her life-long dream of running her own restaurant. Ashley's employees know that she has high expectations in her kitchen. However, they adore her for her kindness and upbeat personality. Ashley is secretly concerned because she has recently begun forgetting recipes and appointments. One week she had to change the entire menu because she forgot to place an order with her seafood distributor for the third time. Communication in the kitchen is becoming a problem as Ashley tries to hide her slurred speech. She jokes, claiming that she tasted a little too much of the cooking wine. Ashley tries to deny it, but she has been making several mistakes when her arms seem to move involuntarily. She has also become easily agitated. Three of her employees quit because they could no longer deal with her angry outbursts.

Ashley has begun to have difficulty walking. She could no longer deny that something is wrong when her stumbling resulted in a kitchen fire that injured her and her sous-chef. At the hospital, Ashley confides in her mom about the symptoms she has been experiencing. Her mom tells her that her father exhibited similar symptoms before he was diagnosed. Ashley agrees to make an appointment with her doctor to diagnose her condition.

What would be the correct disorder? What are the specific symptoms or criteria that led you to this diagnosis?

_____
_____
_____
_____

What specific behaviors caused you to diagnose the disorder?

_____
_____
_____
_____

What other possible disorders might you diagnose Ashley with and why?

_____
_____
_____
_____

Scenario 2

Lou is a 45-year-old male who enjoys golfing with his college and work friends. He also adores spending time with his wife and five children. The have family dinner every Sunday night that he takes pride in. He always makes a big meal so that his children in college have enough food to take back with them. They also have many family traditions, including family vacations to the beach where they go on a new adventure every year. Some of their adventures have included surfing lessons, swimming with the dolphins, kayaking in the ocean, and parasailing.

Over the past 6 months, Lou's family and friends have started to notice a change in him. He has become very irritable. His children describe him as "touchy," and they are afraid to talk to him. His friends say that he started throwing his clubs in anger after just a few shots, even though he has never been the best golfer. His wife became even more worried when he began talking about not having a reason to live anymore.

More recently, Lou has become indifferent about making plans because he has trouble remembering he made them at all. He is normally planning the family vacation from the end of the previous one, but it is a month away, and he has not begun planning it. Although it is not enough yet for his family to notice, Lou is noticing himself that he is having a lot of trouble standing up straight when he gets out of bed. He is worried about what is happening to him.

What would be the correct disorder? What are the specific symptoms or criteria that led you to this diagnosis?

_____
_____
_____
_____

What specific behaviors caused you to diagnose the disorder?

_____
_____
_____
_____

What other possible disorders might you diagnose Lou with and why?

_____
_____
_____
_____

Scenario 3

Janet is a 20-year-old woman who recently returned from being deployed in the Middle East. She talks about always being tired, not being able to concentrate, being irritable, and having headaches frequently. She also mentions that while she was in the Middle East, she was knocked unconscious for less than 10 minutes when she hit her head on a rock after coming across an improvised explosive device. She originally came to you to work through post-traumatic stress disorder symptoms.

What other disorder might Janet have and why?

_____
_____
_____
_____

What types of treatment options would you suggest for Janet?

_____
_____
_____
_____

Web-Based and Literature-Based Resources

Alzheimer's Society video on dementia: https://www.youtube.com/watch?v=6q-H1-XwCZA

Alzheimer's Association: alz.org

Family Caregiver Alliance: caregiver.org

Huntington's Disease Society of America: hdsa.org

Traumatic Brain Injury: traumaticbraininjury.com

References

Alexander, M. & Larson, E. B. (2016). *Patient information: Dementia (including Alzheimer's disease) (Beyond the basics)*. UpToDate. http://www.uptodate.com/contents/dementia-including-alzheimer-disease-beyond-the-basics?view=print

Alzheimer's Association. (2016). *Major milestones in Alzheimer's and brain research*. http://www.alz.org/research/science/major_milestones_in_alzheimers.asp

American Psychiatric Association (APA). (2013). *Diagnostic and statistical manual of mental disorders* (5th ed.).

Beach, T. G., Monsell, S. E., Phillips, L. E., & Kukull, W. (2012). Accuracy of the clinical diagnosis of Alzheimer's disease at National Institute on Aging Alzheimer Disease Centers, 2005–2010. *Journal of Neuropathology Experimental Neurology, 71,* 266–273.

Duthey, B. (2013). *Update on 2004 background Paper 6.11: Alzheimer's disease and other dementias.* World Health Organization. http://www.who.int/medicines/areas/priority_medicines/BP6_11Alzheimer.pdf

Fainaru-Wada, M., Avila, J., & Fainaru, S. (2013). *Doctors: Junior Seau's brain had CTE.* ESPN. http://espn.go.com/espn/otl/story/_/id/8830344/study-junior-seau-brain-shows-chronic-brain-damage-found-other-nfl-football-players

Flaskerud, J. H. (2015). Mental health implications of concussion and brain injury. *Issues in Mental Health Nursing, 36*(3), 239–242. https://doi.org/10.3109/01612840.2014.953279

Greenhow, A., & East, J. (2015). Custodians of the game: Ethical considerations for football governing bodies in regulating concussion management. *Neuroethics, 8*(1), 65–82. https://doi.org/10.1007/s12152-014-9216-1

Huntington's Disease Society of America. (2016). *What is Huntington's disease?* http://hdsa.org/what-is-hd/

Lee, A. Y. (2011). Vascular dementia. *Chonnam Medical Journal, 47*(2), 66–71.

Mayo Clinic. (2015, September). *Diseases and conditions: Delirium.* http://www.mayoclinic.org/diseases-conditions/delirium/basics/symptoms/con-20033982

National Football Hall of Fame. (2016). *Junior Seau.* http://www.profootballhof.com/players/junior-seau/

National Institute on Aging (NIA). (2015a). *Alzheimer's disease genetics fact sheet.* U.S. Department of Health and Human Services. https://www.nia.nih.gov/alzheimers/publication/alzheimers-disease-genetics-fact-sheet

National Institute on Aging (NIA). (2015b). *Types of frontotemporal disorders.* U.S. Department of Health and Human Services. https://www.nia.nih.gov/alzheimers/publication/frontotemporal-disorders/types-frontotemporal-disorders

National Institute on Aging (NIA). (2016, August). *Alzheimer's disease fact sheet.* Department of Health and Human Services. https://www.nia.nih.gov/alzheimers/publication/alzheimers-disease-fact-sheet

National Institute of Neurological Disorders and Stroke. (2015). *Dementia: Hope through research.* U.S. National Library of Medicine. Retrieved from http://www.ninds.nih.gov/disorders/dementias/detail_dementia.htm

National Institute of Neurological Disorders and Stroke (NINDS). (2016a). *Dementia.* U.S. National Library of Medicine. https://www.nlm.nih.gov/medlineplus/dementia.html

National Institute of Neurological Disorders and Stroke (NINDS). (2016b). *NINDS frontotemporal dementia information page.* U.S. National Library of Medicine. http://www.ninds.nih.gov/disorders/picks/picks.htm

National Institute of Neurological Disorders and Stroke (NINDS). (2016c). *NINDS Parkinson's disease information page.* U.S. National Library of Medicine. http://www.ninds.nih.gov/disorders/parkinsons_disease/parkinsons_disease.htm

National Institute of Neurological Disorders and Stroke (NINDS). (2016d). *NINDS Traumatic brain injury information page.* U.S. National Library of Medicine. http://www.ninds.nih.gov/disorders/tbi/tbi.htm

Ortman, J. M., Velkoff, V. A., & Hogan, H. (2014). *An aging nation: The older population in the United States* (Current Population Reports, P25-1140). U.S. Census Bureau.

Sauer, A. (2016, August). How lifestyle changes can help reduce the risk of dementia. Alzheimer's Treatments. *Alzhemiers.net.* http://www.alzheimers.net/7-22-15-lifestyle-changes-help-reduce-risk-of-dementia/

Sevigny, J., Chiao, P., Bussiere, T., Weinreb, P. H., Williams, L., Maier, M., Dunstan, R., Salloway, S., Chen, T., Ling, Y., O'Gorman, J., Qian, F., Arastu, M., Li, M., Chollate, S., Brennan, M. S., Quintero-Monzon, O., Scannevin, R. H., Arnold, M. H...Sandrock, A. (2016). The antibody aducanumab reduces Aβ plaques in Alzheimer's disease. *Nature, 537,* 50–56. https://doi.org/10.1038/nature19323

U.S. National Library of Medicine. (2016, August 23). *Huntington's disease.* https://ghr.nlm.nih.gov/condition/huntington-disease#synonyms

U.S. National Library of Medicine. (n.d.) *Delirium.* http://www.ncbi.nlm.nih.gov/pubmedhealth/PMHT0027314/

Werner, C. A. (2011). *The older population: 2010* (2010 Census Brief). U.S. Census Bureau. https://www.census.gov/prod/cen2010/briefs/c2010br-09.pdf

World Health Organization (WHO). (2015, September). *Ageing and health* (Fact sheet No.404). WHO Media Centre. http://www.who.int/mediacentre/factsheets/fs404/en/

World Health Organization (WHO). (2016). *International statistical classification of diseases and related health problems, 10th revision (ICD-10).*

Yates, L. A., Ziser, S., Spector, A., & Orrell, M. (2016). Cognitive leisure activities and future risk of cognitive impairment and dementia: Systematic review and meta-analysis. *International Psychogeriatrics.* https://doi.org/:10.1017/S1041610216001137

Credits

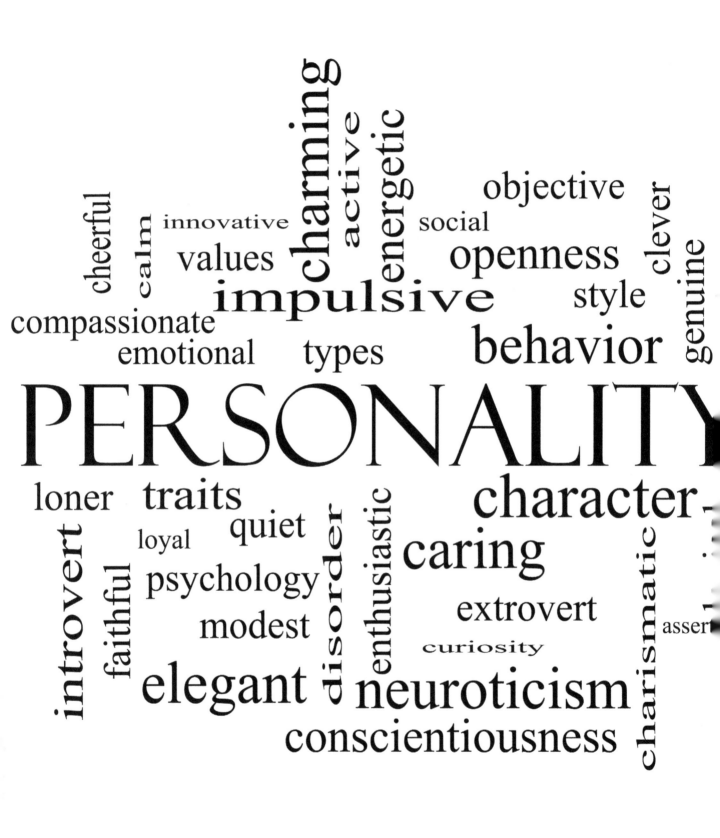

CHAPTER FIFTEEN

PERSONALITY DISORDERS

Chadwick Royal and David A. Scott

CASE STUDY 15.1 Reagan, 30, feels an inability in dealing with her intense emotional pain. She will often cut her arms and upper thighs to give her pain an outlet. What is even worse than the emotional pain is the emptiness that she feels. Reagan has been in five relationships in the past year. All of them she thought to be serious, but each ended because of her boyfriends' claims of her being "needy," "emotional," and "a drama queen." Whenever Reagan feels a partner begin to pull away, she tells them how much she loves and needs them. She tells them she doesn't know what she would do without them. Sometimes she will even threaten to kill herself if they leave. Reagan realizes that her anger can also push others away. She has physically attacked several family members and one of her partners in the past. Reagan will often binge eat when she is stressed, and she also spends impulsively.

Overview

The World Health Organization defines personality disorders as "deeply ingrained and enduring behavior patterns, manifesting as inflexible responses to a broad range of personal and social situations" (World Health Organization [WHO], 2016). These enduring behavior patterns can begin in adolescence and continue throughout a person's life. This pattern is manifested in multiple areas: cognitively, affectively, and interpersonally. In the cognitive realm, ways of perceiving and interpreting the self, others, and events are affected. In the affective realm, range, intensity, lability, and appropriateness of emotional response are impacted. In the interpersonal realm, we see the cognitive and affective realms influencing impulse control and relationships (Candel & Constantin, 2017). Personality disorders are so pervasive that they are risk factors for other mental, social, and physical problems (Bach et al., 2017; Lotfi et al., 2018).

The idea of personality disorder diagnosis is probably one of the more controversial topics among mental health professionals. How are personality disorders conceptualized, and at what point are behaviors associated with personality disorders considered clinically significant or a "disorder"? There are two general models in which personality disorders are currently viewed: a categorical model and a dimensional model. The categorical model is presented in section 2 of the *DSM-5* (American Psychiatric Association [APA], 2013) and has historically been used more by clinicians. It is based on a "medical model" and assumes that normality and abnormality are two quantitatively different client presentations or states (Candel & Constantin, 2017). Using the

Did You Know?

- The prevalence of personality disorders worldwide is 7.8% (Winsper et al., 2020).

- The common term *sociopath* is actually not a diagnosis in the *Diagnostic and Statistical Manual of Mental Disorders, 5th Edition (DSM-5)*. The *DSM-5* uses the term *antisocial* for this disorder.

- The common misperception is that borderline personality disorder is a White female diagnosis. Borderline personality affects all genders and all races.

- Obsessive-compulsive *personality* disorder is not the same as obsessive-compulsive disorder.

categorical model, it is estimated that 6% of the world's population and 12% of the population of Western countries meet the criteria for a personality disorder (Bach et al., 2017; Lotfi et al., 2018).

There are two methods typically used to assess clients for personality disorders: personality tests (formal) and clinical observation and interviews (informal; Candel & Constantin, 2017). Formal personality tests or assessments have a history of difficulty. The instruments are known for low levels of test-retest reliability and construct validity (Disney, 2013) and typically require a good deal of training to be able to administer and interpret the tests. If possible, a combination of testing, client self-report, and a structured (or semi-structured) interview are recommended to be used to overcome problems that are associated with personality disorder assessment (Disney, 2013). Without training in formal personality assessment, most counselors in practice tend to prefer methods of clinical observation and semi-structured interviews anyway.

Can you think of an assessment you could use with Reagan?

There has been much discussion about how personality disorders should be diagnosed (Skodol, 2014). Some researchers claim that some personality disorder diagnoses are rarely used in practice with clients, there is insufficient cross-cultural validity, and there is little evidence of construct validity in clinical practice (Bach et al., 2017; Lotfi et al., 2018; Mulder et al., 2016). The descriptions of behavioral disturbances (the criteria that must be met for diagnosis) are what has been most debated over time (Mulder et al., 2016). Because there isn't a consensus on diagnostic thresholds between normal and abnormal, being able to confidently diagnose a personality disorder is problematic (Lotfi et al., 2018). One clinician may recognize a client with problematic behaviors, and another may not see a clinically significant problem. In addition, there are questions related to the reliability and validity of the categorical presentations of personality disorders (Lotfi et al., 2018). It is believed that categories overlap.

Despite the criticisms and flaws of the categorical model of personality disorders, it is still regarded as the primary method of diagnosing a personality disorder—and is

---

CLINICIAN'S CORNER 15.1

As a new clinician, I remember being intimidated by the idea of working with clients diagnosed with personality disorders. I had been taught about the deeply "engrained patterns" and intense symptoms many with personality disorders experience and wondered how my skill set could possibly make a difference in their lives. One of my clients diagnosed with borderline personality disorder quickly taught me the intensity she often felt was not always a negative trait. For example, my client shared that she was able to become absorbed in the color nuances of rainbows, she could deeply appreciate nature, and she could find reasons to celebrate every life milestone. I challenge my fellow clinicians to remember the intensity experienced with personality disorders, when channeled in a healthy way, can bring clients a source of hope. Using this lens with our clients can be a true gift to clinicians.

Michelle Grant Scott, LISW-CP(S)

included in section II (diagnostic criteria and codes) of the *DSM-5* with all of the other disorders already mentioned in this text (APA, 2013). Many clinicians in practice still use the clinical language related to the categorical model, even if they don't always assign an official personality disorder diagnosis. Therefore, the model is worthy of inclusion in this text. The World Health Organization and the American Psychiatric Association have both proposed new dimensional (trait) oriented models of personality disorders, but they are not yet widely endorsed in Western countries (Lotfi et al., 2018). We will cover the dimensional models a bit later in the chapter, but we will first review the categorical model.

Categorical Model

The *DSM-5* groups personality disorders into three different clusters (A, B, and C); the clusters are grouped based on similarities of diagnosis descriptions (APA, 2013). Cluster A disorders are grouped together because individuals with these personality disorders are known for their odd or eccentric behavior and their lack of social relationships (Candel & Constantin, 2017). Cluster B disorders are grouped together because individuals with these personality disorders are known for their erratic, emotional, or overly dramatic behavior (Candel & Constantin, 2017). Cluster C disorders are grouped together because individuals with these personality disorders will present as anxious or fearful (APA, 2013). The *International Classification of Diseases (ICD-10)* does not group any personality disorders into clusters, but they do group all of the personality disorders into section F60-F69: disorders of adult personality and behavior. Table 15.1 provides a quick snapshot of the clusters and personality disorders.

We will now look at each of the three clusters a bit more in-depth.

Cluster A

Clients diagnosed with one or more Cluster A disorders are characterized by their odd and eccentric behavior and tend to not have too many social relationships (APA, 2013). There are three disorders grouped together within Cluster A:

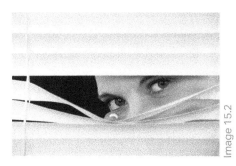

Image 15.2

1. Paranoid personality disorder
2. Schizoid personality disorder
3. Schizotypal personality disorder

It is worthy of mentioning that all three of the disorders in Cluster A correlate with a high rate of schizophrenia in the client's family of origin (Candel & Constantin, 2017).

Would Reagan's possible diagnosis fall within any of the disorders in Cluster A?

PARANOID PERSONALITY DISORDER (301.0) (F60.0)

In paranoid personality disorder, there is a consistent attitude of distrust and suspicion of other people. Other's motives are suspected to be hostile or malicious. It is assumed by someone with this disorder that other people seek to exploit or take advantage of

TABLE 15.1 Personality Disorders from the *DSM-5* and *ICD-10*

DSM-5		
CLUSTER A	**CLUSTER B**	**CLUSTER C**
Paranoid personality disorder	Antisocial personality disorder	Avoidant personality disorder
Schizoid personality disorder	Borderline personality disorder	Dependent personality disorder
Schizotypal personality disorder	Histrionic personality disorder	Obsessive-compulsive personality
	Narcissistic personality disorder	disorder

ICD-10

- Paranoid personality disorder
- Schizoid personality disorder
- Dissocial personality disorder
- Amoral
- Antisocial
- Asocial
- Psychopathic
- Sociopathic
- Emotionally unstable personality disorder
- Aggressive
- Borderline
- Explosive
- Histrionic personality disorder
- Hysterical
- Psychoinfantile
- Anankastic personality disorder
- Complusive
- Obsessional
- Obsessive compulsive
- Anxious (avoidant) personality disorder
- Dependent personality disorder
- Asthenic
- Inadequate
- Passive
- Self-defeating
- Other specific personality disorders
- Eccentric
- "Haltlose type"
- Immature
- Narcissistic
- Passive aggressive
- Psychoneurotic
- Personality disorder, unspecified
- Character neurosis, not otherwise specified
- Pathological personality, not otherwise specified

Sources: ICD-10 (WHO, 2016) and DSM-5 (APA, 2013)

them. They are hesitant to confide in others, and clients with paranoid personality disorder may prove to be difficult in a counseling session—unwilling to answer personal questions. Individuals with this personality disorder are known to hold grudges and may be unwilling to forgive situations in which they have felt slighted (APA, 2013).

Clients with paranoid personality disorder are likely to have problems with relationships, whether it is an intimate relationship (suspecting unfaithfulness) or general relationships (with argumentativeness, suspiciousness, or hostility that gets expressed toward others). However, clients with paranoid personality disorder may form relationships with others who share their paranoid belief systems. It is suggested that this personality disorder has a national prevalence of anywhere from 2.3% to 4.4% of the general population (APA, 2013). The diagnostic criteria between the *DSM-5* and *ICD-10* are very similar, and the nomenclature are identical. Both are labeled as paranoid personality disorder.

SCHIZOID PERSONALITY DISORDER (301.20) (F60.1)

Schizoid personality disorder is explained as a pattern of social detachment that is characterized by a low range of emotional expression in an interpersonal context (Candel & Constantin, 2017). Clients with schizoid personality disorder may have no interest in relationships or intimacy, including being a part of a family, and they will typically choose individual or solitary activities. They may not appear to enjoy many things and will perhaps be indifferent to any praise or criticism from others. They will likely present with a flat affect and not have much emotional reactivity.

Schizoid personality disorder can be differentiated from other disorders, such as delusional disorder, schizophrenia, or other disorders with psychotic features because all of these other disorders are characterized by an onset of psychotic symptoms. Psychosis is not present in schizoid personality disorder. However, there may be some difficulty in distinguishing between schizoid personality disorder and milder forms of autism spectrum disorder, which clinically present very similarly. Clients with autism spectrum disorder, however, are said to have more severely impacted social interactions and stereotyped interests or behaviors (APA, 2013). It is suggested that schizoid personality disorder has a national prevalence of anywhere from 3.1% to 4.9% of the general population (APA, 2013). The nomenclature between the *DSM-5* and *ICD-10* are identical. Both are labeled as schizoid personality disorder.

SCHIZOTYPAL PERSONALITY DISORDER (301.22) (F21)

Schizotypal personality disorder was first introduced in the *DSM-III* in 1980 and has been categorized as a personality disorder in all editions of the *DSM*. The *ICD-10* labels it schizotypal disorder (not a personality disorder) and categorizes it under schizophrenia spectrum disorders. This is one of the primary categorical differences of any personality disorder between the *DSM* and *ICD*. The World Health Organization characterizes schizotypal personality disorder by eccentric behaviors and changes in thinking and affect similar to those with schizophrenia (Kirchner et al., 2018).

In the *DSM-5*, schizotypal personality disorder is described as general impairments in personality and interpersonal functioning, disorder-specific pathological personality traits (unusual perceptual experiences, ideas of reference, eccentricity, unusual beliefs, odd thinking or speech), detachment with restricted affect and withdrawal, and negative affectivity characterized by suspiciousness (Kirchner et al., 2018).

As indicated by the different classification by the *ICD*, it is difficult to differentiate between schizotypal personality disorder and something like schizophrenia. In fact, the personality disorder is phenomenologically and genetically linked to schizophrenia (Hazlett et al., 2015). In distinguishing between schizotypal personality disorder and something like schizophrenia, the clients with the personality disorder are typically not medicated, nor have they been hospitalized for chronic mental illnesses. They will rarely present with acute psychotic symptoms (this is more characteristic of individuals with a psychotic disorder). Individuals with schizotypal personality disorder show less sensory abnormalities than schizophrenia (Hazlett et al., 2015). It is suggested that schizotypal personality disorder has a prevalence of anywhere from 0.6% to 4.6% of the population (APA, 2013).

Cluster B

Clients with a Cluster B disorder appear dramatic, emotional, or erratic (APA, 2013). There are four disorders grouped together within Cluster B:

1. Antisocial personality disorder
2. Borderline personality disorder
3. Histrionic personality disorder
4. Narcissistic personality disorder

Cluster B disorders tend to receive the most attention from clinicians and researchers, and clients with a Cluster B disorder tend to present the most challenge to new clinicians. Challenges arise from clients simply because of the nature of the disorders themselves—these clients can be overly dramatic, highly emotionally reactive, and demonstrate erratic behavior between (and within) sessions.

Would Reagan's possible diagnosis fall within any of the disorders in Cluster B?

ANTISOCIAL PERSONALITY DISORDER (301.7) (F60.2)

The initial *DSM*, published in 1952, first included "sociopathic personality disturbance." The second edition, published in 1968, labeled the condition "antisocial personality." It wasn't until the third edition, published in 1980, that the term "antisocial personality disorder" first appeared (Baliousis et al., 2019; Candel & Constantin, 2017). Antisocial personality disorder is characterized as a pattern of behavior that demonstrates a disregard for and violation of the rights of others, occurring since around the age of 15 (APA, 2013; Candel & Constantin, 2017). The diagnostic criteria for this disorder has typically emphasized observable behavior that has lacked a corresponding (or expected) emotional feature. Individuals with antisocial personality disorder are sometimes described as callous, lacking empathy, and having a certain degree of grandiosity (Baliousis et al., 2019).

In the *ICD*, the World Health Organization labels this condition "dissocial personality disorder," and it is additionally described as individuals having a disregard for social obligations and a lack of concern for the feelings of others (Candel & Constantin, 2017). Clients with antisocial personality disorder may behave in an aggressive way—and may not be influenced by feelings of guilt or any type of punishment. They may not follow any social norms and blame others for things that occur by their hand (Candel & Constantin, 2017). Baliousis et al. (2019) reported that it is understood that

TRUE LIFE 15.1

Ted Bundy—Antisocial Personality Disorder

In the Pacific Northwest, college women were disappearing in the states of Washington and Oregon, and no one was able to figure out who or what was responsible for their disappearances. Who would expect a clean-cut law student with no adult criminal record to be a serial killer? It only made sense after a sketch artist drawing of the suspect was identified by his professor, ex-girlfriend, and a coworker as Ted Bundy that he was identified as a suspect. After all, he did not fit the profile. A man who described himself as "the most cold-hearted son of a bitch you'll ever meet" (Paoletti, 2019), Ted Bundy is one of the most renowned serial killers of the United States.

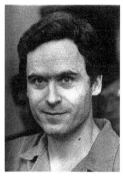

Image 15.3

Ted Bundy was born in Burlington, Vermont, on November 24, 1946. By his teen years, he exhibited behaviors of conduct disorder that showed what was to come in his adult future. A female family member recalled waking up to find Bundy had arranged knives around her body (Jitchotvisut, 2019). On top of watching violent porn, he would scope out the neighborhoods in search of an empty window to peep on women with no regard for their privacy. He was described as charming, articulate, and intelligent (CrimeMuseum, 2007). After all, he graduated from college, and many believed he would have a prosperous future in law or politics. However, a change in interests steered him in the direction of deception of young women. He was an attractive young man and would use this to his advantage when targeting victims. Bundy would pose as a disabled gentleman whether walking on crutches or wearing a sling to persuade victims to carry his belongings to his car. Another tactic of Bundy's was to mask himself as an authority figure to secure the trust of his victims. Once he had the victims' trust, he usually strangled or beat them to death. To take it several steps further, he would revisit the sites of their dumped corpses or take them home with him to gain further sexual gratification (CrimeMuseum, 2007). Upwards of 30 women suffered such cruel and unusual punishment at the hands of Bundy, and he was hardly considered a suspect. So what do psychologists think of this man who never saw a therapist?

In 2007, a group of 73 psychologists studied the mental health of Bundy, and an overwhelming majority agreed he was the prototype for antisocial personality disorder (Gainsburg, 2019). In addition, Bundy exhibited symptoms of psychopathy, which was portrayed through his charm and pathological lying. In the words of clinical and forensic psychologist Darrel Turner, PhD, Ted Bundy was basically the textbook definition of a "prototypical" psychopath (Gainsburg, 2019). Bundy never saw a therapist, and he did not receive a psychiatric evaluation until the court required one to determine his aptitude for violence (Gainsburg, 2019), so it is difficult to pinpoint what disorder he had. Some psychologists suspected he had narcissistic personality disorder, borderline personality disorder, schizoid personality disorder, and even Machiavellianism, an extreme form of narcissism. Dorothy O. Lewis, a psychiatrist who attempted to save Bundy from death row, argued that he may have suffered from bipolar personality disorder.

It was not until after the murders of five Florida State students, an apprehension for a traffic violation, and several escapes from the law that Bundy was sentenced to death by the electric chair on January 24, 1989 (CrimeMuseum, 2007). At the time of his execution, Bundy had confessed to 30 murders, although the actual number of his victims remains unknown.

there is a small group of people with this personality disorder who are responsible for a disproportionate amount of crimes committed in society.

The terms *antisocial* and *psychopathy* are sometimes used interchangeably by some clinicians. However, Baliousis et al. (2019) claimed that these two terms are distinct. Most people with a label of "psychopath" meet criteria for antisocial personality disorder, but the reverse is not always the case (i.e., an individual with antisocial personality disorder may not be labeled a "psychopath"). The more severe offending characteristics relate more to psychopathy, and it represents a more severe end of antisocial personality disorder. Psychopathy is considered a risk factor for violent recidivism (Baliousis et al., 2019).

The *DSM-5* emphasizes that to be given a diagnosis of antisocial personality disorder, the individual must be at least 18 years old. However, they need to have displayed symptoms of the disorder since age 15—and that there is evidence of conduct disorder with onset *before* age 15. The WHO (*ICD*) comments that the presence of conduct disorder during childhood and adolescence support the idea of a diagnosis of dissocial personality disorder but are not required for the diagnosis. In addition to the traits mentioned earlier, some additional symptoms include deceitfulness, impulsivity, a low frustration tolerance and history of aggressiveness and fighting, consistent irresponsibility, a lack of remorse, and an incapacity to maintain enduring relationships (despite being able to easily establish relationships; APA, 2013; WHO, 1993). It is reported that antisocial personality disorder has a prevalence of anywhere between 0.2% and 3.3% in the general population but greater than 70% in samples of people in prisons or forensic settings (APA, 2013).

BORDERLINE PERSONALITY DISORDER (301.83) (F60.3)

Borderline personality disorder is commonly considered one of the more difficult diagnostic issues to deal with in counseling. Clients with this personality disorder typically have unstable and intense interpersonal relationships with most people in their lives, including their therapists. They display symptoms of impulsivity, a persistent unstable self-image or sense of self, inappropriate and/or intense anger, chronic feelings of emptiness, stress-related paranoid ideation, and affective/emotional instability. Some of their behaviors consist of frantic efforts to avoid real or imagined abandonment and suicidal or self-harm behavior. Borderline personality disorder (BPD) tends to be associated with ongoing or pervasive social and occupational dysfunction (McMahon et al., 2019); there is typically a lot of "push-and-pull" in relationships, whether personal or work related. Clients with this disorder often make use of mental health/counseling services, sometimes going in and out of therapy and "firing" therapists; they can be clients at a high risk for attempting suicide (McMahon et al., 2019).

The WHO labels this disorder (in the *ICD*) as "emotionally unstable personality disorder" with two possible subtypes: F60.30—impulsive type and F60.31—borderline type. The borderline type description in the *ICD* first requires that the criteria for the impulsive type be met—and then additional symptoms specific to the borderline type must be met before assigning the borderline diagnosis (WHO, 1993). Symptoms for the impulsive type and bipolar type together (in the *ICD*) are equal to the symptoms indicated earlier and align with the *DSM* version of the same name.

Differentiating borderline personality disorder from other disorders, such as bipolar disorder, can be a bit tricky. Characteristics such as emotional dysregulation (instability) and impulsivity are common to both borderline personality disorder and bipolar disorder. Sometimes, borderline personality disorder is misdiagnosed as bipolar disorder, and vice versa (Bayes & Parker, 2017). There are other features of each that complicate the client's presentation. A symptom of "chronic dysphoria" in bipolar can resemble "chronic emptiness" of borderline personality disorder. Both bipolar and borderline personality disorder share a common temperament—a trend of mood swings—which makes diagnostic clarity difficult (Bayes & Parker, 2017). A clinician should consider a wide range of variables when conducting their assessment (whether it is an initial assessment—or an ongoing one). Counselors should pay attention to the client's lifetime history of mood and relationships and their narrative during sessions.

One particular element to consider when attempting to differentiate diagnoses is the interaction between the counselor and client. Clients with borderline personality disorder tend to have fairly consistent difficulty with relationships (most relationships, including with their counselors). For example, a rapid overvaluing or devaluing interaction (and potential resulting transference) between the client and the counselor might be more indicative of an attachment disturbance that is more characteristic of borderline personality disorder than bipolar (Bayes & Parker, 2017).

McMahon et al. (2019) report that borderline personality disorder affects somewhere between 0.7% to 2.7% of the general United States' population. However, the *DSM-5* indicates that the prevalence of borderline personality disorder in the population is somewhere between 1.6% and 5.9%. If looking only at the population who are receiving outpatient counseling services, the prevalence is stated to be at about 10% (i.e., one out of 10 clients). This prevalence number raises to 20% among clients in an inpatient setting (i.e., one out of five).

HISTRIONIC PERSONALITY DISORDER (301.50) (F60.4)

Histrionic personality disorder, historically speaking, has evolved over time. The root word "hysteria" is considered a classical term in the profession, one of the first conditions indicated by early mental health theorists and professionals. Over time, hysteria has been used to describe a wide variety of psychopathological states (Novais et al., 2015). This personality disorder made its first appearance in the second edition of the *DSM* (APA, 1968), and since the DSM-III (APA, 1980), it is the only modern diagnosis left that has retained a derivative of the old classical term of hysteria.

The modern version of histrionic personality disorder is generally described as an extensive pattern of behavior of attention seeking and excessive emotionality (APA, 2013). A person with histrionic personality disorder is reported to be uncomfortable with situations in which they are not the center of attention. They may have mood swings with a shallow expression of emotion, but on the other hand, they may dramatize or have a theatrical overexpression of emotion to get attention. If not the center of attention, they may do something dramatic to gain attention. They may be overly concerned with their appearance and consistently use it to gain attention, whether seductive in nature or through other means. Individuals with histrionic personality disorder tend to be easily influenced by others or their circumstances (APA, 2013; WHO, 1993). It is believed that individuals with this disorder are at an increased risk for suicidal gestures (or threats) to get attention (APA, 2013).

The WHO (1993) also uses the term histrionic personality disorder, and the criteria necessary for a diagnosis are nearly identical. The APA claims that the prevalence of histrionic personality disorder in the general population is 1.84%. Novais et al. (2015) cite a 0.4% prevalence—but it has a high comorbidity with borderline, narcissistic, and dependent personality disorders. In the current day and time of social media, the concept of prevalence of histrionic personality disorder can be a bit ambiguous.

NARCISSISTIC PERSONALITY DISORDER (301.81) (F60.81)

Narcissistic personality disorder is described as a pervasive pattern of grandiosity (in their behavior or in fantasy), a need for admiration, and a lack of empathy (Hinrichs, 2016; Hoertel et al., 2018). Clinicians tend to focus on the symptoms of grandiosity and feelings of entitlement as defining features. However, clinicians should understand that clients with this personality disorder also tend to have cycling feelings of self-esteem (high to low and back again). There are fluctuating feelings of esteem, inadequacy, anxiety, envy, shame, boredom, emptiness, reactivity, perfectionism, and rage (Hinrichs, 2016). Displays of grandiosity act as a shield to protect the person with narcissistic personality disorder from experiencing feelings of inferiority, hatred, envy, and rejection.

Some of the negative behavioral consequences of narcissistic personality disorder include contempt, argumentativeness, verbal/physical confrontation, dissatisfaction in relationships, infidelity, drug/alcohol/process addictions, depression, anxiety, and suicidality (Hinrichs, 2016). Clients with narcissistic personality disorder present with symptoms such as vanity, self-absorption, and envy. Males are more likely to display symptoms of entitlement, a lack of empathy, fantasies of power and success, and a grandiose sense of self-importance. They may attempt to exploit others and believe they are special and deserve certain privileges. Females are more likely to exhibit greater concern with physical appearance and have a higher reactiveness to perceived slights from others (Hoertel et al., 2018).

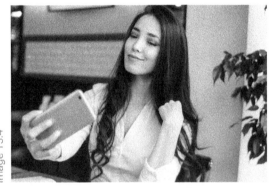

Image 15.4

With the explosion of "selfies," is this narcissistic or just the new norm?

In working with clients with narcissistic personality disorder, a counselor may be devalued during or after a session, with the client claiming that the therapist doesn't know anything or have anything to offer. Clients with this disorder display insecure attachment styles and resist therapeutic attempts at interpersonal support, minimizing the difficulty they may be experiencing or vulnerability that they may be feeling (wanting to project more perfectionistic self-concepts). Even though a client with narcissistic personality disorder may have sought out treatment as a self-growth experience, they may have only done so to satisfy a need for admiration or recognition from someone. Clients with narcissistic personality disorder often end treatment prematurely (Hinrichs, 2016).

The *ICD* (WHO) categorizes this condition under "other specific personality disorders," which falls under the banner of F60.8. This code is used when the general criteria for a personality disorder is met but does not meet any other criteria for a specific personality disorder. For the specific code, F60.81, the "1" in the hundredths place is used to identify this specific personality disorder and is referenced in Annex 1 (WHO, 1993). The *DSM-5* indicates that the prevalence of narcissistic personality disorder in the general population is anywhere from 0% to 6.2%. Hoertel et al. (2018) report that there are prevalence rates of up to 7.7% of males and 4.8% of females.

Cluster C

Clients with a Cluster C disorder appear anxious or fearful (APA, 2013). In general, the development of personality disorders is often attributed to either genetic, temperamental, or childhood factors—or a combination of any or all three (Weinbrecht et al., 2016). Regarding childhood factors, childhood trauma and parental maltreatment have been well documented as risk factors for adult personality disorders (Eikenaes et al., 2015). Someone raised in an environment where there is substantiated abuse or neglect is 4 times more likely than someone not abused or neglected to be diagnosed with one or more personality disorders by early adulthood (Eikenaes et al., 2015). One can easily understand how growing up in an abusive or neglectful environment might lead someone to a personality disorder characterized as anxious or fearful. Self-reported childhood experiences of abuse or neglect have been linked to all Cluster C personality disorders (Eikenaes et al., 2015):

1. Avoidant personality disorder
2. Dependent personality disorder
3. Obsessive-compulsive personality disorder

Would Reagan's possible diagnosis fall within any of the disorders in Cluster C?

AVOIDANT PERSONALITY DISORDER (301.82) (F60.6)

Avoidant personality disorder is described as a pervasive pattern (across time and situations) starting by early adulthood and characterized by social inhibition, feelings of inferiority and inadequacy, persistent feelings of tension and apprehension, hypersensitivity to negative evaluation or criticism, and avoidance of social or occupational activities that may bring opportunities for criticism, disapproval, or rejection (APA, 2013; Eikenaes et al., 2015; Weinbrecht et al., 2016; WHO, 1993). Avoidant personality disorder is described using the term "behavioral inhibition," which means clients with this personality disorder tend to avoid strangers and newness. They are shy, have a heightened emotional sensitivity, and are known to be very reactive, specifically with an anxious reactivity (Eikenaes et al., 2015).

Clients with avoidant personality disorder tend to have low self-efficacy, suffer ongoing mental distress, have lower levels of education, lower income, may not be in paid work, and have other somatic symptoms—all from the symptoms of the personality disorder. In comparison to other personality disorders, clients with avoidant personality disorder are considered to have the highest level of impairment in daily functioning (Weinbrecht et al., 2016). Their fears tend to be more ingrained and internalized and, therefore, interfere with decisions and life roles. Clients with avoidant personality disorder may be more emotionally guarded, have less self-esteem, and have significant difficulty expressing honest feelings in their relationships (Weinbrecht et al., 2016).

The WHO labels this disorder slightly differently (than the *DSM*) as "anxious [avoidant] personality disorder," but the criteria to meet this diagnosis in the *ICD* are nearly identical to the *DSM-5*. The prevalence of this disorder is anywhere from 1.7% to 2.4% of the general population but makes up roughly 14.7% of clients in outpatient therapy (as a comorbid disorder; APA, 2013; Weinbrecht, 2016).

Social anxiety disorder is the most common comorbid disorder of avoidant personality disorder. It is estimated that a diagnosis of social anxiety disorder (also known as social phobia) co-occurs with avoidant personality disorder anywhere from 40% to close to 90% of the time (Weinbrecht et al., 2016). There is an ongoing debate as to whether this personality disorder and social anxiety disorder are actually different conditions (Eikenaes et al., 2015). There are some who believe that the two disorders are on the same continuum; it is just that clients with avoidant personality disorder experience more severe symptoms and impairment than those clients with social anxiety disorder (Weinbrecht et al., 2016). Clients with avoidant personality disorder show higher impairments across work, social, and family environments (Weinbrecht et al., 2016).

DEPENDENT PERSONALITY DISORDER (301.6) (F60.7)

Although early versions of the *DSM* did not contain a specific diagnosis of dependent personality disorder, the disorder has historical roots all the way back to Freud's description of the oral stage of development (Disney, 2013). The disorder has evolved over time, and it first appeared in the *DSM-III* (APA, 1980), which was also the first volume to place personality disorders on axis II (which, by the way, axis II no longer appears in the *DSM-5*). Dependent personality disorder was almost deleted from the *DSM-5* based on a recommendation from the personality disorders work group. But the disorder was eventually included when the APA's board of trustees chose not to approve proposed changes (Disney, 2013). The primary defining element of this disorder is that individuals with dependent personality disorder view themselves as helpless and inept; they view others as strong and competent; they are passive in interpersonal relationships; they lack self-confidence (Disney, 2013). They tend to have a pervasive pattern of submissive dependence on others.

The symptoms of someone with dependent personality disorder include the following: unable to make everyday decisions without advice or reassurance from others, allows others to make decisions for them (particularly important life decisions), submits to and agrees with others to obtain their approval, has difficulty initiating projects, dislikes being alone and fears being left to care for themselves, fears being abandoned, and feels devastated when close relationships end (APA, 2013; Disney, 2013; WHO, 1993). With respect to this last item, an individual with dependent personality disorder may immediately and urgently seek another (new) relationship when a significant (old) relationship ends (APA, 2013).

It is believed that most clinicians are able to accurately identify this personality disorder's criteria the majority of the time and distinguish it from other disorders (Disney, 2013). The *ICD* carries the same name for the disorder, and the criteria overlap quite a bit but are not exactly identical. The *ICD* contains an additional criterion that specifies that individuals with dependent personality disorder may have an unwillingness to make even reasonable demands of the people they depend on (WHO, 1993).

Family environment, social learning, severe childhood illness, and genetics have all been indicated as playing a role in the etiology of dependent personality disorder. However, early traumatic childhood events and attachment style are the best predictors of this disorder (Disney, 2013). A fearful attachment style, a lack of assertiveness, and overprotective or authoritarian parenting styles are linked to dependent personality disorder. Separation anxiety disorder in childhood has also been indicated as a risk factor for the development of adult dependent personality disorder (Disney, 2013). It is estimated that dependent personality disorder has a prevalence in the general community of anywhere from 0.49% to 0.6% (APA, 2013).

OBSESSIVE-COMPULSIVE PERSONALITY DISORDER (301.4) (F60.5)

Obsessive-compulsive personality disorder was first recognized and labeled more than a century ago (Diedrich & Voderholzer, 2015). It was included in the first edition of the *DSM* (APA, 1952) and has been included in every revision since then, including the *DSM-5*. It is considered the most common personality disorder in the general population (Diedrich & Voderholzer, 2015) and is characterized by the following personality traits: preoccupation with details, rules, lists, order, and organization; perfectionism; excessive devotion to work and productivity; overconscientiousness; an inability to throw out worn-out or worthless items; a reluctance to delegate tasks; miserliness; and rigidity and stubbornness (APA, 2013; Diedrich & Voderholzer, 2015, WHO, 1993).

Clinicians may find it difficult to distinguish between obsessive-compulsive personality disorder and obsessive-compulsive disorder, and they are not alone. The differences between the two disorders have long been a source of debate (Diedrich & Voderholzer, 2015; Pinto et al., 2014). The overlap of some symptoms in obsessive-compulsive disorder can look like "perfectionism" in obsessive-compulsive personality disorder. The primary difference is that individuals with obsessive-compulsive personality disorder *lack* obsessive thoughts (APA, 2013; Diedrich & Voderholzer, 2015). Pinto et al. (2014) indicated that the obsessive-compulsive personality disorder and obsessive-compulsive disorder can be differentiated by the presence of obsessions in obsessive-compulsive disorder and by an excessive capacity to delay gratification/reward in the personality disorder. In addition, individuals with obsessive-compulsive disorder may find their symptoms and behaviors intrusive and distressing. Individuals with obsessive-compulsive personality disorder may think of their symptoms and behaviors as appropriate and correct (Pinto et al., 2014).

The *ICD* labels this disorder as "anankastic personality disorder" but acknowledges that it is often referred to as obsessive-compulsive personality disorder (WHO, 1993). The symptoms and criteria in the *ICD* are nearly identical in wording to the *DSM*. It is agreed that obsessive-compulsive personality disorder is one of the most prevalent personality disorders in the general population (APA, 2013; Diedrich & Voderholzer, 2015), but there is some discrepancy in how prevalent it is. The *DSM-5* (2013) claims prevalence rates between 2.1% to 7.9% of the general population, but other researchers claim anywhere from 1% to 7% (Pinto et al., 2014) to 3% to 8% (Diedrich & Voderholzer, 2015).

Dimensional Model

As mentioned earlier, there are problems and concerns related to the reliability and validity of the categorical model (used in section 2 of the *DSM-5*). One of the main problems with the categorical model of personality assessment is a lack of clarity—how differently clinicians may view problematic symptoms. In the *DSM*, the primary point of delineation between "normal" and "abnormal" are criteria in the disorders that are expressions of "little if any" or "almost always" (Candel & Constantin, 2017). Clinicians make decisions and render a diagnosis (the presence versus the absence of a personality disorder) from a relatively vague description of what qualifies as disordered behavior (Mulder et al., 2016). There has been much discussion and disagreement related to where the point is that moves a person from "personality difficulties" to a "personality disorder" (Mulder et al., 2016).

Consequently, there is a current trend of attempting to integrate the classification of personality disorders into a more dimensional model of personality traits (Candel & Constantin, 2017). It is a shift away from thinking traditionally about categories and pathological personalities to an idea that all personalities exist as traits on a continuum across multiple domains (Candel & Constantin, 2017; Skodol, 2014). It is the idea that all personalities, normal or abnormal, are related at the etiological level. The domains of personalities are identical, regardless of whether you are looking at a clinically significant sample of people or not (Candel & Constantin, 2017). Personality disorders are simply extreme versions (on certain domains) of an average personality (Candel & Constantin, 2017).

Both the APA (the *DSM*) and WHO have proposed a trait-based dimensional model of personality pathology (Bach et al., 2017), but their domains are slightly different (Lotfi et al., 2018). In the *DSM-5* (2013), the five trait domains considered are as follows:

1. Negative affectivity versus emotional stability
2. Detachment versus extraversion
3. Antagonism versus agreeableness
4. Disinhibition versus conscientiousness
5. Psychoticism versus lucidity

The first four domains (negative affectivity, detachment, antagonism, and disinhibition) are also found in the *ICD-11* (2018), but the domain of "anankastia" replaces "psychoticism."

The *ICD-11* (WHO, 2018), and its trait-based dimensional model is due to come into effect on January 1, 2022. In the *DSM-5* (2013), the alternate, trait-based model was originally intended for section 2 (diagnostic criteria and codes) of the *DSM-5* but ended up being included in section 3 (emerging measures and models; Skodol, 2014). Because the WHO is the official world classification for all diseases, including personality disorders (Bach et al., 2017), it is very possible that the next version of the *DSM* will have the trait-based dimensional model move out of the "emerging models" section and be listed as a part of section 2 of the manual. So far, there has been scientific support regarding the structural validity of the trait-based models (Lotfi et al., 2018).

Treatment Options

Treating personality disorders can, at times, be difficult. Childhood trauma and parental maltreatment are risk factors for adults who are developing personality disorders (Eikenaes et al., 2015). A family's environment, social learning that occurs in childhood, and severe childhood illnesses have all been linked to the development of a personality disorder (Disney, 2013). In particular, clients who have a history of childhood abuse or neglect are 4 times more likely to be diagnosed with a personality disorder during adulthood (Eikenaes et al., 2015). Specific early traumatic events, such as childhood sexual abuse, are often indicated in the literature regarding the etiology of personality disorders (Disney, 2013).

Some of the primary treatments for personality disorders include pharmacology (i.e., medications), cognitive therapy, and cognitive-behavioral therapy (specifically, dialectical behavioral therapy). It may be worth your time to seek out specialized training in dialectical behavioral therapy. Studies investigating the efficacy of these therapies (cognitive and cognitive behavioral) indicate that they are effective in reducing symptoms of a personality disorder (Diedrich & Voderholzer, 2015). In addition, there can be clinical improvement if the therapeutic alliance between the therapist and client is handled well (Diedrich & Voderholzer, 2015). The cognitive branch of these therapies take the stance that childhood experiences and the schemas that are developed during childhood are the foundation for maladaptive emotions and behaviors. It is important to focus on restructuring thoughts of the self and develop healthier thoughts and behaviors during this process (Disney, 2013).

When seeing adults who have long dealt with their own childhood history (sometimes never discussed or addressed), there can be a lot to unpack as their counselor. They have perhaps developed specific unhealthy mechanisms and skills that have helped them to cope over time. In general, I tend to recommend that your work with a client with a personality disorder be taken one slow step at a time and considered a longer term endeavor. Look for smaller incremental improvements over time rather than quick, great strides. In other words, if someone has been dealing with a childhood trauma for 20 years, it may take a while to unravel what has been knotted during all that time.

I would like to suggest the following metaphor:

Therapy, sometimes, is like working on an ice sculpture. You start with a large, rough block of ice. The ice has just been plucked from a frozen tundra or some large deep freezer—where it would have been isolated for an extended period of time and left to harden. If the ice had feelings, it would be in shock regarding the change in environment.

The block is then plopped down on a workbench for the sculptor or sculptress to start working on it. The workbench is likely located in a fairly cool environment so that the block of ice won't melt while the artist works on it. Turn up the heat too much, and the block may start to quickly melt. This will make it difficult to work on the ice and create the sculpture.

The sculptor or sculptress likely has multiple tools to work with, which all involve shaping the ice in one way or another. The likely tools are a hammer and different types of picks and chisels. The artist selects one of the tools and starts to "tap-tap" here and "tap-tap" there. Try to tap too hard or tap in the wrong place a little too forcefully, and the block will fracture and crumble—creating something undesirable. The artist needs to be patient. Tap a little here and little there—all within the overall plan for the sculpture. Chip away a little bit here where some of the ice needs to shaped ... chip away a little bit there to remove a bulge in the ice. Just don't chip too hard or too fast.

Keep a plan for the sculpture in your mind as you work. It might be a very clear plan for what you are trying to create—or it could be a little more of an abstract (or unknown) design for the sculpture that you will fine-tune and know it when you see it. Some sculptors may not have a plan—and claim that they are working to uncover what the ice was "meant to be."

You may need to turn up the heat just a little bit to make the ice a little easier to work with ... or maybe make the environment in which you work a little more comfortable ... but only just a little bit. The ice can't handle a high degree of heat. It would melt into a puddle—again, something you don't want to happen.

In therapy, sometimes you need to work slowly; chip away at some of the large issues a little bit at a time. For some of our more difficult and challenging clients, some issues need to be approached slowly. Move too fast, and they could "fracture" and move into a fairly dangerous area. They may not be ready for that much change at one time, or you may be addressing past trauma that is a little too scary to deal with in a short amount of time.

Turn up the heat too soon in the therapeutic process, and they can "melt" a little faster than is healthy for them. They can slip away from therapy. You want your client to change over time into a more desirable behavior or cognitive place—but in some cases, this needs to be in a very deliberate and intentional manner. Direct your client in a productive direction (turn up the heat) to make it a comfortable environment with which to work and make progress in therapy, but don't push them to go too far, too fast.

You might have a clear idea of the direction you are headed in therapy. You might have an abstract, or general, idea of the direction you are headed. You may feel that your client is leading the way. To me, this depends on your foundation and training as a therapist.

It takes time for clients to process significant events in their lives (ones that may not have been processed before). Work in ways that help to create change but allow time for your client to process what is happening and settle into a new equilibrium—before pushing them to change again. You don't want them to fracture, and you don't want them to melt.

Case Study Summary

This chapter's case study reviewed the behaviors of Reagan. As you process the story and examine possible diagnostic criteria, take a few minutes to answer the following questions:

1. What would be the correct diagnosis for Reagan?

   _____

   _____

2. What are the specific symptoms or criteria that led you to this diagnosis?

   _____

   _____

3. What other possible disorders might you diagnose Reagan with and why?

   _____

   _____

4. Briefly discuss what types of treatment may be beneficial for Reagan. Could you see using a certain counseling theory and/or medication?

   _____

   _____

Guided Practice Exercises

Scenario 1

Josiah, 52, tells himself he doesn't care what other people think. In reality, what other people think runs his life. He knows that his coworkers envy him. They know that Josiah's skill set is so vast that they could never make it to "his level." He is a reporter and claims to have a "unique take" on articles. His boss describes him as insubordinate;

he never follows instructions for a story and has little work ethic. Josiah says that his boss wants him to "dumb down" his articles for readers, which he refuses to do. Others describe Josiah as contemptuous and intense. Josiah has few friends because of his behavior. He attributes this to the fact that he is brutally honest, and few people are able to handle the truth. Whenever something goes array, Josiah blames the world for the problem. He is the victim.

What would be the correct disorder? What are the specific symptoms or criteria that led you to this diagnosis?

_____
_____
_____
_____

What specific behaviors caused you to diagnose the disorder?

_____
_____
_____
_____

What other possible disorders might you diagnose Josiah with and why?

_____
_____
_____
_____

Scenario 2

Bella, 26, has been through 15 jobs in the last 5 years. She will work somewhere for several months, but anytime she feels as if she is not the center of attention in the office, she quits. She comes to the counselor to discuss her employment issues. She strongly requests a male counselor. During her initial session with the therapist, Bella discloses that she has been married and divorced twice. When asked about her marital situations, she says that her husbands were both always suspicious that she was cheating on them with another man. They always claimed that she was overly flirty and seductive toward other men. Bella admits that she does flirt with other men but claims she never cheated on either man. She sees no problem with being flirty and even tries to seduce the therapist during the session.

What would be the correct disorder? What are the specific symptoms or criteria that led you to this diagnosis?

_____
_____
_____
_____

What specific behaviors caused you to diagnose the disorder?

_____
_____
_____
_____

What other possible disorders might you diagnose Bella with and why?

_____

_____

_____

_____

Web-Based and Literature-Based Resources

American Psychiatric Association: Help with Personality Disorders: https://www.psychiatry.org/patients-families/personality-disorders

Dialectical Behavioral Therapy Worksheets via Therapist Aid: https://www.therapistaid.com/therapy-worksheets/dbt/none

Dialectical Behavioral Therapy: About, worksheets, skills: https://positivepsychology.com/dbt-dialectical-behavior-therapy/

Lineham, M. (1993). *Cognitive-behavioral treatment of borderline personality disorder.* Guilford Press.

Lineham, M. (2015). *DBT skills training manual* (2nd ed.). Guilford Press.

Lineham, M. (2015). *DBT skills training handouts and worksheets* (2nd ed.). Guilford Press.

National Alliance on Mental Illness: http://www.nami.org

National Education Alliance for Borderline Personality Disorders: https://www.borderlinepersonalitydisorder.org/

National Institute of Mental Health: https://www.nimh.nih.gov/health/topics/index.shtml

Personality Disorder Awareness Network: http://www.pdan.org

References

American Psychiatric Association (APA). (1952). *Diagnostic and statistical manual of mental disorders.*

American Psychiatric Association (APA). (1968). *Diagnostic and statistical manual of mental disorders* (2nd ed.).

American Psychiatric Association (APA). (1980). *Diagnostic and statistical manual of mental disorders* (3rd ed.).

American Psychiatric Association (APA). (2013). *Diagnostic and statistical manual of mental disorders* (5th ed.).

Bach, B., Sellbom, M., Kongerslev, M., Simonsen, E., Krueger, R. F., & Mulder, R. (2017). Deriving ICD-11 personality disorder domains from DSM-5 traits: Initial attempt to harmonize two diagnostic systems. *Acta Psychiatrica Scandinavia, 136,* 108–117. https://doi.org/10.1111/acps.12748

Baliousis, M., Duggan, C., McCarthy, L., Huband, N., & Vollm, B. (2019). Executive function, attention, and memory deficits in antisocial personality disorder and psychopathy. *Psychiatry Research, 278*(2019), 151–161. https://doi.org/10.1016/j.psychres.2019.05.046

Bayes, A. J., & Parker, G. B. (2017). Clinical vs. DSM diagnosis of bipolar disorder, borderline personality disorder and their co-occurrence. *Acta Psychiatrica Scandinavia, 135,* 259–265. https://doi.org/10.1111/acps.12678

Candel, O. S., & Constantin, T. (2017). Antisocial and schizoid personality disorder scales: Conceptual bases and preliminary findings. *Romanian Journal of Applied Psychology, 19*(1), 10–16. https://doi.org/10.24913/rjap.19.1.02

CrimeMuseum. (2017). *Ted Bundy: Serial killers: Crime library.* www.crimemuseum.org/crime-library/serial-killers/ted-bundy/

Diedrich, A., & Voderholzer, U. (2015). Obsessive-compulsive personality disorder: A current review. *Current Psychiatry Reports, 17*(2), 1-10. https://doi.org/10.1007/s11920-014-0547-8

Disney, K. L. (2013). Dependent personality disorder: A critical review. *Clinical Psychology Review, 33*, 1184–1196. https://doi.org/10.1016/j.cpr.2013.10.001

Eikenaes, I., Egeland, J., Hummelen, B., & Wilberg, T. (2015). Avoidant personality disorder versus social phobia: The significance of childhood neglect. *PLoS ONE, 10*(3), 1–14. https://doi.org/10.1371/journal.pone.0122846

Gainsburg, M. (2019, May 06). This list of Ted Bundy's potential mental health disorders is bizarrely fascinating. *Women's Health Magazine.* https://www.womenshealthmag.com/life/a27346043/ted-bundy-mental-health-disorders-antisocial-behavior-personality/

Hazlett, E. A., Rothstein, E. G., Ferreira, R., Silverman, J. M., Siever, L. J., & Olincy, A. (2014). Sensory gating disturbances in the spectrum: Similarities and differences in schizotypal personality disorder and schizophrenia. *Schizophrenia Research, 161*(2015), 283–290. https://doi.org/10.1016/j.schres.2014.11.020

Hinrichs, J. (2016). Inpatient therapeutic assessment with narcissistic personality disorder. *Journal of Personality Assessment, 98*(2), 111–123. https://doi.org/10.1080/00223891.2015.1075997

Hoertel, N., Peyre, H., Lavaud, P., Blanco, C., Guerin-Langlois, C., Rene, M., Schuster, J., Lemogne, C., Delorme, R., & Limosin, F. (2018). Examining sex differences in DSM-IV-TR narcissistic personality disorder symptom expression using Item Response Theory (IRT). *Psychiatry Research, 260*, 500–507.

Jitchotvisut, J. (2019, January 28). *How Ted Bundy got away with so many murders, according to a forensic psychologist.* Insider. https://www.insider.com/ted-bundy-case-explained-forensic-psychologist-2019-1#meanwhile-bundys-longtime-girlfriend-elizabeth-kloepfer-was-one-of-four-people-who-had-suggested-bundys-name-to-police-as-a-suspect-3

Kirchner, S. K., Roeh, A., Nolden, J., & Hasan, A. (2018). Diagnosis and treatment of schizotypal personality disorder: Evidence from a systematic review. *npj Schizophrenia, 4*(20), 1–18. https://doi.org/10.1038/s41537-018-0062-8

Lotfi, M., Bach, B., Amini, M., & Simonsen, E. (2018). Structure of DSM-5 and ICD-11 personality domains in Iranian community sample. *Personality and Mental Health, 12*, 155–169. https://doi.org/10.1002/pmh.1409

McMahon, K., Hoertel, N., Peyre, H., Blanco, C., Fang, C., & Limosin, F. (2019). Age differences in DSM-IV borderline personality disorder symptom expression: Results from a national study using item response theory (IRT). *Journal of Psychiatric Research, 110*, 16–23. https://doi.org/10.1016/j.jpsychires.2018.12.019

Mulder, R. T., Horwood, J., Tyrer, P., Carter, J., & Joyce, P. R. (2016). Validating the proposed ICD-11 domains. *Personality and Mental Health, 10*, 84–95. https://doi.org/10.1002/pmh.1336

Novais, F., Araujo, A., & Godinho, P. (2015). Historical roots of histrionic personality disorder. *Frontiers in Psychiatry, 6*(1463), 1–5. https://doi.org/10.3389/fpsyg.2015.01463

Paoletti, G. (2019, May 16). *"The very definition of heartless evil": The story of Ted Bundy.* All That's Interesting. https://allthatsinteresting.com/ted-bundy

Pinto, A. Steinglass, J. E., Greene, A. L., Weber, E. U., & Simpson, H. B. (2014). Capacity to delay reward differentiates obsessive-compulsive disorder and obsessive-compulsive personality disorder. *Biological Psychiatry, 75*, 653–659. https://doi.org/10.1016/j.biopsych.2013.09.007

Skodol, A. E. (2014). Personality disorder classification: Stuck in neutral, how to move forward? *Current Psychiatry Reports, 16*(480), 1–10. https://doi.org/10.1007/s11920-014-0480x

Weinbrecht, A., Schulze, L., Boettcher, J., & Renneberg, B. (2016). Avoidant personality disorder: A current review. *Current Psychiatry Reports, 18*(29), 1–8. https://doi.org/10.1007/s11920-016-0665-6

Winsper, C., Bilgin, A., Thompson, A., Marwaha, S., Chanen, A. M., Singh, S. P., Wang, A., & Furtado, V. (2020). The prevalence of personality disorders in the community: A global systematic review and meta-analysis. *British Journal of Psychiatry: The Journal of Mental Science, 216*(2), 69–78. https://doi.org/10.1192/bjp.2019.166

World Health Organization (WHO). (1992). *International classification of diseases and related health problems* (10th rev., ICD-10).

World Health Organization (WHO). (1993). *ICD-10 classification of mental and behavioural disorders: Diagnostic criteria for research.*

World Health Organization (WHO). (2016). *International statistical classification of diseases and related health problems, 10th revision (ICD-10).*

World Health Organization (WHO). (2018). *International classification of diseases and related health problems* (11th rev., ICD-11).

Credits

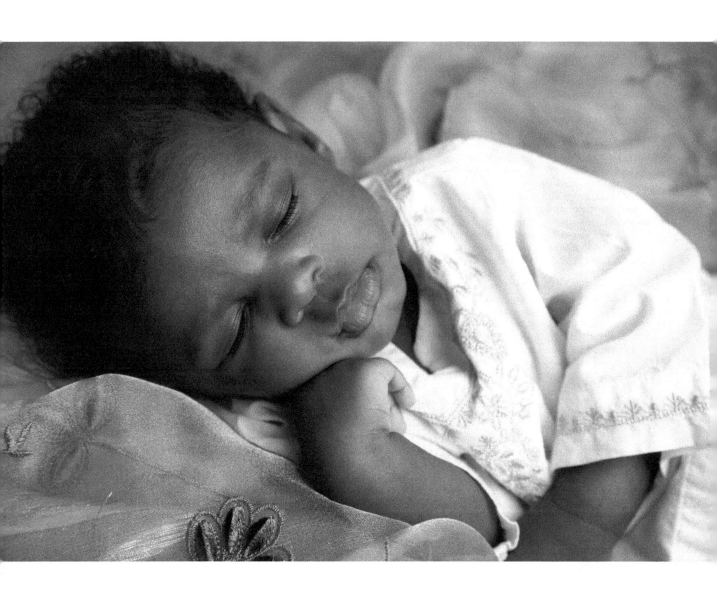

CHAPTER SIXTEEN

SLEEP-WAKE DISORDERS

David A. Scott and Michelle Grant Scott

CASE STUDY 16.1 Jardin, 56, has been a nurse for the last 30 years. She enjoys her work at the hospital and finds it incredibly rewarding. Six months ago, the hospital administration voiced an exaggerated need for night nurses. Jardin readily volunteered. After all, the pay was better, and Jardin has always been a model employee. Unfortunately, the change has had a negative effect on Jardin's health. She has found herself tired for most of her shift and has had to catch herself when she begins to doze off. Jardin finds it impossible to sleep during the day. The light streaming in through the window makes it feel as if it is time to get up. Initially, Jardin thought that her body just needed time to adjust, but now she is concerned there may be a greater problem. She decides to make an appointment at the hospital's sleep clinic.

Did You Know?

- One in five adults don't get enough sleep (American Academy of Sleep Medicine, 2008).
- There are close to 100 different types of sleep disorders.
- Americans will spend around $52 billion on sleeping aids by the year 2020.

Overview

How much sleep is enough sleep? Why did I toss and turn all night? Why am I so sleepy during the day? I can't go to sleep until very late. All statements that we have probably said at some point in our lives. Sleep is such a vital part of our lives, yet we seem to put sleep concerns (and getting enough sleep) on the back burner until it is affecting our lives in a negative way. Research continues to support the idea that quality sleep is a critical component to our mental and physical health. Around 30%–50% of the population has trouble sleeping. Sleep issues can also be very dangerous. The National Sleep Foundation (2016) reported that 37% of American drivers have fallen asleep while driving. Drowsy driving is a term used to describe how sleep deprivation can have similar effects on your body as driving while intoxicated. Shift workers (working at night) can also be affected by sleep problems (Could Jardin's work as a nurse be impacted when she moved to the night shift?). Exploring sleep patterns is also a part of a thorough mental health evaluation. We are doing our clients a disservice if we don't check in on their sleep patterns. This chapter will explore the current sleep-wake disorders and possible treatment modalities.

Sleep research started to gain interest in the 1950s. Until then, most people thought that sleep was needed just to help us recharge our internal batteries, not really understanding how sleep can affect our physical and mental well-being. Our brain regulates sleep by the use of serotonin and norepinephrine while we are awake and then neurons switching off these neurotransmitters to signal sleep time. A chemical called adenosine is also believed to play a role in causing drowsiness (National Institute of Neurological

TABLE 16.1 Phases of Sleep

PHASES OF SLEEP	CHARACTERISTICS OF PHASE
Stage 1	Light sleep, can be awakened easily, slow eye movements
Stage 2	Brain waves slow and eye movements stop
Stage 3	Delta brain waves (extremely slow) mixed with smaller, faster waves Considered deep sleep
Stage 4	Difficult to wake up, almost all delta brain waves Considered deep sleep
REM	Rapid eye movements Irregular and rapid breathing Muscles become temporarily paralyzed Occurs typically around 70 to 90 minutes after falling asleep

Note: Adapted from NINDS (2014).

Disorders and Stroke [NINDS], 2014). Sleep typically consists of five phases. Table 16.1 provides a quick look at each phase.

In 1979, the *Diagnostic Classification of Sleep and Arousal Disorders* was published and provided a framework in which to assist in the diagnosing of sleep disorders (Association of Sleep Disorders Centers, 1979). This first classification system enabled the development of the currently used *International Classification of Sleep Disorders* (ICSD) manual that is now in its third edition (American Academy of Sleep Medicine, 2014). The manual places sleep disorders into seven major categories that include the following:

- Insomnia
- Sleep-related breathing disorders
- Central disorders of hypersomnolence
- Circadian rhythm sleep-wake disorders
- Sleep-related movement disorders
- Parasomnias
- Other sleep disorders

The International Statistical Classification of Diseases (*ICD-10*; World Health Organization [WHO], 2016) and *Diagnostic and Statistical Manual of Mental Disorders, 5th Edition* (*DSM-5*; American Psychiatric Association [APA], 2013) also include and categorize sleep-wake disorders. Table 16.2 provides the *ICD-10* and *DSM-5* sleep-wake disorder comparisons. The *DSM-5* (2013) lists 10 conditions within the sleep-wake disorder chapter. Many professionals find that using both the *DSM-5* and *ICSD-3* has caused some confusion because of the inconsistencies between the two systems.

Insomnia

Insomnia is one of the most common and well-known sleep disorders. The basic definition of insomnia is a disorder where people have problems falling asleep and/or

TABLE 16.2 *ICD-DSM* Sleep-Wake Disorder Comparisons

ICD-10 CODES	DSM-5 CODES
NONORGANIC SLEEP DISORDERS (F51.X)	*SLEEP-WAKE DISORDERS*
Nonorganic insomnia (F51.0, G47.0) Unsatisfactory sleep that impacts a person's daily activities. Can include problems with going to sleep, staying asleep, and early wakening	Insomnia disorder (780.52)
Nonorganic Hypersomnia (F51.1) Greater than normal sleepiness or trouble waking up after sleep	Hypersomnolence disorder (780.54)
Nonorganic disorder of the sleep-wake schedule (F51.2) Problems with a person's sleep-wake schedule resulting in either insomnia or hypersomnia *Delayed sleep phase syndrome and irregular sleep-wake pattern (G47.2)*	
Sleepwalking (somnambulism) (F51.3) Walking or performing other "awake" tasks during sleep.	
Sleep terrors (night terrors) (F51.4) Nighttime episodes of terror and panic. Person can get up and sometimes scream. Very little recall of the event	
Nightmares (51.5) Vivid dreams, including fear and anxiety. Person can recall very detailed amounts of the nightmare	
Sleep apnea (G47.3)	
Narcolepsy and cataplexy (G47.4)	
Nonorganic sleep disorder, unspecified (F51.9)	

Note: Adapted from ICD-10 (WHO, 2016); DSM-5 (APA, 2013)

staying asleep. Insomnia can be either primary (a distinct disorder with no specific cause) or secondary (a symptom of another problem). The National Heart, Lung, and Blood Institute (NHLBI, 2014) lists several factors that could contribute to secondary insomnia. They include the following:

• Complications with a person's thyroid
• Chronic pain
• Menopause
• Gastrointestinal problems
• Asthma and other conditions that make breathing difficult

Insomnia can also be either chronic (lasting for a month or longer) or acute (lasting several days or weeks). Acute insomnia can be the result of a traumatic event, stress, or crisis situations. Chronic insomnia can be the result of various medical conditions, substance abuse, or issues with certain medications (NHLBI, 2014). Caffeine close to bedtime, decongestants, and some diet pills can interfere with our ability to go to sleep. For some, insomnia can occur with mental health disorders, such as depression or anxiety. Typically, insomnia is more common in women and older adults. Older adults are also at higher risk of cognitive problems, falls, memory lapses, and stroke if they are struggling with insomnia (Alessi et al., 2016).

Would Jardin experience insomnia created by the sudden move to working night shift?

Treatment for insomnia can include lifestyle changes, medications, and cognitive behavioral therapy (CBT). CBT (and other mental health techniques) can help a client address issues related to stress/anxiety and/or possible depressive symptoms that can disrupt normal sleep. By focusing on thoughts and behaviors related to sleep, clients can effectively address the issues that are impacting their ability to have quality sleep. Typically, most medications for sleep have mixed results. While they may increase the amount of sleep, their possible side effects (habit forming, lack of quality sleep, sedation lasting into the morning) can be worrisome. Alessi et al. (2016) also reported a higher risk of falls, fractures, and even death in elderly adults who use sedatives for sleep. An over-the-counter medication, melatonin, has been increasing in popularity to help treat insomnia. Some people can dramatically reduce their episodes of insomnia by completing the following:

- Engaging in regular exercise
- Reducing the amount of caffeine and other stimulants, especially reducing/eliminating use after lunchtime
- Reducing/eliminating external stimuli at night (e.g., television in the bedroom, cell phone use, leaving a "night-light" on in bedroom)

CASE STUDIES 16.2 Edna Mae, 73, presents to her primary care physician with complaints of headaches and lack of sleep. Upon further questioning, the doctor finds that Edna Mae lost her husband 8 months earlier and since then has been struggling to get restful and lasting sleep. She reports some depression but overall seems to be coping well with the loss of her husband. Edna Mae confides that her racing thoughts keep her awake late into the night and the absence of her husband next to her makes her more anxious. She has tried several over-the-counter sleep aids but does not like how groggy they make her feel in the morning. Lately, she has been drinking a glass of wine to help her relax and sleep. Unfortunately, she has had to increase the amount she drinks to three or four glasses to be able to fall asleep.

Samuel

Samuel, 24, is finding it difficult to complete his work and school responsibilities. He is working at a local auto factory and takes night classes at a community college. Samuel has always had a high amount of anxiety, but lately it feels difficult to manage. His anxious thoughts will keep him awake most of the night, and he has to consume a huge amount of caffeine the next day to be able to work. He does not have any time during the day to take naps. One day last week, he almost fell asleep at work. His manager left him with a warning, but because of the dangerous equipment around, Samuel will be let go the next time it happens. His school performance has also been suffering. His girlfriend has always noticed the ill effects of Samuel's lack of sleep. She notes that he appears to have a lack of energy and has given up going to the gym.

Questions

- What are some easy tips a physician could give a patient in regard to helping them fall asleep (e.g., less caffeine)?

_____
_____
_____
_____

- Explain the difference between situational insomnia and chronic insomnia. Which one does Edna Mae have? Samuel?

_____
_____
_____
_____

- Have you ever been unable to fall asleep? Describe your experience. What would it be like to be unable to sleep every night?

_____
_____
_____
_____

Sleep-Related Breathing Disorders

Sleep-related breathing disorders are listed in several categories, including obstructive sleep apnea, central sleep apnea, sleep-related hypoventilation, and sleep-related hypoxemia (Sateia, 2014). Treatment usually involves the use of a continuous positive airway pressure machine (CPAP). This machine uses air pressure to keep the airway from being blocked during sleep. The most common of the sleep-related breathing disorders is *obstructive sleep apnea*. This disorder occurs when a person's airway is blocked, and they stop breathing during sleep. This is typically caused by tissue in the throat relaxing and/or the tongue falling back into the throat during sleep. Common symptoms include snoring, breathing pauses (can be observed by sleeping partner), and waking from sleep with a feeling of suffocation.

The causes of central sleep apnea are located in the brain or heart and not the result of a blocked airway. This disorder is divided into five categories (American Academy of Sleep Medicine, 2016a) for adults:

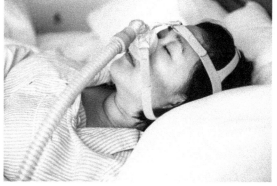

Image 16.2

1. *Primary Central Sleep Apnea.* Cause is unknown.
2. *Cheyne-Stokes Breathing Pattern.* Heart failure, stroke, or kidney failure.
3. *Medical Condition Not Cheyne-Stokes.* Heart and kidney problems but without the Cheyne-Stokes breathing pattern.
4. *High-Altitude Periodic Breathing.* Sleeping above 15,000 feet and no history of heart or kidney problems.
5. *Drug or Substance Use.* Caused by substance use, including opioids.

Sleep-related hypoventilation and *hypoxemia* occurs when a person has an insufficient exchange of gases (carbon dioxide and oxygen) during sleep (hypoventilation) or abnormally low oxygen levels in the arterial blood (hypoxemia). This can increase in seriousness (higher levels of carbon dioxide in the body) when a person is also diagnosed with sleep apnea. Factors for sleep-related hypoventilation include natural airway obstructions, other medical conditions (emphysema, bronchitis, chronic obstructive pulmonary disease, and diseases of the lungs), and smoking (American Sleep Association, 2007). The use of a CPAP machine is one of the most common treatment options.

CASE STUDIES 16.3 Sleep Apnea

Charley

Charley, 56, does not understand why he constantly feels tired. He tries to get a full 8–9 hours of sleep a night but always wakes exhausted. He usually will wake up three to four times during the night. On top of his exhaustion, his wife complains that he snores at night. Charley feels bad but cannot help it. He is overweight and has extremely high blood pressure, despite being put on four different blood pressure medications. The doctor suggests that Charley exercise, but his energy level is so low that he does not feel as if he can. He barely has the energy to go to work.

Lyle

Lyle, 60, presents to her primary care physician with complaints of fatigue and a low energy level. Lyle explains that she easily falls asleep and stays asleep for most of the night, yet she will wake feeling exhausted. She used to go fishing and camping on a regular basis with her husband but now feels that she doesn't have the energy. She has cut back her hours at work to have more time to rest. This has meant that her husband has had to pick up more overtime at his job, and Lyle does not see him often. Lyle's husband has told her that she often snores loudly in her sleep. He is concerned that her sleep might not be restful.

Questions

- Describe the two different types of sleep apnea.

  _____
  _____
  _____
  _____

- Biologically, why do people with sleep apnea feel tired even when they have slept a sufficient number of hours?

  _____
  _____
  _____
  _____

- Describe the treatment options for someone with sleep apnea.

  _____
  _____
  _____
  _____

Central disorders of hypersomnolence are characterized by extreme daytime sleepiness that is not the result of another sleep disorder. The two main categories are narcolepsy (type 1 and 2) and idiopathic hypersomnia. Khan and Trotti (2015) reported that the exact cause of narcolepsy type 2 and idiopathic hypersomnia still remain unknown. Narcolepsy is a nervous system disorder (hypothalamus) that is typically chronic and involves sudden episodes of sleep that can last a few seconds or even several minutes. These *sleep attacks* can occur at any time, even while driving. Many times, cataplexy (sudden muscle weakness without losing consciousness), is common with narcolepsy. While there is no known genetic cause, most people with narcolepsy have low levels of the neurotransmitter hypocretin. The first reported case of narcolepsy was by Dr. Jean Gelineau in 1880. Dr. Gelineau discussed his work with a 38-year-old male who was falling asleep up to 200 times a day (Schenck et al., 2007). The man would usually fall asleep, on average, every 30 minutes and needed constant care from his son to awaken him.

Narcolepsy type 2 is differentiated by the absence of cataplexy. Idiopathic hypersomnia is severe daytime sleepiness despite normal sleep amounts. A person with sleep disorder will typically not have the sleep attacks as with narcolepsy but will remain extremely sleepy throughout the day. Their nighttime sleep is usually described as very deep, and they have trouble waking up in the morning.

While there is no known cure, treatment for central disorders of hypersomnolence usually start with the person undergoing testing, which includes overnight polysomnography (sleep study that records brain waves and oxygen levels), multiple sleep latency tests (how fast you fall asleep during the day), and, if needed, a cerebrospinal fluid test to measure hypocretin levels. Medications such as Modafinil (Provigil), sodium oxybate, and stimulants (methylphenidate) have been approved for the treatment of narcolepsy. Antidepressants (tricyclics and selective serotonin reuptake inhibitors) have been found effective in treating cataplexy. In 2016, The NINDS suggested various behavioral strategies to help with these disorders, such as keeping a regular sleep schedule, avoiding smoking, and avoiding alcohol and caffeine several hours before bedtime.

CASE STUDY 16.4 Central Disorders of Hypersomnolence
Erin

Erin, 26, is a computer programmer in a large urban area. She lives in a small apartment with her boyfriend, but neither of them are there much because of their jobs. The biggest problem that Erin has is falling asleep at inopportune times. It seems like no matter how much of the night she is able to sleep, she still suffers during the day. Her boss has threatened to fire her if she continues falling asleep on the clock. The first time he found her sleeping, he thought that maybe she had just had a rough night, but finding her asleep seems to have become a norm. Erin usually falls asleep on the train to and from work as well. Erin has noticed that if something makes a loud noise, such as a door slamming, her legs seem to give out. If Erin laughs too hard or is surprised, she will feel as if she is going to fall down. Erin finally decides to go to a sleep clinic after having a near accident because of falling asleep at the wheel.

Questions

- Define cataplexy. Does this condition have to be present for someone to meet the *DSM* criteria for insomnia?

_____
_____
_____
_____

- Often, others mistakenly label those with narcolepsy as lazy. What can this teach us about working with clients who appear to be lazy?

  _____
  _____
  _____
  _____

- Should people diagnosed with narcolepsy be allowed to drive alone? Defend your position.

  _____
  _____
  _____
  _____

Circadian rhythm sleep-wake disorders are characterized by clinically significant disturbances in a person's sleep-wake cycle relative to the day-night cycle. People with these disorders have trouble going to sleep and/or waking at "normal" times. These can be caused by biological factors and external factors, such as jet lag and working during a normal sleep time (i.e., working second or third shift on a regular basis). The *ICD-10* (WHO, 2016) lists six types of circadian rhythm sleep-wake disorders:

Could this be Jardin's diagnosis?

1. Delayed sleep phase type
2. Free-running type
3. Advanced sleep phase type
4. Irregular sleep-wake type
5. Shift-work type
6. Jet lag type

A type that has been in the news more lately, is the free-running type, non-24-hour, sleep-wake disorder (Non-24). Typically, this neurological disorder is mostly seen in individuals who are blind, but there are cases of sighted people with Non-24. It is important to note that the causes of Non-24 in blind and sighted people are different (Circadian Sleep Disorders Network, 2016). Non-24 occurs when a person struggles to keep a consistent sleep/wake cycle. One night they may fall asleep at 11 p.m., the next day midnight, the day after that 1 a.m., and so on. The length of sleep stays relatively the same, but since they are going to sleep later and later, it affects the daily wake time and daily activities.

For those individuals who have traveled by plane across several time zones, many would say that they have experienced jet lag. Simply put, jet lag results in a disturbance in the sleep/wake cycle. A person with jet lag will feel sleepy during the day, have trouble falling asleep at their normal home time, and experience fatigue. Eventually, the person's internal clocks will adjust to the new time zone without any medical treatment. People who work nights also struggle with their bodies adjusting to the different sleep times. These people can also have higher rates of heart problems, emotional problems, and digestive problems (NINDS, 2014). Gathering information concerning a person's sleep history is the first step in treating someone with a circadian rhythm sleep-wake disorder. Typically, making changes to a person's sleep habits, use of melatonin, focusing on light/dark exposure, and using behavioral techniques are the most common forms of treatment for circadian rhythm sleep-wake disorders (Zhu & Zee, 2012).

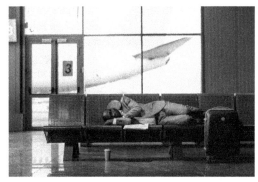

Image 16.3

CASE STUDY 16.5 Circadian Rhythm Sleep Disorder
Gordon, Delayed Sleep Phase Type

Gordon, 22, is a senior in college at a medium-sized public university. He has had significant trouble lately waking and sleeping at the correct time of day, especially since he started college. Gordon reports not being able to fall asleep until 5 or 6 a.m. and then typically sleeping until 1 p.m. His quality of sleep and length of sleep are normal, and Gordon feels rested after he sleeps. The problem is that he has an 8 a.m. class that he has only attended once the entire semester. Gordon has tried to go to bed earlier in anticipation of getting up for the class in the morning. Unfortunately, he will just toss and turn in his bed, unable to fall asleep until 5 or 6 a.m. Gordon is afraid that once he graduates, he will not be able to work a regular job because of his difficulty sleeping at regular times.

- What differentiates circadian rhythm sleep disorders from insomnia or narcolepsy?

———————————————————————————————
———————————————————————————————
———————————————————————————————
———————————————————————————————

- Often, it is common for college students to have unhealthy sleep schedules. For example, staying up late into the night and then waking early for an exam is usually a common occurrence. How would you be able to tell that a college student has a delayed sleep phase type of a circadian disorder and is not just conforming to the norm of sleep for college students?

———————————————————————————————
———————————————————————————————
———————————————————————————————
———————————————————————————————

Parasomnias are sleep disorders that involve unwanted experiences or behaviors, such as sleep terrors, sleepwalking, nightmares, bedwetting, sleep talking, and sleep-related eating episodes. Sleep (or night) terrors differ from nightmares in that sleep terror clients usually do not remember the dream and wake up violently (screaming, thrashing, and/or kicking). A person suffering from nightmares experiences disturbing dreams that wake them from their sleep without the physical outbursts related to sleep terrors. Antidepressants and antihypertensives can be a factor in nightmares. Sleepwalking is probably one of the most popular parasomnias and is portrayed in movies and television shows. Clients who sleepwalk actually get out of bed (while still asleep) and move about their residence. Sometimes the client will even have their eyes open and become aggressive if someone tries to restrain them.

Most parasomnias do not require medical attention. Typically, making adjustments in sleep routines will help in a reduction of parasomnias. Fleetham and Fleming (2014) reported that the research on how to effectively treat parasomnias still needs to be expanded.

There are two parasomnias that may require help from a medical professional: the *REM sleep behavior disorder* and the *sleep-related eating disorder*. In *REM sleep behavior disorder*, the client will flail around in bed to the point of injuring themselves and/or their sleep partner. Parents of children with this disorder are usually encouraged to remove sharp objects from their bedroom and ensure that the child cannot easily access stairs or windows. *Sleep-related eating disorder* is a type of parasomnia in which a person engages in binge eating while they are only partially awake. Many times the food is high-calorie and ingested in a hurried manner (Fleetham & Fleming, 2014). This could lead to the person accidently eating or drinking a toxic substance (American Academy of Sleep Medicine, 2016b). Most psychopharmalogical treatment for these disorders include the use of benzodiazepines, opiates, or other sleep medications.

CASE STUDIES 16.6 Parasomnias

January, Sleep Terrors

January, 6, is generally well behaved but has a rebellious side. She often gets in trouble for talking too much during class and disrupting her classmates. Her parents argue with January, insisting she behave, and it was common for January to throw tantrums after these confrontations. For the last 2 months, January has been waking in the middle of the night screaming. Her mother, Sharee, tries to comfort her during these episodes, but nothing seems to calm her down. January is fearful and yells, "Don't get me! Please don't let them get me!!" January has rapid and shallow breathing, and she is covered in sweat during these episodes. Even stranger, January has no memory of the event after waking. Sharee does not know what to do about the issue. January's screams keep the family awake for a significant portion of the night.

Justin, Sleepwalking

Justin, 35, presents at the sleep clinic with complaints of exhaustion and chronic sleepwalking. His wife, Alesha, explains that Justin will often jump up from the bed and begin walking or running in the middle of the night. Sometimes he will yell, "I don't want to die!" or "Help!" as he tries to run from the bed. Alesha cannot wake Justin when he is sleepwalking. He will walk around with a blank stare on his face during these episodes, unable to be awakened. He has even fallen down the stairs once in his sleep, not remembering afterward what had happened. The constant sleepwalking has caused a significant rift in the couple's marriage, with each of them being drowsy during the day.

Questions

• Why do you think sleepwalking and night terrors are so common in childhood?

_____

_____

_____

_____

• Sleepwalking and REM sleep disorder (nonparalysis of muscles during REM sleep resulting in acting out one's dreams) have both been used as criminal defenses successfully (e.g., *Massachusetts v. Tirrel*, *R. v. Parks*). Do you believe that someone can unknowingly murder someone in their sleep?

_____

_____

_____

_____

Another well-known sleep disorder falls into the category of *sleep-related movement disorders*: restless legs syndrome. Sleep-related movement disorders involve some type of movement prior to or during sleep that disturbs normal sleep. The sleep-related movement disorders include the following (Thorpy, 2012):

- *Restless Legs Syndrome.* Urge to move legs during the night. Around 12 million people in the United States have restless legs syndrome
- *Periodic Limb Movement.* Repetitive arm and leg movements during sleep
- *Sleep-Related Leg Cramps.* Leg cramps during sleep
- *Sleep-Related Bruxism.* Clenching of teeth during sleep. Can lead to a wearing down of the teeth
- *Sleep-Related Rhythmic Movement Disorder.* Large, rhythmic movements of the head, body, and/or limbs

While there is no cure for sleep-related movement disorders, there are some treatments that may help with the symptoms. Decreasing caffeine, tobacco, and alcohol intake is recommended, along with the possible use of benzodiazepines, anticonvulsants, and opioids.

Treatment Options

Sleep-wake disorder treatment continues to expand as more and more research is conducted on these topics. Sleep studies, brain imaging, and more specific uses of psychopharmacological medications are trying to improve the quality of sleep for individuals suffering with sleep-wake issues. Also, it is critically important to educate clients concerning good sleep hygiene, the use of appropriate behavior modifications, and recognizing the need to seek help early on when they encounter sleep problems.

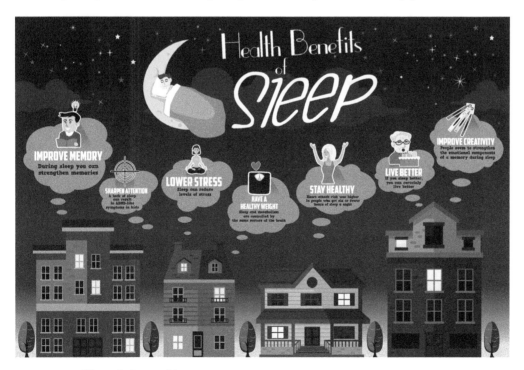

FIGURE 16.1 Sleep Infographic

Case Study Summary

One of this chapter's case studies reviewed the behaviors of Jardin. As you process the story and examine possible diagnostic criteria, take a few minutes to answer the following questions:

1. What would be the correct diagnosis for Jardin?

   _____

   _____

2. What are the specific symptoms or criteria that led you to this diagnosis?

   _____

   _____

3. What other possible disorders might you diagnose Jardin with and why?

   _____

   _____

4. Briefly discuss what types of treatment may be beneficial for Jardin. Could you see using a certain counseling theory and/or medication?

   _____

   _____

5. What are some tips that may be helpful for people who work third-shift jobs to be able to sleep during the day?

   _____

   _____

Guided Practice Exercises

Scenario 1

Wendy is a 16-year-old Asian American female. Her mother, Cindy, brought her into the clinic after noticing an increase in complaints from Wendy's teachers about her falling asleep in class. Cindy has also noticed that Wendy is no longer interested in outdoor activities, spending time with friends, or being a part of any of her extracurricular activities. Wendy reports that she often feels incredibly weak and finds herself having vivid, frightening visions upon falling asleep. She states that her severe daytime sleepiness prevents her from getting through the day without taking "random naps." Although many of these symptoms have followed Wendy through most of adolescence, she explains that they have become more difficult to deal with, as they often hinder her from completing tasks and interfere with daily life. Wendy states that she wants to go to college after graduating high school but is afraid that she will be unable to do so based on how her sleepiness has interfered with her academics. Cindy explains that she and Wendy's father have never had Wendy see a specialist because of the idea that she would simply grow out of this problem.

What would be the correct disorder? What are the specific symptoms or criteria that led you to this diagnosis?

_____
_____
_____
_____

What specific behaviors caused you to diagnose the disorder?

_____
_____
_____
_____

What other possible disorders might you diagnose Wendy with and why?

_____
_____
_____
_____

Scenario 2

Quentin, 16, does not know exactly when his trouble with sleep started. He remembers always struggling to stay awake in school. Teachers would question his parents about the apparent lack of sleep, but they were always confused when Quentin or his parents explained that he sleeps 8 hours a night. During high school, it seems that the symptoms have worsened. Quentin feels his legs are going to give whenever he is surprised or he laughs too hard. It is not uncommon for Quentin to fall asleep suddenly and wake up an hour later, not remembering what happened. His grades have suffered from his inability to stay awake in class. His teachers label him as lazy, even when he tries to explain his situation. His parents take him to the school counselor when they realize that he is in danger of failing out.

What would be the correct disorder? What are the specific symptoms or criteria that led you to this diagnosis?

_____
_____
_____
_____

What specific behaviors caused you to diagnose the disorder?

_____
_____
_____
_____

What other possible disorders might you diagnose Quentin with and why?

_____
_____
_____
_____

Web-Based and Literature-Based Resources

National Sleep Foundation: https://sleepfoundation.org

American Sleep Association: https://www.sleepassociation.org

All about sleep: KidsHealth.org

References

Alessi, C., Martin, J. L., Fiorentino, L., Fung, C. H., Dzierzewski, J. M., Tapia, J. C., Song, Y., Josephson, K., Jouldjian, S., & Mitchell, M. N. (2016). Cognitive behavioral therapy for insomnia in older veterans using nonclinician sleep coaches: Randomized controlled trial. *Journal of the American Geriatrics Society, 64*, 1830–1838. https://doi.org/10.1111/jgs.14304

American Academy of Sleep Medicine. (2008). *Sleep deprivation*. http://www.aasmnet.org/resources/factsheets/sleepdeprivation.pdf

American Academy of Sleep Medicine. (2014). *International classification of sleep disorders* (3rd ed.).

American Academy of Sleep Medicine. (2016a). *Central sleep apnea—overview & facts*. http://www.sleepeducation.org/sleep-disorders-by-category/sleep-breathing-disorders/central-sleep-apnea/overview-facts/

American Academy of Sleep Medicine. (2016b). *Parasomnias*. http://www.sleepeducation.org/essentials-in-sleep/parasomnias/symptoms

American Sleep Association. (2007). *Hypoventilation*. https://www.sleepassociation.org/patients-general-public/hypoventilation/

Association of Sleep Disorders Centers. (1979). Diagnostic classification of sleep and arousal disorders. Prepared by the Sleep Disorders Classification Committee. *Sleep, 2*, 1–137.

American Psychiatric Association (APA). (2013). *Diagnostic and statistical manual of mental disorders* (5th ed.).

Circadian Sleep Disorders Network. (2016). *Non-24-hour sleep-wake disorder*. http://www.circadiansleepdisorders.org/docs/N24-QandA.php

Fleetham, J. A., & Fleming, J. A. E. (2014). Parasomnias. *Canadian Medical Association Journal, 186*(8), 273–280. https://doi.org/10.1503/cmaj.120808

Khan, Z., & Trotti, L. M. (2015). Central disorders of hypersomnolence: Focus on the narcolepsies and idiopathic hypersomnia. *Chest, 148*(1), 262–273. http://doi.org/10.1378/chest.14-1304

National Heart, Lung, and Blood institute (NHLBI). (2014). *Insomnia*. https://www.ncbi.nlm.nih.gov/pubmedhealth/PMH0063022/

National Institute of Neurological Disorders and Stroke (NINDS). (2014, July). *Brain basics; understanding sleep*. http://www.ninds.nih.gov/disorders/brain_basics/understanding_sleep.htm

National Institute of Neurological Disorders and Stroke (NINDS). (April, 2016). *Narcolepsy fact sheet*. NIH Publication No. 13-1637. http://www.ninds.nih.gov/disorders/narcolepsy/detail_narcolepsy.htm

National Sleep Foundation. (2016). *Sleep in America*. https://sleepfoundation.org/sleep-topics/drowsy-driving

Sateia, M. J. (2014). International classification of sleep disorders-third edition: Highlights and modifications. *Chest, 146*, 1387–1394. https://doi.org/10.1378/chest.14-0970

Schenck, C. H., Bassetti, C. L., Arnulf, I., & Mignot, E. (2007). English translations of the first clinical reports on narcolepsy and cataplexy by Westphal and Gatineau in the late 19th century, with commentary. *Journal of Clinical Sleep Medicine: JCSM: Official Publication of the American Academy of Sleep Medicine, 3*, 301–311.

Thorpy, M. J. (2012). Classification of sleep disorders. *Neurotherapeutics, 9*, 687–701.

World Health Organization (WHO). (2016). *International statistical classification of diseases and related health problems, 10th revision (ICD-10)*.

Zhu, L., & Zee, P. C. (2012). Circadian rhythm sleep disorders. *Neurologic Clinics, 30*(4), 1167–1191. https://doi.org/1016/j.ncl.2012.08.011

Credits

INDEX

ABOUT THE EDITORS

Michelle Grant Scott, LISW-CP(S) is a Licensed Independent Social Worker–Clinical Practitioner and approved clinical supervisor in the state of South Carolina.

Michelle completed her graduate work at the University of North Carolina at Chapel Hill and undergraduate work at UNC–Greensboro. She currently serves as a lecturer and the coordinator of the human services program at Lander University, as well as a visiting lecturer in the University of South Carolina College of Social Work. She previously served as an instructor and site coordinator for USC's Master of Social Work program. Michelle has served as a guest lecturer at multiple universities since 2001. She also has over 20 years of clinical experience, including practice in mental health counseling and private practice, college campus counseling services, evaluation of children, home health, and hospice work.

David A. Scott, PhD, LPC is a quantitative researcher, Licensed Professional Counselor, and associate professor in Clemson's Counselor Education program. Dr. Scott is a member of ACA, NCDA, and AMHCA. He has served as the president of the South Carolina Counseling Association and was the program coordinator for the clinical mental health counseling program at Clemson. His areas of interest include identity development, at-risk youth, career counseling, and clinical counseling. Dr. Scott has worked in a variety of settings over the past 20 years, which include an inpatient hospital, outpatient counseling center, and in private practice with his wife. Before entering academia, he was one of the directors for a large nonprofit agency that provided a continuum of care services for at-risk youth and their families.

ABOUT THE CONTRIBUTORS

Theresa C. Allen, PhD, NCC, LPC, is a licensed professional counselor in the state of South Carolina and has a PhD in counselor education and supervision. Theresa is a cognitive behavioral therapy therapist who primarily works from a developmental and attachment theory framework. She has been in private practice since 2014. In addition, Theresa is an assistant professor of counseling at Liberty University and an adjunct professor for Colorado Christian University and Piedmont International University. Dr. Allen has also served as the women's director for a nonprofit, faith-based residential program for men and women with drug and alcohol addictions.

T'Airra Belcher, PhD, LPC(VA), NCC, is a native of Richmond, Virginia. She earned her bachelor's degree from James Madison University (2012), a master's degree in clinical mental health counseling from Old Dominion University (2014), and a doctoral degree in education with a concentration in counselor education and supervision from Old Dominion University (2019). Dr. Belcher's research interests include meta-analysis, interprofessional collaboration, multisystemic therapy, teaching practices, teen suicide, LGBT development, and experiences of African Americans in higher education. Currently, Dr. Belcher is an assistant professor at Loyola University New Orleans in the Counseling Department. Dr. Belcher has a private practice, offering teletherapy and providing outpatient therapy to individuals, families, and couples. Clinically, Dr. Belcher has experience working with children and teens on topics associated with development, gender and sexuality, trauma, depression, anxiety, attention deficit hyperactivity disorder, and adjustment disorder, as well as adults with serious mental health disorders, relationships, anxiety, and communication skills.

Taheera Blount, PhD, NCC, LCMHC (NC), is an assistant professor of counselor education at North Carolina Central University. She earned her PhD in counseling and counselor education from North Carolina State University. Prior to transitioning to higher education, Dr. Blount worked as a professional school counselor and as a licensed professional counselor serving children and adolescents with mental health disorders. Dr. Blount's research agenda focuses on school counselors implementing data-driven comprehensive school counseling programs, career and college readiness among urban youth, and dropout prevention strategies for school counselors. Currently, Dr. Blount serves on the editorial board for *Professional School Counseling* and the *Journal of Mental Health Counseling*.

Liz Boyd, PhD, is a clinical assistant professor of counselor education at Clemson University. She earned her PhD in counselor education and supervision from Old Dominion University. Dr. Boyd has more than 10 years of college-level teaching experience, including master's level mental health and school counseling courses and undergraduate human services courses. Her research interests include grief and trauma specifically related to women's health, as well as cultural competency and counselor education.

Jennifer Barrow, PhD, NCC, LCMHCS, is a licensed clinical mental health counselor supervisor, a national certified counselor, and veteran professional school counselor. Dr. Barrow serves as assistant professor in the Department of Allied Professions at North Carolina Central University, where she directs the school counseling program. Dr. Barrow's research and practice interests focus on depression, anxiety, counseling children and adolescents, and enhancement of school counseling, in particular professional development and role advancement.

Melanie Burgess, PhD, is an assistant professor of counseling and the co-coordinator of the counselor education and supervision PhD program in the Department of Counseling, Educational Psychology, and Research at the University of Memphis. She earned her PhD in counselor education and supervision and an MSEd in counseling with a concentration in school counseling from Old Dominion University. Dr. Burgess has experience working with a diverse PK–12 students, including those in Title-I schools, military-affiliated students, international students, and students with disabilities. She has taught doctoral students, master's school counseling and mental health counseling courses, and undergraduate human services courses. Her research interests include school counselor preparation and supervision, data-driven, evidence-based practices in PK–12 settings, and instrument creation and validation. She has presented national conferences, published qualitative and quantitative articles in peer-reviewed journals, and received national, regional, and state-level grants to support her research. She currently serves as an editorial board fellow for *Counselor Education & Supervision*, co-chair of the Association for Child and Adolescent Counseling Research Grant Committee, and one of the recipients of the 2020 American Counseling Association's Research Award.

Andy J. Flaherty, MSW, is a doctoral candidate at the College of Social Work (University of South Carolina). Andy has specialized in substance use recovery, mental health, and positive youth development. Andy spent 4 years as a mental health clinician after completing his MSW at the California State University at Chico. He currently serves as an instructor for Austin Peay State University in Clarksville, Tennessee, and is a program evaluator for a statewide agency in California. Andy seeks to explore ways that interventions for substance use can be used to positively impact clients' lives and studies the intersection of social work, spirituality, and congregations as they pertain to mental health.

Christopher J. Hipp, PhD, EdS, LPC, NCC, is an adjunct professor at the University of South Carolina, Augusta University, and Grand Canyon University. He has 9 years of counseling practice in elementary, middle, and high schools, a college counseling center, and a nonprofit agency working with individuals experiencing homelessness and severe mental illness. His research interests involve technology use within romantic relationships and the influence of relationship dynamics on relationship and sexual satisfaction among couples.

Sonja Lund, PhD, LPC-R, is an assistant professor of counseling and human services at the University of Scranton. She earned her doctorate in counseling education and supervision from Old Dominion University. Currently, she is licensed as a resident counselor in the state of Virginia. She is a board member of the Northeast Pennsylvania Counseling Association and holds memberships in the American College Counseling Association; the Society for Sexual, Affectional, Intersex, and Gender Expansive Identities; the Association for Counselor Education and Supervision; and the Association of Counseling Sexology and Sexual Wellness. Sonja is passionate about her work with the college student-athlete population. She has presented at various regional, state, national, and international conferences on college student-athlete mental health issues, including the coach-athlete relationship, attitudes toward help seeking, counseling interventions, and student-athlete diversity considerations. She was recognized as an emerging leader by the American College Counseling Association and as an outstanding practitioner by the Omega Delta chapter of Chi Sigma Iota at Old Dominion University. Her other areas of interest include issues in sexual wellness, empathy, career counseling, and experiential learning in the higher education setting.

Robin Moody, PhD, LPCS, began her work as a licensed professional counselor after earning a bachelor's degree in Christian counseling from Toccoa Falls College and a master's degree in counseling and guidance from Clemson University. Her passion for nonprofit agencies led her to acquire a position as assistant director of crisis ministries, a 24-hour walk in and mobile crisis center. She specialized in suicidal/homicidal intervention and stabilization and began a teen pregnancy and parenting class that infiltrated the local high schools. While serving at the crisis center, she also earned a PhD in Christian counseling from Christian Bible College. She is also a cognitive behavioral and rational emotive therapist and is certified in hypnotherapy. Dr. Moody also has a PhD in clinical psychology and industrial organizational psychology from Walden University. Her private practice is located in several upstate South Carolina cities. Her specialty is neurocognitive testing with an emphasis on brain trauma. She became a certified brain health coach through the Amen Clinic and serves as a licensed professional counselor supervisor for the state of South Carolina. Dr. Moody contracts with several state agencies and performs various clinical diagnostic and neurocognitive evaluations.

Chadwick Royal, PhD, LCMHCS, has been a counselor for more than 25 years. He has worked in public and private mental health settings with children, families, and adults, and he is a licensed clinical mental health counselor supervisor in North Carolina. He currently serves as a professor of counselor education and chair of the Department of Allied Professions at North Carolina Central University. In addition to his work as an academic, he maintains a small private practice, providing counseling and supervision.

Kyla Maria Sawyer-Kurian, PhD, LCMHC, is an assistant professor in the counseling program at North Carolina Central University, in the Research Triangle. She is the coordinator of the clinical mental health program and teaches Assessment and Advanced Assessment in Counseling, along with Multicultural and Gender Issues in Counseling, Internship in Counseling, Introduction to Substance Abuse and Research Methods. She has served as both an outpatient therapist and a clinical director within mental health agencies. She was a National Institute on Drug Abuse postdoctoral fellow, and her training focused on the impact of a Women's focused HIV intervention on risky sex practices, intimate partner violence, pregnancy, and employment among African American crack-using women. From this training, Dr. Kurian received a University of North Carolina Center for AIDS Developmental Award in which she adapted the women's focused intervention for African American college women who used drugs and alcohol. Dr. Kurian's areas of expertise include preparing counselors in training for diverse cultural contexts and clinical mental health counselor identity and training. Most recently, Dr. Kurian is developing expertise in infertility counseling.

Regina Gavin Williams, PhD, NCC, LCMHC-NC, is a counselor educator at North Carolina Central University. She received her PhD in counseling and counselor education from North Carolina State University. Her research focuses on the career and college readiness and adult self-sufficiency of adolescents aging out of the foster care system, training therapeutic foster caregivers, and assisting adolescents with postsecondary education and career decision making. Dr. Williams has experience working in educational and clinical mental health settings and is the 2019–2020 recipient of the Chi Sigma Iota Distinguished Alumni Award for the North Carolina State-Nu Sigma Chi Chapter.

Brooke Wymer, PhD, MSW, LISW-CP/S, is a clinical assistant professor in the counselor education program at Clemson University. She has a PhD in counselor education and a master of social work from the University of South Carolina. She has academic experience teaching in the discipline of both counseling and social work. She is a clinically licensed social worker and supervisor who specializes in providing and supervising trauma treatment services for children and families. Most of Dr. Wymer's clinical work and specialized training has been in child sexual trauma treatment and parenting support interventions. She is currently the co-owner of a clinical consulting business where she provides professional clinical consultation services regarding trauma-informed communities, organizations, supervision, and treatment. Her research interests include trauma-focused clinical supervision, improving child trauma treatment outcomes, counselor wellness, and child abuse prevention through parenting support programs.